ADVANCED CONCEPTS
IN
ARRHYTHMIAS

ADVANCED CONCEPTS IN ARRHYTHMIAS

Henry J. L. Marriott, M.D., F.A.C.P., F.A.C.C.

Director of Clinical Research, Rogers Heart Foundation,
St. Petersburg, Florida; Clinical Professor of
Medicine (Cardiology), Emory University,
Atlanta, Georgia

Mary H. Conover, R.N., B.S.

Instructor and Education Consultant,
California Hospital Medical Center, Los Angeles;
Instructor of Intermediate and Advanced Arrhythmia Workshops,
West Hills Hospital, Canoga Park, California;
Education Consultant, Center for Diagnosis and Treatment
of Cardiac Arrhythmias, Holy Cross Hospital,
Mission Hills, California

with 733 illustrations

The C. V. Mosby Company

ST. LOUIS   TORONTO   1983

MOSBY

A TRADITION OF PUBLISHING EXCELLENCE

Editor: Thomas Allen Manning
Assistant editor: Bess Arends
Manuscript editor: George B. Stericker, Jr.
Book design: Susan Trail
Cover design: Suzanne Oberholtzer
Production: Judy England, Ginny Douglas

The C.V. Mosby Company
11830 Westline Industrial Drive, St. Louis, Missouri 63141

Library of Congress Cataloging in Publication Data

Marriott, Henry Joseph Llewellyn, 1917-
  Advanced concepts in arrhythmias.

  Bibliography: p.
  Includes index.
  1. Arrhythmia. I. Conover, Mary Boudreau,
1931-   II. Title. [DNLM: 1. Arrhythmia.
WG 330 M342a]
RC685.A65M369   616.1'2807   82-3447
ISBN 0-8016-3110-6   AACR2

AC/VH/VH 9 8 7 6 5 4 3   03/C/345

To
George

Preface

This book was written in reponse to the many requests that both of us have received over the years for "something more advanced." It is therefore intended for those who have the basics well in hand and who wish to enhance their diagnostic skills with a broader background in arrhythmogenic mechanisms and a firm, consistent approach to the differential diagnosis of arrhythmias.

It is our intention to bridge the gap between the basic arrhythmia text and the voluminous highly technical books written for those involved in research. For example, in the chapter on electrophysiology we first explain the simple physical laws governing the behavior of all semipermeable membranes and ionic solutions. This information is then easily applied to the human cell by simply adding the concept of special "pumps" and gated membrane channels for "fast" and "slow" currents.

In other chapters we explain and illustrate sinus node and His bundle electrograms, phase 3 and phase 4 block, concealed conduction, accessory pathways, all of the known arrhythmogenic mechanisms, and the embryology of the conduction system. We report on the latest findings in the differential diagnosis between aberrancy and ectopy; present a new approach to the diagnosis of AV block, and a time-tested, dependable method of tackling arrhythmias; explain the sick sinus syndrome, all forms of reentry, and the theories currently proposed for protection of the parasystolic focus; and illustrate the arrhythmias common in digitalis toxicity.

We are grateful to the Williams & Wilkins Company, Baltimore, for permission to use many of the tracings from Marriott, H.J.L.: Contemporary Electrocardiography, 1979.

Henry J. L. Marriott
Mary H. Boudreau Conover

Contents

CHAPTER 1

Development of the conduction system

The conduction system is made up of highly specialized muscle tissue peculiar to the heart. We briefly present its fascinating embryology here in the belief that some knowledge of the development of the conduction system will facilitate an understanding of its normal and abnormal function.

The primitive straight cardiac tube is illustrated in Fig. 1-1 at 3 weeks of intrauterine development. Five segments are recognized: the truncus, bulbus, ventricle, atrium, and sinus venosus (sinus horn). Each is separated from adjacent segments by a slightly constricted ring, named for the segments it separates—the sinoatrial (S-A), atrioventricular (A-V), bulboventricular (B-V), and bulbotruncal (B-T) rings. These rings of specialized tissue are believed to form the conducting tissues.

The S-A ring, separating the sinus venosus from the atrium, is destined to form the sinus node. The B-V ring is destined to become the right bundle branch (RBB) and contribute to the left bundle branch (LBB) along with the A-V ring.

The origin of the AV node is controversial. Anderson[1] believes the node has multiple origins whereas others[2,3] believe that it is derived from the left horn of the sinus venosus while the sinus node comes from the right horn.

As the tube begins to loop, the sinus venosus is absorbed into the right atrium so that the S-A ring is in the posterior wall of the right atrium. One end of each of the remaining three rings is now in close apposition, as shown in Fig. 1-2.

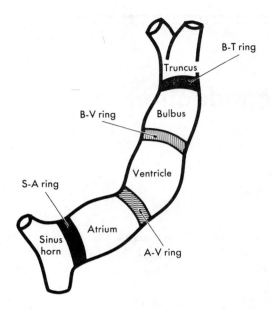

Fig. 1-1. The primitive straight cardiac tube. (From Anderson, R.H., and others: In Roberts, N.K., and Gelband, H., editors: Cardiac arrhythmias in the neonate, infant, and child, New York, 1977, Appleton-Century-Crofts.)

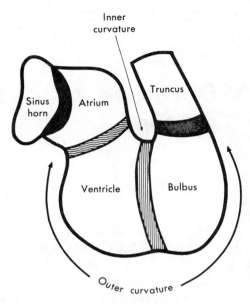

Fig. 1-2. The primitive straight cardiac tube begins to loop, bringing the three rings into close apposition. (From Anderson, R.H., and others: In Roberts, N.K., and Gelband, H., editors: Cardiac arrhythmias in the neonate, infant, and child, New York, 1977, Appleton-Century-Crofts.)

Development of the sinus node

After 11 weeks of intrauterine life the SA node can be recognized. Its formation begins with a thickening of the junction between the superior vena cava and the sinus venosus in the region of the S-A ring cells. This thickening is confined to the antero-medial quadrant of the junction between the superior vena cava and the atrium. By 11 weeks the thickening has aggregated around a prominent artery and is recognizable as the SA node, generally called simply the sinus node. The embryonic origin of the sinus node is illustrated in Fig. 1-3.

Blood supply. The large central sinus node artery is a branch of the right coronary artery in 55% of people, and of the left in 45%.

Ultrastructure. A wax model of the human sinus node as reconstructed from longitudinal sections is shown in Fig. 1-4.[4]

Note how nodal tissue blends with atrial tissue. These perinodal fascicles have a different refractory period from that of the sinus node and the atrial tissue. Thus they may provide reentry pathways for arrhythmias and the anatomic substrate for SA nodal blocks.

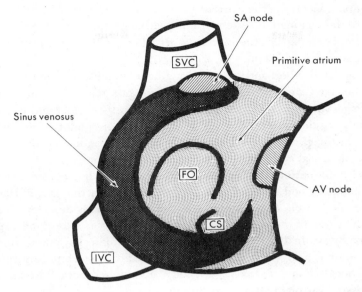

Fig. 1-3. The sinus node begins with a thickening of the junction between the superior vena cava and the sinus venosus. (From Anderson, R.H., and others: In Roberts, N.K., and Gelband, H., editors: Cardiac arrhythmias in the neonate, infant, and child, New York, 1977, Appleton-Century-Crofts.)

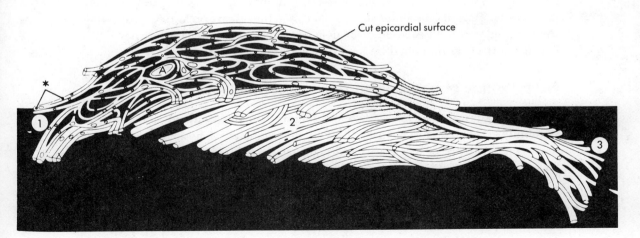

Fig. 1-4. A wax model of the human sinus node. (From Truex, R.C.: In Wellens, H.J.J., Lie, K.I., and Janse, M.J., editors: The conduction system of the heart, Hingham, Mass., 1976, Martinus Nijhoff, Publishers.)

Specialized internodal pathways

Controversy concerning the existence of specialized internodal tracts is "as old as the history of the conduction system itself,"[5] although the existence of preferential conduction implemented by the *geometric structure* of the muscle bundles of the right atrium is well established.[5-8]

On the one hand, Sherf and James,[9] using light and electron microscopic studies of atrial tissue, have described six different types of atrial cells, with morphologic evidence of specialization that, according to Hoffman,[10] is "clear and compelling."

Conversely, Anderson and Becker[5] in 1980 "strongly endorse the opinion that there are *no* histologically discrete tracts of specialized conduction tissue extending between the sinoatrial and atrioventricular nodes."

We will briefly outline the historical development of this controversy. In 1906 Wenckebach[11] described a muscle bundle extending from the area of the superior vena cava to the muscle of the right atrial appendage. This description was made before the discovery of the sinus node. He did not, therefore, describe a specialized *internodal* pathway. In 1910 Thorel described "Purkinje cells" connecting the two nodes and running along the crista terminalis.[12] This was refuted by the German Pathological Society[13] and by Koch,[13] Aschoff,[14] and Mönckeberg,[15] who said that the internodal tissue was plain atrial myocardium.

In 1916 Bachman[16] described an interatrial bundle, and in 1963 James[17] proposed that there were specialized fibers within Bachman's bundle that divided at the crest of the interatrial septum to continue down the septum and enter the top of the AV node (the anterior internodal tract). At this time James also described the middle (Wenckebach's muscle bundle) and posterior (Thorel's "specialized" pathway) internodal tracts. The impetus for his studies came from the discovery, in 1961, that cells of the atria differed from each other in their electrophysiologic characteristics.[18] The internodal tracts as described by James are illustrated in Fig. 1-5.

No evidence of specialized internodal pathways

Most modern investigators[2,5-7] except James[17] feel that, without ruling out the possibility of the existence of atrial cells with different electrophysiologic properties, there is no evidence of specialized internodal conduction tissue, although preferential conduction exists via muscle bundles (Fig. 1-6).

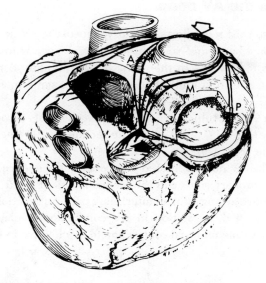

Fig. 1-5. The internodal tracts as described by James. (From James, T.N.: In Hurst, J.W., editor: The heart, ed. 5, New York, 1982, McGraw-Hill Book Co.)

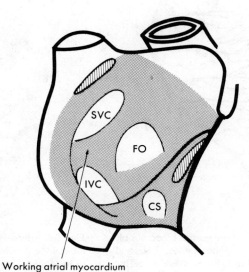

Working atrial myocardium

Fig. 1-6. Diagram illustrating the results of Anderson's investigations concerning the nature of the internodal atrial myocardium. Geometry, rather than specialized tissue, favors preferential conduction. (From Anderson, R.H., and Becker, A.E.: In Mandel, W.J., editor: Cardiac arrhythmias; their mechanisms, diagnosis, and management, Philadelphia, 1980, J.B. Lippincott Co.)

Development of the AV node

Controversies also exist regarding the embryology of the AV node and the bundle of His.[1,3,19] Anderson[20] has found specialized tissue analogous to the AV node and bundle as early as 5 to 6 weeks in the embryo and therefore considers that these structures develop in situ from multiple origins and are not a migration of tissue as proposed by some.

Blood supply. In 90% of subjects the AV node receives its blood supply from the right coronary artery (Figs. 1-7 and 1-8). In the remaining 10% the circumflex artery supplies the AV node (Fig. 1-9).

Ultrastructure. The AV node is located just beneath the endocardium in the right atrium between the coronary sinus and the medial leaflet of the tricuspid valve. The fibers of the AV node are arranged in an interlacing pattern, functioning as a triage for atrial impulses and as a delay station in AV conduction. Delay is an important function since it allows time for atrial contraction to be effective in filling and stretch-

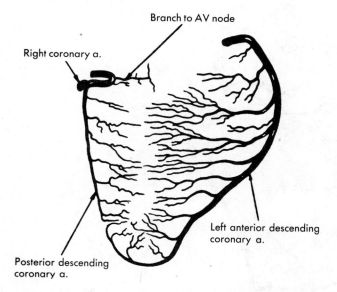

Fig. 1-7. Drawing from a vinylite cast of the normal blood supply of the human interventricular septum. (From James, T.N., and Burch, G.E.: Circulation **17:**391, 1958. By permission of the American Heart Association, Inc.)

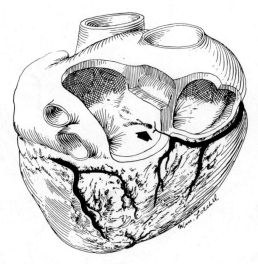

Fig. 1-8. Arterial supply to the diaphragmatic surface of the human heart as it occurs in about 90% of instances. (From James, T.N.: Anatomy of the coronary arteries, New York, 1961, Hoeber Medical Division, Harper & Row, Publishers.)

ing the ventricles. A diagrammatic representation of the ultrastructure of the AV node and bundle of His is presented in Fig. 1-10.

As the AV node begins to penetrate the central fibrous body (the central core of fibrous tissue dividing atria and ventricles), its cells become more and more longitudinally oriented until they become the parallel pathways of the bundle of His and, as such, descend along the posterior border of the membranous ventricular septum.

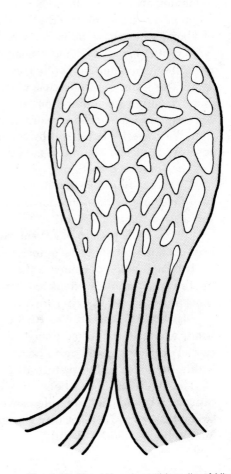

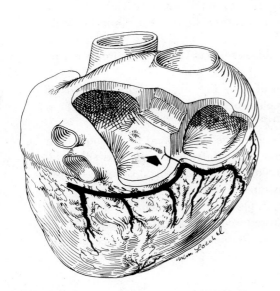

Fig. 1-9. The arterial supply to the diaphragmatic surface of the human heart as it occurs in about 10% of instances. (From James, T.N.: Anatomy of the coronary arteries, New York, 1961, Hoeber Medical Division, Harper & Row, Publishers.)

Fig. 1-10. The AV node and bundle of His.

Branching portion of the bundle of His

At approximately 6 weeks in the embryonic heart the bundle branches can be seen cascading down both sides of the septum with ramifications into the trabeculated pouches.[1] At 18 weeks the LBB is recognizable as a fanlike structure and the RBB as cordlike.[1]

Left bundle branch. The main LBB lies on the left side of the ventricular septum beginning at the level of the commissure formed by the aortic cusps and extending for about 1 to 2 cm before it divides. Here the bundle of His gives off a "fine stream"[20] of fibers, which have been described by James[21] as "a virtual sheet," that forms a large posterior radiation and a smaller anterior one. A third midseptal radiation was noted by Demoulin and Kulbertus[22,26] in 33 out of 49 normal hearts (type I, Fig. 1-11). This lesser-known fascicle was readily identified by these investigators and was found to originate either from the common left bundle or from the anterior or posterior fascicle. In the remaining 16 cases the septum was supplied by radiations from the posterior fascicle or by combined radiations from both the anterior and the posterior fascicles. The findings of these investigators are illustrated in Fig. 1-11.

They observed that

1. There are three main interconnecting fascicles in the left ventricle rather than two. One supplies the anterior (superior) wall, another the posterior (inferior) wall, and a third the midseptum.

2. The ECG pattern of left anterior hemiblock reflects LBB disease but is hardly ever confined solely to the anterior fascicle.

It is interesting to compare the drawings of these investigators with that in 1906 by Tawara,[23] who also depicted *three* fascicles in the left ventricle (Fig. 1-12), a concept supported by other investigators.[5,24-26]

Right bundle branch. The RBB proceeds along the septal band to the moderator band, where it divides and fans out into the right ventricular wall. It is subendocardial at its origin and again before it fans out. The middle portion travels deeper within the muscle. The mature RBB is illustrated in Fig. 1-13.

The difference in size between the right and left bundle branches is striking and explains why the right bundle can be compromised with a lesser lesion than the larger LBB can. This fact may account for the frequent clinical innocence of right bundle-branch block (RBBB).

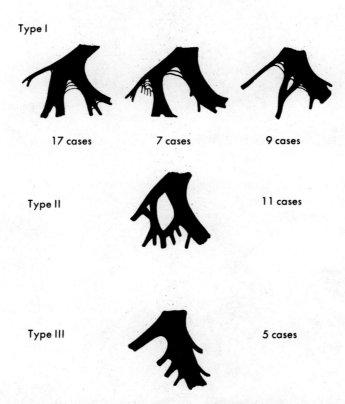

Type I

17 cases   7 cases   9 cases

Type II   11 cases

Type III   5 cases

Fig. 1-11. Distribution of the left bundle branch fibers in 49 human hearts. (From Kulbertus, H.E., and Demoulin, J.: In Wellens, H.J.J., Lie, K.I., and Janse, M.J., editors: The conduction system of the heart, Hingham, Mass., 1976, Martinus Nijhoff, Publishers.)

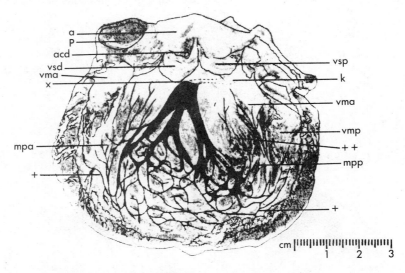

Fig. 1-12. Human LBB anatomy as depicted by Tawara in 1906.

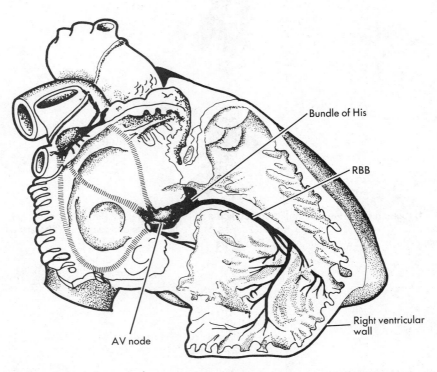

Fig. 1-13. The right bundle branch. Note the division supplying the right ventricular wall and the septal division. (From Marriott, H.J.L.: Workshop in electrocardiography, Oldsmar, Fla., 1972, Tampa Tracings.)

References

1. Anderson, R.H., Becker, A.E., Wenink, A.C.G., and Janse, M.J.: The development of the cardiac specialized tissue. In Wellens, H.J.J., Lie, K.I., and Janse, M.J., editors: The conduction system of the heart, Philadelphia, 1976, Lea & Febiger.
2. Retzer, R.: Some results of recent investigations on the mammalian heart, Anat. Rec. **2**:149, 1908.
3. Patten, B.M.: The development of the sino-ventricular conduction system, Univ. Mich. Med. Bull. **22**:1, 1956.
4. Truex, R.C.: The sinoatrial node and its connections with the atrial tissues. In Wellens, H.J.J., Lie, K.I., and Janse, M.J., editors: The conduction system of the heart, Philadelphia, 1976, Lea & Febiger.
5. Anderson, R.H., and Becker, A.E.: Gross anatomy and microscopy of the conducting system. In Mandel, W.J., editor: Cardiac arrhythmias; their mechanisms, diagnosis, and management, Philadelphia, 1980, J.B. Lippincott Co.
6. Chuyaqui, B.J.: Uber die Ausbreitungsbündel des Sinusknotens. Eine kritische Analyse der wichtigsten Arbeiten, Virchows Arch. [Pathol. Anat.] **335**:179, 1972.
7. Spach, M.S., Liebermen, M., Scott, J.G., Barr, R.C., Johnson, E.A., and Kootsey, J.M.: Excitation sequences of the atrial septum and A-V node in isolated hearts of the dog and the rabbit, Circ. Res. **29**:156, 1971.
8. Spach, M.S., King, T.D., Barr, R.C., Boaz, D.E., Morrow, M.N., and Herman-Giddens, S.: Electrical potential distribution surrounding the atria during depolarization and repolarization in the dog, Circ. Res. **24**:857, 1969.
9. Sherf, L., and James, T.N.: Fine structure of cells and their histologic organization within internodal pathways of the heart; clinical and electrocardiographic implications, Am. J. Cardiol. **44**:345, 1979.
10. Hoffman, B.F.: Fine structure of internodal pathways [Editorial], Am. J. Cardiol. **44**:387, 1979.
11. Wenckebach, K.F.: Beiträge zur Kenntnis der menschlichen Herztätigkeit, Arch. Anat. Physiol. (Physiol. Abth.) 297, 1906.
12. Thorel, C.: Vorläufige Mitteilung über eine besondere Muskel-verbindung zwischen der Cava superior und den Hisschen Bundlein, Munch. Med. Wochenchr. **57**:183, 1910.
13. Bericht über die Verhandlungen der XIV Tagung der deutschen pathologischem Gesellschaft in Erlangen vom 4-6 April 1910, Zentralbl. Allg. Pathol. **21**:433, 1910.
14. Aschoff, L.: Referat über die Herzstörungen in ihren Beziehungen zu den spezifischen Muskelsystem in Herzens, Verh. Dtsch. Pathol. Ges. **14**:3, 1910.
15. Mönckeberg, J.G.: Beiträge zur normalen und pathologischen Anatomie des Herzens, Verh. Dtsch. Pathol. Ges. **14**:64, 1910.
16. Bachmann, G.: The inter-auricular time interval, Am. J. Physiol. **41**:309, 1916.
17. James, T.N.: The connecting pathways between the sinus node and the AV node and between the right and left atrium in the human heart, Am. Heart J. **66**:498, 1963.
18. Paes de Carvalho, A.: Cellular electrophysiology of the atrial specialized tissues. In Paes de Carvalho, A., de Mello, W.C., and Hoffman, B.F., editors: Specialized tissues of the heart, Amsterdam, 1961, Elsevier.
19. Walls, E.W.: The development of the specialized conducting tissue of the human heart, J. Anat. **81**:93, 1947.
20. Anderson, R.H., Becker, A.E., Brechenmacher, C., Davies, M.J., and Rossi, L.: The atrioventricular junctional area of the human heart—a morphological study of the atrioventricular node and bundle, Eur. J. Cardiol. **3**:11, 1975.
21. James, T.N.: Anatomy of the conduction system of the heart. In Hurst, J.W., editor: The heart, ed. 5, New York, 1982, McGraw-Hill Book Co.
22. Demoulin, J.C., and Kulbertus, H.E.: Histopathological examination of concept of left hemiblock, Br. Heart J. **34**:809, 1972.
23. Tawara, S.: Das Reitzleitungssystem des Säugetierherzens, Jena, 1906, Gustav Fischer.
24. Rossi, L.: Histopathology of the conducting system, G. Ital. Cardiol. **2**:484, 1972.
25. Uhley, H.N.: The quadrifascicular nature of the peripheral conduction system. In Dreifus, L.S., and Liboff, W., editors: Cardiac arrhythmias, New York, 1973, Grune & Stratton, Inc.
26. Kulbertus, H.E., and Demoulin, J.: Pathological basis of concept of left hemiblock. In Wellens, H.J.J., Lie, K.I., and Janse, M.J., editors: The conduction system of the heart, Philadelphia, 1976, Lea & Febiger.

CHAPTER 2

Sinus node and His bundle electrograms

Normal cardiac activation is initiated in the sinus node, where pacemaker cells discharge at regular intervals and at a rate dependent upon autonomic influences and the hemodynamic needs of the body.

The action potential generated in the sinus node is conducted to the atrial myocardium and from there across the AV node, bundle of His, and bundle branches into the ventricles. Specialized perinodal fibers connecting the sinus node and the atrium have been identified in the rabbit but not in humans. It is believed that conduction is facilitated between the sinus node and the atrial myocardium either by such specialized connecting fibers or simply because of the anatomic orientation of the atrial myocardial fibers.[1]

Propagation of current through the myocardium is dependent upon the cable properties of myocardium. When the membrane potential changes in one segment of fiber, neighboring segments are affected so that they also depolarize and in turn act as an excitatory stimulus to the adjacent tissue. The current flows through the myocardium longitudinally, along the length of the fibers. If for any reason the current is not strong enough or if the cells themselves have been functionally impaired, the velocity of the depolarization wave may slow considerably or the wave stop altogether.

The discharge of the sinus node is a silent event, in that the magnitude of the electrical activity generated is too small to be picked up by the surface ECG, and indeed it was not recorded directly at all until 1978.[2-4]

The electrical activity generated during depolarization of the AV node and bundle of His is, like the sinus discharge, not strong enough to be recorded on the surface ECG. However, the PR interval offers a time frame for these events that is not available for the sinus node discharge and conduction through the sinus node to the atrial musculature.

Initial activation of the AV node occurs only 0.03 or 0.04 second after the beginning of the P wave, with the bundle of His and bundle branches being activated during the PR segment.

Fig. 2-1 illustrates electrical events in the heart and relates them to what is actually seen on the surface ECG. Note that the discharge of the sinus node occurs before the onset of the P wave and that there is a measurable conduction time between sinus node discharge and the depolarization of atrial myocardium as signaled by the P wave.

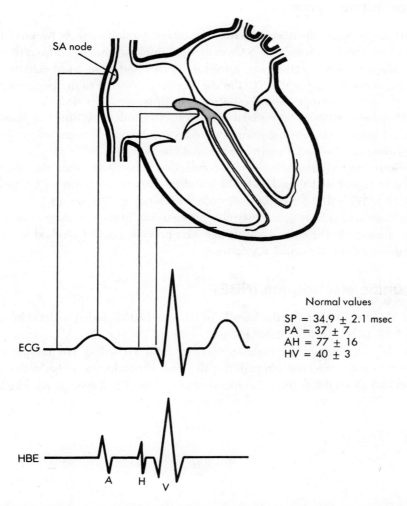

Normal values
SP = 34.9 ± 2.1 msec
PA = 37 ± 7
AH = 77 ± 16
HV = 40 ± 3

Fig. 2-1. Schematic representation of the electrical events in the heart related to the surface ECG and His bundle electrogram (HBE). The approximate relationship of sinus node discharge is also related to the surface ECG. *SP*, SA conduction time; *PA*, intraatrial conduction time; *AH*, AV nodal conduction time; *HV*, His-Purkinje conduction time.

Sinus node electrogram

Direct recording of the electrical discharge of the human sinus node was not available until, at Columbia University in 1978,[2] the electrical potentials of the sinus node in the canine heart were successfully recorded. In 1979 and 1980,[3-5] the same team developed a technique for direct recording of the electrical potentials from the human sinus node.

SA conduction time

During the above-mentioned experiments conduction time between the sinus node and the atrial myocardium (SA conduction time) was measured from the deflection on the SA nodal electrogram, attributed to SA nodal electrical activity, to the beginning of the P wave of the ECG in the bipolar records or to the beginning of the high right atrial electrogram in the unipolar records.

In 15 patients without SA nodal dysfunction, SA conduction time was found to be 34.9 ± 2.1 msec. Accurate measurement of SA conduction time permits differentiation between normal and abnormal SA nodal function.

Clinically an understanding of SA conduction time illuminates the mechanism involved in type I and type II SA block and the difference between SA block and sinus arrest. We will discuss these disorders in detail in Chapter 15.

The sinus node electrogram may also prove useful in cardiac surgery as an aid to avoiding damage to the sinus node. It may also provide a better method for differentiating normal from abnormal SA nodes.

His bundle electrogram (HBE)

The electrical activity in the bundle of His was first recorded in 1960 in Europe[6] and in 1969 in the United States.[7]

The development of the catheter technique for recording His bundle electrograms has enabled the clinician to define the level of conduction delay within the AV junction and to establish the difference between type I and type II AV block.

HBE deflections

The deflections seen in the HBE are illustrated in Fig. 2-1:

The A wave: The first deflection represents atrial activation and is called the A wave. This deflection represents low right atrial activation, since the recording lead is either the bipolar His bundle lead or a low atrial lead.

The H deflection: This deflection follows the A wave and represents His bundle electrical activity as recorded by a catheter lying at the base of the tricuspid valve, close to the His bundle.

The V deflection: The last deflection on the His bundle electrogram represents ventricular activation and is concurrent with the QRS complex on the surface ECG.

HBE intervals and normal values

The HBE divides the PR interval into three components defined by the PA, AH, and HV intervals.

PA interval. This interval is an approximate measurement of intraatrial conduction time from the area around the sinus node to the low right atrium. It is measured from the onset of the P wave on the standard ECG or from the atrial deflection of a high right atrial electrogram to the A wave on the HBE. The normal range is 25 to 45 msec (37 ± 7).

AH interval. This interval represents AV nodal conduction time. It is measured from the A wave on the HBE to the earliest onset of the His bundle potential. The normal range is 50 to 120 msec (77 ± 16).

HV interval. This interval represents the conduction time through the His-Purkinje system (from the bundle of His to the distal Purkinje fibers). The normal range is 35 to 45 msec (40 ± 3).

Sequence of activation through the conduction system

Fig. 2-2 relates the sequence of activation through the conduction system to the ECG. Note that the sinus node is activated before the P wave is inscribed and that the AV node is initially activated well before atrial depolarization is completed.

Activation of most of the His-Purkinje system naturally precedes activation of the working myocardium, as represented by the QRS complex; the QRS therefore begins after most of the conduction system is already depolarized. An appreciation of this helps one to grasp the concept of concealed conduction in the bundle branches, as discussed in Chapter 8.

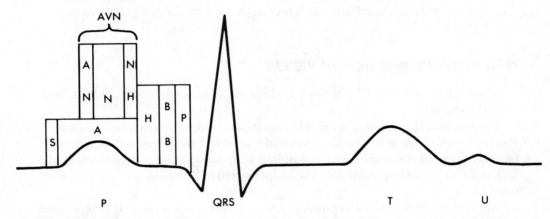

Fig. 2-2. Schematic representation of the sequence of activation through the conduction system related to the surface ECG. Note that the QRS begins only after most of the conduction system has already been activated. *S,* SA conduction; *A,* atria; *AVN,* atrioventricular node; *AN,* atrionodal; *N,* nodal (central); *NH,* nodal-His; *H,* His bundle; *BB,* bundle branches; *P,* Purkinje fibers.

Surface recording of His-Purkinje activity

In 1973[8-10] it was first demonstrated that the electrical activity arising from the His-Purkinje system could be recorded from the body surface. Technical problems limited the success of these and further studies.[11-25] In 1981[26] Flowers and her group developed a new system which records on a beat-to-beat basis but has a portability problem. The advances made since the initial surface recording of His bundle potentials are promising, and the potential for diagnostic and therapeutic applications is important.

Indications for His bundle recordings

The extrapolation of data obtained from His bundle electrograms over the past decade has actually lessened the clinical need to use this technique.

In most cases of AV block the routine ECG and the clinical setting will provide enough information to correctly deduce the site of block. Even when the site of block cannot be so deduced, as when the AV block is associated with a wide QRS complex, a HBE would be necessary only in the asymptomatic patient, since the symptomatic patient should receive a pacemaker, no matter at what level the block, and the treatment for the asymptomatic patient would depend upon whether the pathology was in the AV node (type I) or in the His-Purkinje system (usually type II).

Even a diagnosis of concealed junctional extrasystoles, although not definitive, can generally be made from long continuous tracings.

In the realm of research His bundle electrograms will most certainly continue to contribute to the flow of information about reentrant phenomena, the mechanisms and actions of drugs, and the mechanisms of complex arrhythmias.

References

1. Jordan, J.L., and Mandel, W.J.: Disorders of sinus function. In Mandel, W.J., editor: Cardiac arrhythmias; their mechanisms, diagnosis, and management, Philadelphia, 1980, J.B. Lippincott Co.
2. Cramer, M., Hariman, R.J., Boxer, R., and Hoffman, B.F.: Electrograms from the canine sinoatrial pacemaker recorded in vitro and in situ, Am. J. Cardiol. **42**:939, 1978.
3. Reiffel, J., Gliklich, J., Gang, E., Weiss, M., Davis, J., and Bigger, J.T., Jr.: Human sinus node electrograms: transvenous catheter recorded technique and normal sinoatrial conduction times in adults [Abstract], Circulation **60**:238, 1979.
4. Hariman, R.J., Krongrad, E., Boxer, R.A., Weiss, M.B., Steeg, C.N., and Hoffman, B.F.: Method for recording electrical activity of the sinoatrial node and automatic atrial foci during cardiac catheterization in human subjects, Am. J. Cardiol. **45**:775, 1980.
5. Hariman, R.J., Krongrad, M.D., Boxer, R.A., Bowman, F.O., Jr., Malm, J.R., and Hoffman, B.F.: Methods for recording electrograms of the sinoatrial node during cardiac surgery in man, Circulation **61**:1024, 1980.
6. Giraud, G., Puech, P., Latour, H., and Hertault, J.: Variations de potentiel liées à l'activité du système de conduction auriculo-ventriculaire chez l'homme (enregistrement electrocardiographic endocavitaire), Arch. Mal. Coeur **53**:757, 1960.
7. Scherlag, B.J., Lau, S.H., Helfand, T.H., Berkowitz, W.D., Stein, E., and Damato. A.N.: Catheter technique for recording His bundle activity in man, Circulation **39**:13, 1969.
8. Berbari, E.J., and others: Non-invasive technique for detection of electrical activity during the P-R segment, Circulation **48**:1005, 1973.
9. Flowers, N.C., and others: Surface recording of electrical activity from the His bundle area. Presented at the Annual Meeting of the Cardiac Electrophysiologic Group, Atlantic City, April, 1973.
10. Flowers, N.C., and Horan, L.G.: His bundle and bundle branch recordings from the body surface, Circulation **48**:102, 1973.
11. Flowers, N.C., and others: Surface recording of electrical activity from the region of the bundle of His, Am. J. Cardiol. **33**:384, 1974.
12. Flowers, N.C., and others: Surface recordings of low-level internal signals. In Miller, H.A., and Harrison, D.C., editors: Biomedical electrode technology: theory and practice, New York, 1974, Academic Press, Inc.
13. Berbari, E.J., Lazzara, R., El-Sherif, N., and Scherlag, B.J.: Extracardiac recordings of His-Purkinje activity during conduction disorders and junctional rhythms, Circulation **51**:802, 1975.
14. Berbari, E.J., and others: The His-Purkinje electrocardiogram in man. An initial assessment of its uses and limitations, Circulation **54**:219, 1976.
15. Stopczyk, M.J., and others: Surface recording of electrical heart activity during the P-R segment in man by a computer averaging technique [Abstract]. In Proceedings of the World Congress of Cardiology, p. 162, 1974.
16. Hishimoto, Y., and Sawayama, T.: Non-invasive recording of His bundle potential in man: simplified method, Br. Heart J. **37**:635, 1975.
17. Furness, A., and others: The feasibility of detecting His-bundle activity from the body surface, Cardiovasc. Res. **9**:390, 1975.
18. Takeda, H., and others: Noninvasive recording of His-Purkinje activity in patients with complete atrioventricular block: clinical application of an "automated descrimination circuit," Circulation **60**:421, 1979.
19. Van Den Akker, T.J., and others: Real time method for noninvasive recording of His bundle activity of the electrocardiogram, Comput. Biomed. Res. **9**:559, 1976.
20. Sano, T.: Electrical activity of His bundle, Jpn. Circ. J. **40**:209, 1976.
21. Honda, M., and others: Clinical studies on noninvasive investigation of the His bundle electrogram. In Proceedings of the 5th International Symposium of Cardiac Pacing, p. 19, 1977.
22. Hombach, V., Behrenbeck, D.W., and Hilger, H.H.: Ösophagosternale and ösophagoapikale Ableitungen zur Registrierung von Oberflächen-His-Potentialen, Z. Kardiol. **66**:565, 1977.
23. Denis, J.G., and Cywinski, J.K.: The use of microprocessor for noninvasive recordings of electrical activity from the conduction system of the heart. In Proceedings of the 29th Annual Conference of Engineers in Medicine and Biology, vol. 18, p. 187, 1976.

24. Ishijima, M.: Statistically compensated averaging method for noninvasive recording of His-Purkinje activity. In Proceedings of the 14th Rocky Mountain Bioengineering Symposium, Biomed. Sci. Instrum. **14:**129, 1978.

25. Vincent, R., and others: Noninvasive recording of electrical activity in the PR segment in man, Br. Heart J. **40:**124, 1978.

26. Flowers, N.C., and others: Surface recording of His-Purkinje activity on an every-beat basis without digital averaging, Circulation **63:**948, 1981.

CHAPTER 3

Electrophysiology

The normal cardiac cycle has its origin in the sinus node, where an impulse is regularly generated at a rate consistent with the needs of the body and the age of the individual. This impulse then propagates through the atria, the AV node, His-Purkinje system, and ventricular myocardium in a predictable and orderly fashion.

Just as in any other cardiac cell, the generation of the impulse in cells of the sinus node depends upon the gradient of electrical potential that exists across the membrane at the boundary of the cell. In fact, the impulse reflects a very precise and rapid sequence of changes in this electrical potential across the cell membrane. These changes constitute what is referred to as the cardiac action potential. By means of a microelectrode inserted into the cell interior, the action potential (i.e., the impulse) can be recorded directly. An example is illustrated in Fig. 3-1. The graph shows the voltage recorded by the microelectrode before and after impalement of a cell, when the potential is measured across the cell membrane (transmembrane potential).

The cardiac action potential consists of five phases, which we briefly name here and describe in detail later. With the introduction of the microelectrode into the nonpacemaker cell, the graph reading plunges from 0 to about −90 mV. Phase 0 marks the period on the graph when the cell rapidly depolarizes from −90 to approximately +30 mV (Fig. 3-1, A).

Phases 1 to 3 represent the three stages of repolarization, with phase 2 being referred to as the "plateau." Phase 4 is the period of electrical diastole and differs in pacemaker and nonpacemaker cells. Note that in the nonpacemaker cell phase 4 is flat. The pacemaker cell is essentially the same except that phase 4 gradually slopes upward (Fig. 3-1, B).

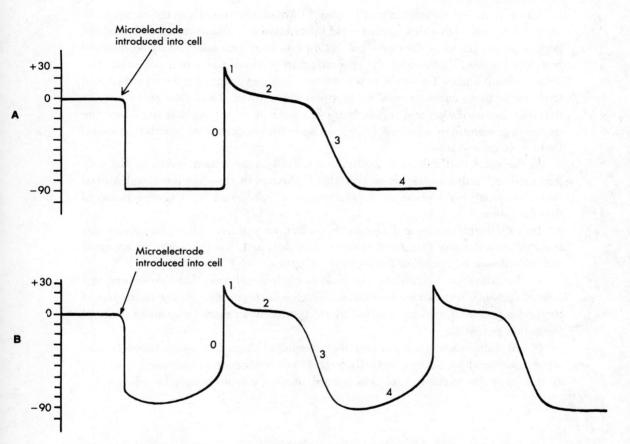

Fig. 3-1. The transmembrane resting and action potentials of (**A**) a myocardial fiber and (**B**) a pacemaker Purkinje fiber. The arrow indicates the point at which the microelectrode was introduced into the cell. Note that the graph suddenly dips to −90 mV as it records the resting, or diastolic, membrane potential.

Historical highlights

In 1949 Hodgkin and Katz[1] demonstrated that a rapid influx of sodium into the cell was responsible for the depolarization of squid nerve cells and that this sudden increase in sodium permeability determined the amplitude and rate of rise of phase 0 of the action potential.

Three years later Hodgkin and Huxley,[2] through the use of voltage-clamp technique, determined that this sudden rapid inward flow of sodium, which underlies the depolarization phase of the nerve cell action potential, was followed by an outward flow of potassium that caused the repolarization phase of the action potential. The voltage clamp makes it possible to set transmembrane voltage at selected values and then study ionic currents relative to time and voltage. Thus they were able to describe depolarization and repolarization in terms of equations that show how the underlying membrane currents of sodium and potassium ions vary with transmembrane voltage and time.

In the years that followed, sodium and potassium were assumed to be the only ions involved in the cardiac action potential,[3] although by this time it was well known that the initial rapid phase of depolarization was followed by a slower phase of depolarization.[4]

In 1966 Neidergerke and Orkand,[5] working with intracellular microelectrodes inserted into strips of frog heart muscle, demonstrated that there was an apparent sodium-calcium competition during depolarization.

In that same year Hagiwara and Nakajima[6] demonstrated that there were two inward currents, one carried by sodium, which was responsible for the initial rise of the action potential, and one carried by calcium, which causes the plateau phase of the action potential.

It was subsequently established that the initial depolarization, caused by the rapid inward sodium current, actually triggered the change in membrane permeability that gave rise to the second slow inward current, carried mainly by calcium.

Cardiac action potential compared to other action potentials

The cardiac action potential has a much longer duration than that of skeletal muscle, nervous tissue, and smooth muscle. This is because the heart must perform as a pump with adequate time to fill and with a contraction that propels the chamber contents with the same force each beat. Whereas skeletal muscle may be stimulated rapidly and repetitively, cardiac muscle needs time to relax for the heart to fill. Moreover, the vigor of force development of skeletal muscle can be altered by changing the number of muscle bundles activated whereas cardiac muscle must be activated in precisely the same sequence each beat and the spread of the impulse must be uniform if arrhythmias are to be avoided.

The cardiac action potential differs markedly from that of skeletal muscle; but even among cardiac action potentials there are characteristic differences, for example:

1. Pacemaker cells possess the property of automaticity; nonpacemaker cells do not. Phase 4 of the action potential reflects this property.

2. The cells of the two nodes (sinus and AV) depolarize because of the relatively slow inward current, which is mainly carried by calcium and probably some sodium to produce what has been called a "slow response action potential."[7] In addition, the sinus node possesses the property of automaticity and the AV node usually does not. All other cells (atrial and ventricular, pacemaker and nonpacemaker) normally depolarize because of the rapid inward sodium current, and that depolarization itself triggers the relatively slower inward calcium current, although under abnormal situations these cells may be depolarized by the slow calcium current alone.

3. Within the ventricles the duration of the action potential, and hence the refractory period, of the intraventricular conduction system becomes progressively longer from the beginning of the bundle branches to their endings and then gets progressively shorter again through the transitional cells to the ventricular muscle, resulting in a mechanism called "gating"[8,9] (Fig. 3-2). This is discussed in detail on p. 42.

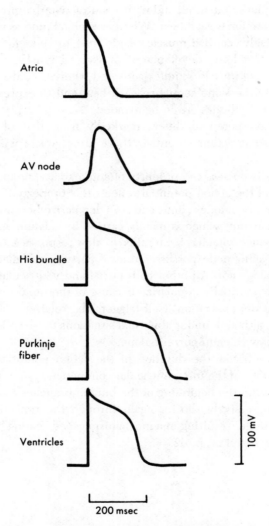

Atria

AV node

His bundle

Purkinje
fiber

Ventricles

100 mV

200 msec

Fig. 3-2. Action potential configuration from different areas of the heart. Note that the action potential gets longer and longer until it reaches its maximum duration in the Purkinje fibers; then in the ventricular myocardium it again decreases. This results in a mechanism called "gating."

Study of the action potential is possible through the use of a glass capillary microelectrode with an infinitesimally small tip inserted into a single cardiac fiber. This impalement does not result in significant cell injury because the microelectrode tip is so small (<1 μm). Thus the normal electrophysiologic properties of the fiber can be studied.

It is most useful in the study of arrhythmogenesis to understand the difference between the properties of fibers with action potentials dependent upon the fast sodium channel and those with slow-response action potentials, as well as the difference between pacemaker and nonpacemaker cells.

These mechanisms are easier to understand with some basic electrophysiologic concepts well in hand, such as concentration gradient, electrical potential gradient, membrane conductance, and equilibrium potential.

CONCENTRATION GRADIENT. A concentration gradient exists across a membrane that separates a high concentration of a particular ion from a low concentration of the same ion. Fig. 3-3 shows a permeable membrane separating two volumes of fluid. On the left side there is a high concentration of ionized potassium (K^+). On the right side the concentration of K^+ is low. By the process of diffusion, K^+ flows across the membrane from the high concentration to the low concentration (in Fig. 3-3 from left to right) until the concentration of K^+ becomes the same on both sides of the membrane. Such a flow of ions down a concentration gradient constitutes an electrical current.

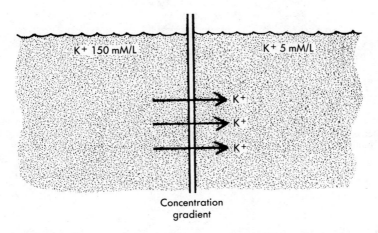

Concentration
gradient

Fig. 3-3. When a concentration gradient exists across a membrane, ions move across the membrane from the region of high concentration to the region of low concentration.

ELECTRICAL POTENTIAL GRADIENT. An electrical potential gradient exists when an electrical voltage difference exists across a membrane. For example, if a voltage is applied across a permeable membrane separating two ionic solutions, there is an electrical potential gradient across this membrane (Fig. 3-4). Let us assume that, at the time the voltage is first introduced across the membrane, the concentration of K^+ is the same on both sides of the membrane (Fig. 3-4); then, in response to this electrical potential gradient, the positive ions (in this case K^+) will move across the membrane to the more negative side. The ions flow from a high voltage to a low voltage, that is, down the electrical potential gradient. Such a flow of ions down the electrical potential gradient constitutes an electrical current.

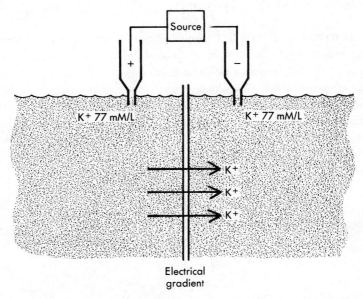

Fig. 3-4. There is an electrical potential gradient across this membrane. At the time the voltage is first applied across the membrane, the concentration of potassium ions is the same on both sides of it. In response to the electrical potential gradient the positive ions move to the negative side.

MEMBRANE CONDUCTANCE. Membrane conductance reflects the degree of permeability of the membrane to particular ions. A membrane that is highly permeable to a particular ion has a "high conductance" for that ion whereas a membrane with a relatively low permeability to a particular ion has a low conductance for that ion. When a decrease in the permeability of membrane to an ion occurs, it is sometimes said that conductance for this ion "falls."

The pumps

So far we have been talking about diffusion of ions in response to electrical and chemical gradients. In order to apply these principles to the cells of the heart, the concept of active transport mechanisms, usually called "pumps," must be introduced.

The Na^+ that enters and the K^+ that leaves the cells during each action potential must be returned in order for the necessary concentration gradients to be maintained. It is known that during diastole Na^+ is pumped out of the cell and K^+ is pumped back in and that more Na^+ is pumped out than K^+ in, generating a small net outward current of sodium ions across the cell membrane.[10] Since the pumping of Na^+ out of the cell (and K^+ into the cell) is against both electrical and concentration gradients, a considerable expenditure of energy is involved. This energy is stored in the form of ATP (adenosine triphosphate) and is released when the ATP is split by the Na^+-dependent and K^+-dependent Mg^{++}-ATPase (adenosinetriphosphatase), which constitutes the Na^+/K^+ pump, and which is located in the sarcolemma.[11]

Resting membrane potential

During diastole, when the heart muscle is at rest, most cardiac cells demonstrate a transmembrane voltage of -85 to -90 mV. This is referred to as the resting membrane potential and means that the inside of the cell is negative with respect to the outside, to the tune of -85 to -90 mV. It is the size of this voltage that determines both the amplitude of the action potential and its velocity of conduction.

The cell membrane at rest is relatively permeable to K^+ and relatively impermeable to Na^+, Ca^{++}, and Cl^- so that only the K^+ is free to migrate back and forth across the cell membrane. Thus it is predominantly the K^+ that determines the resting membrane potential.

Na^+ is pumped out of the cell, creating a large concentration gradient (outside: inside = 15:1). However, since the resting membrane is relatively impermeable to Na^+, very few of these ions leak back into the cell down the concentration gradient (Fig. 3-5).

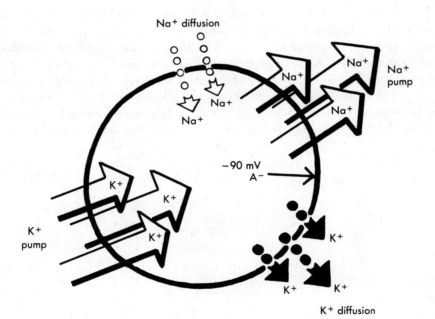

Fig. 3-5. Maintenance of the resting membrane potential by the ionic fluxes of sodium and potassium. The large empty arrows indicate active transport (pumping) and the small dots and arrows indicate passive diffusion (leakage) of ions down their electrochemical potential gradients.

K⁺ is pumped into the cell to maintain a large concentration gradient (outside: inside = 1:30). The membrane is relatively permeable to K⁺, which will therefore diffuse out of the cell down the concentration gradient (Fig. 3-5). The movement of K⁺ out of the cell produces a buildup of negativity on the inside of the cell that reaches some −85 to −90 mV with respect to the outside. This voltage is the resting membrane potential and is thus maintained until there is a change in membrane permeability, for example, during depolarization. One might expect negative ions (anions) inside the cell to diffuse out of the cell in response to the electrical gradient. This, however, does not happen since the majority of the intracellular anions are too large to pass through the membrane "pores." The resting membrane voltage thus created is related to the K⁺ concentration ratio between the inside and the outside of the cell. If this concentration ratio is reduced, the equilibrium resting voltage will also be reduced, roughly in accordance with the Nernst equation, which is discussed in detail elsewhere[11] and briefly summarized here.

The Nernst equation relates the electrical potential across a membrane to the concentration ratio across that membrane of permeable ions; and since resting cardiac cells are predominantly permeable to K⁺, it is the K⁺ gradient across the cardiac cell membrane that determines the resting membrane potential. As the K⁺ gradient decreases or increases in magnitude, so does the membrane potential. This is because with a smaller K⁺ gradient the driving force for K⁺ to leave the cell is smaller; since it is this driving force for K⁺ diffusion across the membrane that generates the intracellular negativity, the resting membrane potential will be less negative. Conversly, a larger K⁺ gradient results in a more negative resting membrane potential.

K⁺ concentration inside the cell might be altered by cardiac disease and thus the resting membrane potential might decrease, possibly resulting in arrhythmias and conduction disturbances. The resting membrane potential would also be reduced if the cell membrane itself became more permeable to Na⁺ or Ca⁺⁺.

In summary, the Na⁺/K⁺ pump maintains a high concentration of intracellular K⁺. The resting cell membrane is highly permeable to K⁺, which therefore diffuses out of the cell down the concentration gradient, thereby creating an electrical gradient. When the electrical gradient is large enough to exactly counter the outward diffusion of K⁺, an electrochemical equilibrium exists (i.e., the sum of the electrical and chemical potential gradients is zero) that maintains the resting membrane potential at approximately −90 mV, depending upon the concentrations of K⁺ inside and outside the cells. As the K⁺ level inside the cell decreases, so does the resting membrane potential, which in turn, as you will see, leads to the depression of conduction velocity.

Threshold potential

The threshold potential is the voltage level to which a cell must be depolarized before it can produce an action potential. This level is −60 to −70 mV for most cardiac fibers except those of the two nodes (SA and AV), where it is −30 to −40 mV. When the threshold is reached, specialized membrane channels open to permit the passage of Na^+ and/or Ca^{++} into the cell.

The threshold potential may vary, not only because of different cell types but also because of various other factors including changes in ionic environment and the level of the resting membrane potential at the time of stimulation.

Depolarization defined

Depolarization is the reduction of the membrane potential to a less negative value. For example, if from a resting membrane potential of −90 mV there is a slow buildup of positive ions on the inside of the cell that eventually brings the voltage to −85 mV, the voltage change would be called depolarization and the positive current responsible a depolarizing current. The cell, of course, can be depolarized rapidly by a fast influx of positive ions, which may actually bring the voltage to +30 mV.

The depolarization process, as you can see, is accomplished at different speeds depending, for example, upon the type of cells involved and whether the process is taking place during phase 0 (the rapid upstroke of the action potential) or phase 4 ("diastolic depolarization") of the action potential.

Except for the cells of the SA and AV nodes, the depolarization during phase 0 occurs rapidly (100 to 1000 V/sec) because the membrane, for a fraction of a second, becomes much more permeable to sodium than to potassium. The resultant flow of sodium ions into the cell down the electrochemical gradient (i.e., the fast sodium current mentioned earlier) produces a reversal in sign of the membrane potential from negative to positive.

For the cells of the SA and AV nodes the depolarization is slower (about 10 V/sec) and is the result of a smaller and slower current, probably carried by Ca^{++} and Na^+ (as described above) through the so-called "slow channels."

Slower still is the spontaneous depolarization that takes place in pacemaker cells during phase 4, termed "diastolic depolarization," which is currently believed to be due to a fall in K^+ conductance. We discuss this under "Automaticity" (p. 34).

Phase 0

Phase 0 is the upstroke of the action potential. In all cells except those of the two nodes this is the result of a sudden increase in Na^+ permeability, which permits a large inward current of Na^+ to flow down the electrochemical gradient (concentration and electrical gradient) into the cell. Two gates are believed to control the sudden increase in Na^+ conductance. One gate activates the fast Na^+ channel and the other inactivates it. A similar kind of mechanism is believed to control the slow Na^+/Ca^{++} channel. This is discussed under "Phase 2."

When the impulse arrives from the sinus node, the cell membrane is depolarized rapidly and driven to threshold potential. Upon reaching threshold potential, an adequate number of the fast Na^+ channels are opened to allow a Na^+ current large enough to depolarize the cell further and thus cause a greater number of fast Na^+ channels to become open. This kind of depolarization is thus regenerative. In order for this process to be initiated, a large enough area of membrane must be depolarized rapidly enough to bring the cell to threshold potential.

Fig. 3-6 illustrates phase 0 from a normal Purkinje fiber. You will note that the fiber was driven to threshold rapidly. This is the result of the depolarizing stimulus from adjacent cells, which opens the activation gates for the fast Na^+ channel. These gates open briskly and the Na^+ rushes into the cell down both concentration and electrical gradients to produce phase 0, which causes the graph to shoot almost vertically up past zero to approximately +30 mV. The attainment of a level above zero is referred to as the "positive overshoot."

The rapid opening of the activation gates for the fast Na^+ channel is immediately followed by the slower closing of different (inactivation) gates, interrupting the influx of Na^+ into the cell. In order for the inactivation gates to reopen again, so that the next action potential can occur, the membrane must be repolarized fully.

Phase 1

Phase 1 is the initial rapid repolarization phase of the action potential, which results in a spike due to the abrupt termination of phase 0. This phase of the action potential has, in the past, been thought to reflect the inactivation of the fast Na^+ current combined with a repolarizing current of Cl^-. More recently the repolarizing current flowing during phase 1 has been shown to be carried mainly by K^+ leaving the cell[12] but also partly by Cl^-.

Phase 2

Before the membrane potential returns to its resting level, another slower inward current is activated, resulting in phase 2, the "plateau" (Fig. 3-6), a characteristic feature of cardiac cells. The slow inward current responsible for this phase of the action potential is probably carried predominantly by Ca^{++}, but possibly also partly by Na^+,[7,13] and is triggered by the depolarization caused by the fast Na^+ current. The channel through which the slow inward current flows is called the *"slow channel"*.[14]

The threshold potential for activation of the slow channel is thought to be −30 to −40 mV. Thus by the time the fast Na^+ channel has been partially inactivated, the slow Na^+/Ca^{++} channel has already been opened so that a relatively slow influx of Na^+ and Ca^{++} into the cell maintains the plateau phase of the action potential. Outward repolarizing currents, at least one of which is probably K^+,[15-17] almost balance out the inward flow of Na^+ and Ca^{++} so that the membrane potential is almost steady for a short time. The Ca^{++} that enters the cell during phase 2 of the action potential is essential to electromechanical coupling.

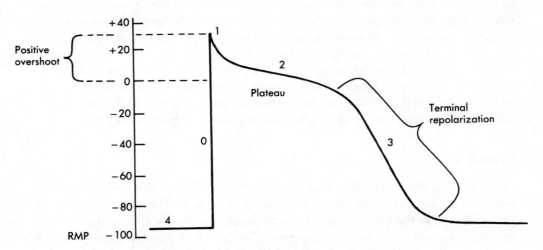

Fig. 3-6. Phases of the cardiac action potential.

Phase 3

Phase 3 is the terminal rapid repolarization accomplished mainly by an outward K^+ current that is activated slowly during the plateau. As the slow inward Na^+/Ca^{++} current diminishes with time and the outward K^+ current increases, the cell rapidly repolarizes.[14-16] After repolarization the Na^+/K^+ pump extrudes the accumulated intracellular Na^+ and pumps the lost K^+ back into the cell.

If for any reason the Na^+ pump is interfered with, there will be a gradual accumulation of intracellular sodium and loss of cellular potassium, since when Na^+ enters the cell K^+ leaves. The resulting decline in the transmembrane concentration gradient for K^+ causes the cell to gradually depolarize. This might result in cardiac arrhythmias.[11]

Membrane potential related to conduction velocity

An important determinant of conduction velocity is the magnitude of the rapid sodium influx, reflected in the speed with which phase 0 rises (dV/dt) and in the level of the positive overshoot.[18,19] The size of the sodium current is, in turn, dependent upon the membrane potential at the time of stimulation. The more negative this potential, the greater will be the number of sodium channels available to be opened to allow sodium to rush into the cell and the faster and higher will phase 0 climb. When the membrane potential just before excitation is about -95 mV, conduction velocity is optimal.[18,20] When the membrane potential is less negative, -70 mV for example, some of the Na^+ channels will be "unavailable" for opening because their inactivation gates remain closed, resulting in a smaller Na^+ current on depolarization. Phase 0 of the resting action potential will, in turn, have a slower rate of rise and a smaller amplitude (Fig. 3-7). Such an action potential might be an inadequate stimulus for neighboring cells in its conduction path, so that the amplitude of phase 0 of the action potential might diminish progressively as the impulse propagates. Such a sequence has been termed "decremental conduction."[4,21] The relationship between the membrane potential at the time of stimulation and the maximal rate of depolarization of the action potential reflects a property known as *membrane responsiveness*.

Other determinants of conduction velocity are the level of the threshold potential, the electrical cable properties of the fibers, and the diameter and structure of the fiber.[22]

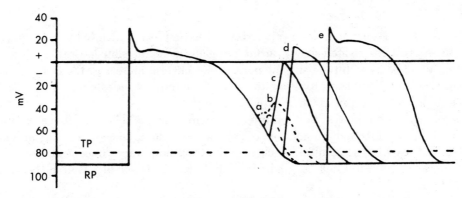

Fig. 3-7. Diagrammatic representation of a normal action potential and the responses elicited by stimuli applied at various stages of repolarization. The amplitude and upstroke velocity of the responses elicited during repolarization are related to the level of the membrane potential from which they arise. The earliest responses (*a* and *b*) arise from such low levels of membrane potential that they are too small to propagate (graded or local responses). Response *c* represents the earliest propagated action potential, but it propagates slowly because of its low upstroke velocity and low amplitude. Response *d* is elicited just before complete repolarization, and its rate of rise and amplitude are greater than those of *c* because it arises from a higher membrane potential. However, it still propagates more slowly than normal. Response *e* is elicited after complete repolarization and, therefore, has a normal rate of depolarization and amplitude and so propagates rapidly. (From Singer, D.H., and Ten Eick, R.E.: Prog. Cardiovasc. Dis. **11:**488, 1969.)

Automaticity

Automaticity is the capability of a cell to depolarize spontaneously, reach threshold potential, and initiate an action potential. This is accomplished through a slow buildup of positive ions inside the cell during diastole (thus the terms "slow diastolic depolarization," "spontaneous diastolic depolarization," or "phase 4 depolarization").

In normal hearts only the cells of the SA node reach threshold potential without an outside stimulus, although cells in other areas are capable of automaticity and are referred to as subsidiary or latent pacemakers. Those potential pacemaking areas are mitral and tricuspid valve muscle, atrial cells near the ostium of the coronary sinus, the distal part of the AV node, and the His-Purkinje system.[11,23,24] Normally before latent pacemakers can reach threshold, they are depolarized by the impulse generated in the SA node.

The pacemaking mechanism of Purkinje fibers has been studied more than that of the SA node, which might have a different ionic mechanism (described on p. 39). The following is a description of the pacemaker phenomenon in Purkinje fibers.

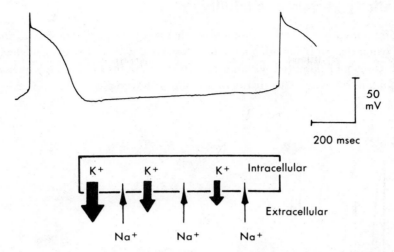

Fig. 3-8. One cycle of an automatic rhythm. Under the record are the transmembrane potassium (outward) and sodium (inward) ionic currents associated with spontaneous phase 4 depolarization. The arrows indicate the directions of these currents. The slowly declining potassium (pacemaker) current allows the steady sodium current to cause gradual depolarization until the threshold potential is reached. (From Rosen, M.R., and Hordof, A.J.: In Roberts, N.K., and Gelband, H., editors: Cardiac arrhythmias in the neonate, infant, and child, New York, 1977, Appleton-Century-Crofts.)

The slow diastolic depolarization results from the gradual shift in the balance between inward and outward current components in the direction of net inward (i.e., depolarizing) current. Earlier studies suggested that the shift reflects a time-dependent decrease in an outward K^+ current, referred to as the "pacemaker current." Fig. 3-8 diagrammatically illustrates the decrease in this outward K^+ current during phase 4 in a cell undergoing spontaneous depolarization.

It is believed that the gates for this special pacemaker current are fully opened by the depolarization during phase 0 and then slowly close following repolarization, during phase 4, causing the slow diastolic depolarization. The cell may reach threshold potential by means of this slow diastolic depolarization, or, as usually happens, it may be rapidly driven to threshold by an impulse emanating from the dominant pacemaker.

Automaticity versus excitability

All normal myocardial cells are excitable; that is, they can all give rise to an action potential when driven by an adequate stimulus. However, only the specialized cells can reach threshold potential without an outside stimulus. These cells possess the property of automaticity. This distinction is illustrated in Fig. 3-9.

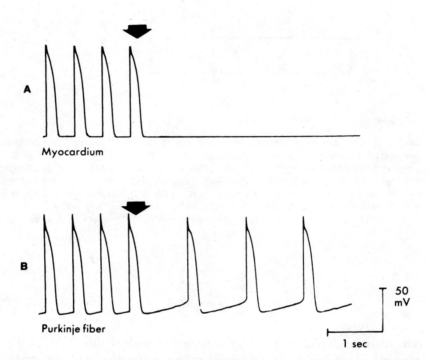

Fig. 3-9. Excitability and automaticity. The fibers in **A** and **B** are being driven by an extracellular electrode. Both types of cells are excitable. At the arrows the stimulus is discontinued. The myocardial fiber (**A**) will not begin to fire again until the stimulus is reinitiated, but the Purkinje fiber (**B**) can depolarize spontaneously during phase 4 until threshold potential is attained and an action potential is initiated (automaticity). (From Rosen, M.R., and Hordof, A.J.: In Roberts, N.K., and Gelband, H., editors: Cardiac arrhythmias in the neonate, infant, and child, New York, 1977, Appleton-Century-Crofts.)

Refractory periods

Refractoriness is the inability of a cell or tissue to respond to a stimulus because it has been too recently activated by a previous stimulus. The *refractory period* is the interval during which the cell or tissue in question remains unresponsive to a second stimulus. Four refractory periods have been described: absolute, relative, effective, and functional.

The first description of the refractory period seems to have been as early as 1850 (Schiff). Classically it has been divided into *absolute* and *relative*, depending upon the response of the myocardium to a stimulus as recorded by electrodes some distance from the stimulating electrode. During the *absolute refractory period* (ARP) no stimulus can evoke a propagated response; during the *relative refractory period* (RRP) a propagated response can result from a strong stimulus. For example, the ARP of the AV node is that interval during which it is impossible for a stimulus to activate and penetrate the node; in the RRP the stimulus can penetrate the node if it is strong enough, but conduction velocity through the node is impaired.

ELECTROPHYSIOLOGY OF REFRACTORINESS. The refractory period itself is determined by the level of the transmembrane potential. Following phase 0 of the action potential the fast sodium channels are inactivated and do not become reactivated until the membrane potential has achieved −60 mV (phase 3 of the action potential). During this time the membrane does not respond with a propagated action potential to even a strong stimulus. When the membrane achieves −60 mV, the fast sodium channels become partially activated; and as the recovery of excitability (repolarization) proceeds, a strong stimulus may elicit a propagated response (relative refractory period). Such a response is characterized by slow conduction.

CONFUSION REGARDING TERMINOLOGY. In 1926 Lewis and Drury[25] differentiated the absolute from the effective refractory period, stating that "the end of the absolute refractory period signals the instant at which the muscle will again respond, at least in part"; and the effective refractory period "signals the first instant at which the muscle will again *transmit a propagated wave* to any distance." The two terms, absolute and effective, have resulted in such confusion that some authors[26,27] have even equated the *relative* with the *effective* and others[28] have equated the *relative* with the *functional* refractory period.

Although the *effective refractory* period does correspond in duration to the *absolute refractory* period, these terms imply different effects at the cellular level. It has been shown that a stimulus which falls too early to propagate still is not without influence; it may cause a prolongation of refractoriness, and thus the muscle is not "absolutely" refractory although it is "effectively" refractory in that it will not respond with a propagated action potential. Thus the term *effective refractory period* best defines the period during which a propagated action potential cannot be evoked (even though the stimulus may produce active responses at the cellular level).[4] Clinically the two terms are interchangeable.

The *functional refractory period* is measured between a basic and a premature impulse and is the shortest time in which an impulse will traverse the tissue in question. It is not applicable to single cells; its measurement is complex, involves and includes conduction through tissue, and is therefore affected by numerous variables (including the length of the tissue, the refractory periods of all cells along the way, the conduction velocity through the tissue, etc.).

REFRACTORINESS OF THE SLOW RESPONSE ACTION POTENTIAL. Fibers with a low resting potential are depolarized by Na^+/Ca^{++} currents flowing through slow channels and are very difficult to stimulate once repolarization is complete because refractoriness far outlasts the action potential duration.[7]

The supernormal period

The supernormal period occurs at the end of phase 3 (Fig. 3-10). During this period a beat can be initiated with a smaller stimulus than is required at normal resting membrane potential.[29] This is thought to be because, at a point when the fiber has almost returned to its resting state, the membrane potential is closer to threshold than it is after full return to the resting potential.

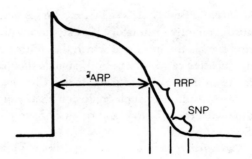

Fig. 3-10. The supernormal period of the action potential related to the refractory periods. *SNP,* Supernormal period; *ARP,* absolute refractory period; *RRP,* relative refractory period.

Action potential of the sinus node

Fig. 3-11 illustrates action potentials from the dominant SA nodal pacemaker as recorded in 1965 by Sano and Yamagishi.[31]

The maximum diastolic potential in the cells of the SA and AV nodes is about 20 mV less negative than the resting membrane potential of other myocardial fibers.[4]

The very steep phase 4 of SA node cells is probably caused by a different ionic mechanism from that of Purkinje cells.[32] The AV node has an action potential similar to that of the SA node, although the property of automaticity has not been observed in AV nodal cells in the in vitro heart.

Phase 0 of SA and AV nodal cells has a slower upstroke and lower amplitude than that of action potentials from other areas of the heart. This upstroke results from activation of a slow inward current thought to be carried by calcium and sodium ions[7,35-37] as opposed to the fast currents underlying the rapid depolarization of other myocardial fibers. Such action potentials are called *slow response action potentials,* and they conduct slowly through the SA and AV nodal tissue (0.01 to 0.1 m/sec). This slow inward positive current is inactivated more slowly than the fast sodium current.

Following phase 0 in nodal cells the slow inward positive current is gradually inactivated and an outward potassium current is turned on, thereby causing repolarization. The slow channel is then only gradually reactivated through diastole, so that even after full repolarization the slow inward channels may still not be ready to respond to another stimulus. This explains the long relative refractory period and slow conduction typical of the two nodes. The long relative refractory period, in turn, causes premature impulses to be conducted through the nodes even more slowly than normal, an important feature in the support of reentry arrhythmias (p. 73).

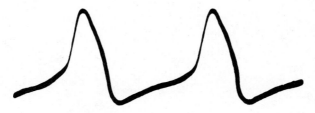

Fig. 3-11. Sinus node action potential. (Modified from Sano, T., and Yamagishi, S.: Circ. Res. **16:**423, 1965.)

Information about the action potential of the SA node is slow in coming because of the difficulties involved in studying that structure.[7] Those difficulties include the facts that

1. The SA node has two types of pacemaker cells, dominant and latent, that differ in their response to changes in ionic environment and drugs.

2. Phase 4 in the SA node cannot easily be studied separately from phase 0 since ions and drugs affecting one usually profoundly affect the other, a feature not shared by Purkinje cells.

3. It is difficult to drive the SA node directly; and when it is driven by retrograde activation, its action potentials are not normal.

4. The dominant pacemaker site within the SA node often shifts when one fiber is being studied, causing the one studied to be retrogradely and thus abnormally activated.

5. Because the SA node is richly innervated, its properties are easily altered by acetylcholine and catecholamines released from the nerve terminals.

Action potential related to the ECG

Because the ventricular depolarizing current begins in the septum and ends in the posterior basal part of the left ventricle, first and last cells depolarize asynchronously (as indicated in Fig. 3-12). Note that as a result of this difference in electrical potential between the first and the last cells to depolarize, the ECG stylus is displaced from the isoelectric line to produce the QRS complex. Thus abnormalities in depolarization are reflected in the QRS; those in repolarization are reflected in the QT interval. During phase 2 the action potential of the first and the last cells to depolarize are at approximately the same potential. With little difference in potential, no current flows and the ECG has an isoelectric ST segment. During rapid repolarization (phase 3) there is again a difference in potential, which produces the T wave. The effects of injury currents on ST and TQ segments are discussed in other publications.[36,37]

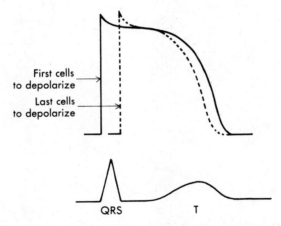

Fig. 3-12. Action potentials from the first and last cells to depolarize related to the ECG. Because of a difference in potential between the first and last cells to depolarize, the QRS is inscribed. The ST segment results when there is no difference in potential and is therefore isoelectric. The T wave reflects the difference in potential during phase 3. (Modified from Surawicz, B., and Saito, S.: Am. J. Cardiol. **41:**943, 1978.)

The gating mechanism

The action potential duration increases progressively from the AV node to the distal Purkinje system, where it reaches its maximum; beyond this its duration decreases.[8,38]

In Fig. 3-13 this trend can be seen. The refractory periods depend upon the durations of the action potentials, being maximal when the action potential is broadest. This region of maximal action potential duration is referred to as the "gate." In order for a premature stimulus to propagate through the entire conduction system, it must arrive at the gate after the gate's effective refractory period is over. If the stimulus arrives while the distal Purkinje fibers are still refractory, it will not propagate into the ventricular myocardium even though that part of the heart is nonrefractory. Hence the functional refractory period for tissue distal to the Purkinje system is determined by the effective refractory period at the gate.

This gate protects the ventricles from premature depolarization during their relative refractory period.

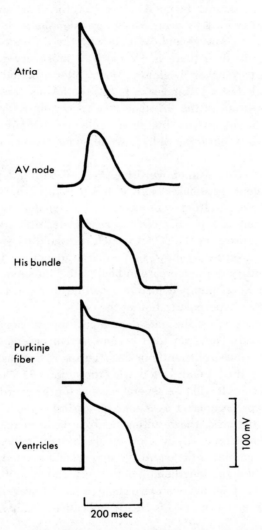

Atria

AV node

His bundle

Purkinje
fiber

Ventricles

100 mV

200 msec

Fig. 3-13. The gating mechanism. Note that the action potential gets longer and longer until it reaches its maximal duration in the Purkinje fibers. Then it decreases in length.

Overdrive suppression

Overdrive suppression is the inhibitory effect of a faster pacemaker on a slower pacemaker. This, along with the successful race to threshold potential exhibited by the SA node, normally assures the node of its role as the dominant pacemaker of the heart. The inhibition exerted by overdrive suppression makes it more difficult for a subsidiary pacemaker to emerge and compete with the SA node.

If the SA node fails or if there is AV block, a subsidiary pacemaker may become the dominant pacemaker, beginning slowly after a period of quiescence and then becoming a little faster but never as fast as the SA node.

Overdrive suppression of the SA node itself generally refers to the inhibitory effect of a period of driven activity (by use of an electrical stimulus) on the automatic activity of the SA node,[39] but it is a well known phenomenon even after a single atrial extrasystole.[40,41]

Mechanism. The mechanism of overdrive suppression is a depression of phase 4 in the dominated, latent, pacemaker cells. In the atria this is believed to involve the release of acetylcholine, resulting in an increase in K^+ conductance so that the fall in pacemaker K^+ current is less effective in causing depolarization. This, in turn, lengthens the time it takes for the cells to reach threshold potential.

In Purkinje fibers overdrive suppression is due to an increase in the activity of the Na^+/K^+ pump secondary to the increase in heart rate.[41] Since more Na^+ is pumped out of the cell than K^+ is pumped in, the resulting increase in net outward Na^+ pump current causes a hyperpolarization of the cells.

During sinus bradycardia the rate-dependent suppression of the subsidiary pacemakers is reduced. They can thus become active pacemakers without much delay if the SA node slows sufficiently or fails. This is in contrast to the effects of a sudden suppression of the SA node or following the sudden development of complete heart block. In such cases it will take several seconds for the overdrive suppression to subside and the escape pacemaker to assume its intrinsic rate. Thus, although vagal stimulation inhibits the atria, the resulting bradycardia secondarily removes an inhibition from the ventricles and may allow escape beats to appear more promptly.

Fig. 3-14 gives examples of the overdrive suppression exerted on the SA node by atrial extrasystoles. In *A* the lengthening of the cycle following the premature atrial beat is a manifestation of normal overdrive suppression. However, in *B* such slowing following the atrial premature beats is clearly indicative of abnormal SA node function.

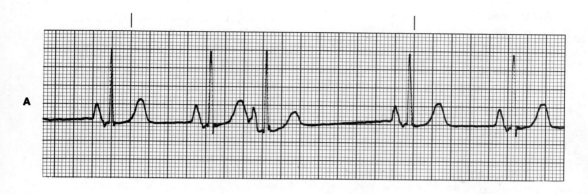

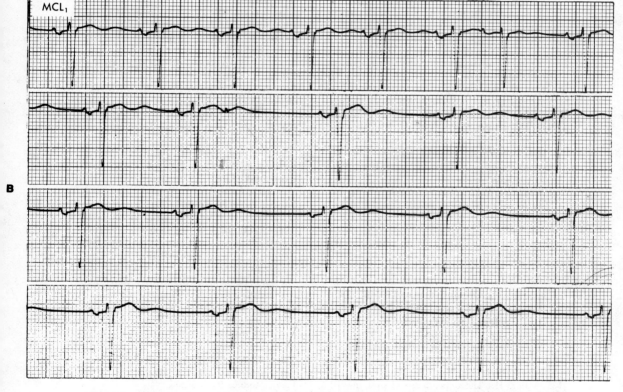

Fig. 3-14. A, Normal manifestation of overdrive suppression. Note the lengthening of the cycle following the atrial premature beat. **B,** Abnormal response by the sinus node to overdrive suppression by
two atrial premature beats.

References

1. Hodgkin, A.L., and Katz, B.: Ionic currents underlying activity in the giant axon of the squid, J. Physiol. **108**:37, 1949.
2. Hodgkin, A.L., and Huxley, A.F.: A quantitative description of membrane current and its application to conduction and excitation in nerve, J. Physiol. **117**:500, 1952.
3. Noble, D.: A modification of the Hodgkin-Huxley equations to Purkinje-fibre action and pacemaker potentials, J. Physiol. **160**:317, 1962.
4. Hoffman, B.F., and Cranefield, P.F.: Electrophysiology of the heart, New York, 1960, McGraw-Hill Book Co.
5. Neidergerke, R., and Orkand, R.K.: The dependence of the action potential of the frog's heart on the external and intracellular sodium concentration, J. Physiol. **84**:312, 1966.
6. Hagiwara, S., and Nakajima, S.: Differences in Na and Ca spikes as examined by application of tetrodotoxin, procaine, and manganese ions, J. Gen. Physiol. **49**:793, 1966.
7. Cranefield, P.F.: The conduction of the cardiac impulse, Mount Kisco, N.Y., 1975, Futura Publishing Co.
8. Myerburg, R.J., Stewart, J.W., and Hoffman, B.F.: Electrophysiological properties of the canine peripheral AV conducting system, Circ. Res. **26**:361, 1970.
9. Myerburg, R.J.: The gating mechanism in the distal AV conducting system, Circulation **43**: 955, 1971.
10. Thomas, R.C.: Electrogenic sodium pump in nerve and muscle cells, Physiol. Rev. **52**:563, 1972.
11. Gadsby, D.C., and Wit, A.L.: Electrophysiologic characteristics of cardiac cells and the genesis of cardiac arrhythmias. In Wilkenson, R.D., editor: Cardiac pharmacology, New York, 1981, Academic Press, Inc.
12. Kenyon, J.L., and Gibbons, W.R.: Effects of low-chloride solutions on action potentials of sheep cardiac Purkinje fibers, J. Gen. Physiol. **70**:635, 1977.
13. Reuter, H.: The dependence of slow inward current in Purkinje fibers on the extracellular calcium concentration, J. Physiol. (Lond.) **192**: 479, 1967.
14. Reuter, H.: Divalent cations as charge carriers in excitable membranes, Prog. Biophys. Mol. Biol. **26**:1, 1973.
15. Trautwein, W.: Membrane currents in cardiac muscle fibers, Physiol. Rev. **53**:973, 1973.
16. Noble, D., and Tsien, R.W.: Outward membrane currents activated in the plateau range of potentials in cardiac Purkinje fibers, J. Physiol. (Lond.) **200**:205, 1969.
17. Isenberg, G., and Trautwein, W.: The effect of dihydro-ouabain and lithium-ions on the outward current in cardiac Purkinje fibers evidence for electrogenicity of active transport, Pfluegers Arch. **35**:41, 1974.
18. Weidmann, S.: The effect of the cardiac membrane potential on the rapid availability of the sodium-carrying system, J. Physiol. **127**:213, 1955.
19. Jack, J.J.B., Noble, D., and Tsien, R.W.: Electric current flow in excitable cells, Oxford, 1975, Clarendon Press.
20. Draper, M.H., and Weidmann, S.: Cardiac resting and action potentials recorded with an intracellular electrode, J. Physiol. **115**:74, 1951.
21. Erlanger, J.: Further studies on the physiology of heart block. The effects of extra systoles upon the dog's heart and upon strips of terrapin's ventricle in the various stages of block, Am. J. Physiol. **16**:160, 1906.
22. Cranefield, P.F., and Hoffman, B.F.: Conduction of the cardiac impulse impulse. 2. Summation and inhibition, Circ. Res. **28**:220, 1971.
23. Wit, A.L., Fenoglio, J.J., Wagner, B.M., and Bassett, A.L.: Electrophysiological properties of cardiac muscle in the anterior mitral valve leaflet and the adjacent atrium in the dog. Possible implications for the genesis of atrial dysrhythmias, Circ. Res. **32**:731, 1973.
24. Bassett, A.L., Wit, A.L., and others: Ectopic impulses originating in the tricuspid valve and contiguous atrium, Fed. Proc. **33**:445, 1974.
25. Lewis, T., and Drury, A.N.: Revised views of the refractory period, in relation to drugs reputed to prolong it and in relation to circus movement, Heart **13**:95, 1926.
26. Goldman, M.J.: Principles of clinical electrocardiography, ed. 10, Los Altos, Calif., 1979 Lange Medical Publications.
27. Shine, K.: Ionic basis of excitation and of excitation-contraction coupling. In Roberts, N.K., and Gelband, H., editors: Cardiac arrhythmias in the neonate, infant, and child, New York, 1977, Appleton-Century-Crofts.

28. Pick, A., and Langendorf, R.: Interpretation of complex arrhythmias, Philadelphia, 1979, Lea & Febiger.

29. Spear, J.F., and Moore, E.N.: Supernormal excitability and conduction in the His-Purkinje system of the dog, Circ. Res. **35**:782, 1974.

30. Rosen, M.R., and Hordof, A.J.: Mechanisms of arrhythmias. In Roberts, N.K., and Gelband, H., editors: Cardiac arrhythmias in the neonate, infant, and child, New York, 1977, Appleton-Century-Crofts.

31. Sano, T., and Yamagishi, S.: Spread of excitation from the sinus node, Circ. Res. **16**:423, 1965.

32. Noma, A., and Irisawa, H.: A time- and voltage-dependent potassium current in the rabbit sinoatrial node cell, Pfluegers Arch. **366**:251, 1976.

33. Paes de Carvalho, A., Hoffman, B.F., and de Paula Carvalho, M.: Two components of the cardiac action potential. I. Voltage time course and the effect of acetylcholine on atrial and nodal cells of the rabbit heart, J. Gen. Physiol. **54**:607, 1969.

34. Zipes, C.P., and Mendez, C.: Action of manganese ions and tetrodotoxin on atrioventricular nodal transmembrane potentials in isolated rabbit hearts, Circ. Res. **32**:447, 1973.

35. Wit, A.L., and Cranefield, P.F.: Effect of verapamil on the sinoatrial and atrioventricular nodes of the rabbit and the mechanism by which it arrests reentrant atrioventricular nodal tachycardia, Circ. Res. **35**:413, 1974.

36. Surawicz, B., and Saito, S.: Exercise testing for detection of myocardial ischemia in patients with abnormal electrocardiograms at rest, Am. J. Cardiol. **41**:943, 1978.

37. Conover, M.H.: Understanding electrocardiography, ed. 3, St. Louis, 1980, The C.V. Mosby Co.

38. Myerburg, R.J., Gelband, H., and others: Electrophysiology of endocardial intraventricular conduction: the role and function of the specialized conducting system. In Wellens, H.J.J., Lie, K.I., and Janse, M.J., editors: The conduction system of the heart, Philadelphia, 1976, Lea & Febiger.

39. Vassalle, M.: The relationship among cardiac pacemakers: overdrive suppression, Circ. Res. **41**:269, 1977.

40. Katz, L.N., and Pick, A.: Clinical electrocardiography. I. The arrhythmias, Philadelphia, 1956, Lea & Febiger.

41. Paulay, M.K.L., Varghese, P.J., and Damato, A.N.: Atrial rhythms in response to an early atrial premature depolarization in man, Am. Heart J. **85**:323, 1973.

CHAPTER 4

The reentry mechanism

"Reentry" is well named: it implies that an impulse, after activating a segment of tissue once, returns and activates it again. Obviously the impulse cannot double back on its tracks and retrace its steps since tissue in its wake is refractory; there must be a separate return pathway. Equally as obvious, it must not return too soon or the just-activated tissue will still be refractory. Therefore prerequisites for reentry include a second approach to the involved segment (which implies the existence of a circuit) and slow enough conduction.

However, there is a third requirement as well: there must be unequal responsiveness in two segments of the dual circuitous path; otherwise, the spreading impulse would synchronously activate all in its path and there would be no opportunity for it to turn back and reactivate the tissue it had previously depolarized. This third requirement is often described as "unidirectional block"; and, of course, such block would and does favor reentry. However, unidirectional block—implying that conduction is possible in only one direction—is essential only when the block is permanent. When the block is transient (due to refractoriness), the difference in the refractory periods of two limbs of the circuit suffices.

In Fig. 4-1 the segment of tissue, X, is initially activated from left to right (continuous line). If the impulse finds that path Y is still refractory after path Z has recovered from a previous activation, the impulse will traverse Z but will be unable to enter Y. If, however, Y has recovered by the time the impulse approaches its other end, the impulse will be able to activate it from right to left; and if, in turn, the impulse has traveled slowly enough that X or Z has had time to recover, the impulse will reenter X and/or Z to initiate a single reentry (reciprocal, echo) beat or a run of reciprocating tachycardia.

When the circuit involved is tiny, as in the AV node or a distal Purkinje circuit, the phenomenon is *"micro*reentry." When the circuit includes long tracts, as in the WPW tachycardias or the fascicular divisions of the LBB, the term *"macro*reentry" is appropriate.

We can summarize the requirements for reentry as follows:

1. An available circuit
2. Unequal responsiveness in two segments of the circuit
3. Slow conduction

Thus it is that one of the factors favoring reentry is delayed conduction; and, in fact, the existence of such conduction delay may be the decisive clue to the fact that the underlying mechanism is reentry. It is therefore true to say that rhythms which depend upon reentry for their development or perpetuation are disorders of conduction rather than of impulse formation.

Among the disturbances of rhythm known to be due to reentry are

1. Some extrasystoles
2. Some ventricular tachycardias
3. Most supraventricular tachycardias
4. WPW tachycardias
5. Reciprocal rhythms (atrial and ventricular echoes)

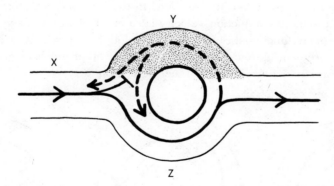

Fig. 4-1. Reentry. The segment of tissue *(X)* is initially activated from left to right (continuous line). One path *(Y)* is still refractory and the impulse cannot enter. The other path *(Z)* has recovered partially and the impulse travels slowly through it, by which time the *Y* path has recovered. The impulse then travels retrogradely in *Y* to reenter *X* and *Z*.

History of reentry

Reentry was mentioned as early as 1887[1]; but first proof of its existence was adduced by Mayer in 1906[2] and 1908[3] through his work with jellyfish, an animal that also provided early researchers with an understanding of the concepts of cardiac rhythmicity, pacemaker function, and conduction block.[4-7]

The concepts of reciprocating rhythms and reciprocal or "echo" beats arose from the experiments of Mines in 1913[8] and 1914,[9] using portions of the atria and ventricles of the frog and electrical ray.

The original jellyfish studies by Mayer are worth recounting here since the results of his experiments can be applied to atrial, ventricular, and Purkinje fibers in the human heart.

Fig. 4-2 represents the subumbrella tissue of the jellyfish, which Mayer cut into a ring. Note in *A* that when the ring was stimulated at one point the excitation waves traveled in opposite directions around the ring to meet and cancel each other out. When pressure was applied (the shaded area in *B*) on one side of the ring near the point of origin, the impulse was blocked there and traveled only in the opposite direction. When the impulse was on its one-way journey around the ring, the pressure was released and the impulse was able to continue around and around (*C*). The impulse continued to propagate because it traveled in only one direction and because the ring was long enough to allow the point of stimulation to recover before the impulse arrived from the opposite direction. In the human heart more than this is necessary since normal conduction velocity is so fast that it is unlikely that such a circuit could exist in functional isolation.[10] In the following pages we will discuss the additional requirement of *slow conduction* as well as other mechanisms involved in reentry, such as summation, inhibition, and reflection.

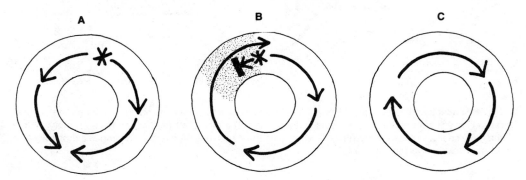

Fig. 4-2. Diagrammatic representation of the first studies by Mayer proving reentry. In **A** the impulses travel from the stimulus in opposite directions around the ring to meet and cancel each other out. In **B** pressure has been applied at the shaded area in the ring, at which point the impulse is blocked and travels only in the opposite direction. Pressure is then removed and the impulse continues around and around (**C**) on its one-way journey as long as refractory tissue is not encountered.

Slow conduction

You will recall from Chapter 3 that one of the determinants of conduction velocity is the level of the resting membrane potential at the time of stimulation. The more negative the resting membrane potential, the more sodium channels are available and the quicker these channels open to allow sodium to rush into the cell. This mechanism has been referred to as the "fast response" action potential.[11] It occurs in fibers in which the resting membrane potential is optimal (−80 to −90 mV) and, in the Purkinje system, results in conduction velocity of 1 to 4 m/sec.[12,13]

DEPRESSED FAST RESPONSE.[14] When the resting membrane potential is between −60 and −70 mV, only about half the fast sodium channels are available and consequently the upstroke velocity and amplitude of phase 0 of the action potential are less than normal and conduction velocity decreases. Such an action potential is the result of both sodium and calcium influxes into the cell, which are slower and of less magnitude than at a more negative resting membrane potential.

SLOW RESPONSE.[15,16] When the resting membrane potential is less than −55 or −60 mV, the action potential is mainly the result of a relatively slow influx of calcium along with some sodium, since the fast sodium channels are completely inactivated at approximately −50 mV.[12] A strong depolarizing current may initiate the slow upstroke velocity and low amplitude. This type of action potential results in slow conducton, and may result in one-way conduction block,[17] or with further reduction of the resting membrane potential the action potential no longer acts as a stimulus for the fibers ahead of it and conduction will be blocked in both directions.

Both the depressed fast response and the slow response action potentials have been shown to occur in the diseased human heart.[18,19] Therefore in a sufficiently long segment conduction can proceed slowly enough to still be traveling when the normal tissue has completed its effective refractory period. This impulse can then reenter the newly repolarized normal tissue and produce an ectopic beat. Actually the slow response action potentials are conducted so slowly that the length of depressed tissue may be short indeed and still support a current until the surrounding tissue has recovered.

Fig. 4-3 illustrates and compares the normal fast response action potential with the depressed fast response and the slow response action potentials. Note that as the resting membrane potential decreases (becomes less negative) so do the upstroke velocity and height of phase 0.

Within minutes following a coronary occlusion the resulting anoxia produces continuous localized electrical activity, the action potential duration shortens, and the resting membrane potential decreases.[20-22] Thus the depressed fast response and the slow response are the rule in infarcted tissues.

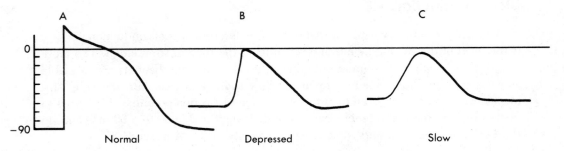

Fig. 4-3. Comparison of the normal fast response action potential (*A*) with the depressed fast response (*B*) and the slow response (*C*) action potentials.

Unidirectional block

Unidirectional block, as mentioned above, is one of the conditions that favor reentry and may result from a lowered resting membrane potential.

When bundles of myocardial tissue (atrial, ventricular, or Purkinje) are stimulated at both ends, the impulse travels at almost equal velocities in both directions. If the resting membrane potential is so reduced that the upstroke velocity and amplitude of phase 0 are less (a depressed fast response), conduction is slower in both directions. If the resting membrane potential is reduced even further to produce a slow response action potential, conduction may proceed slowly in only one direction and not at all in the other.[12]

Summation

Summation has been mentioned by Cranefield[15] as a possible cause of one-way conduction block. It requires a particular arrangement of fibers: if two fibers converge to form one, it is possible that two impulses, both traveling toward the convergence, could meet and form a stronger current.

If the segment is depressed, then conduction may actually depend upon this convergence and the resulting "summation," as illustrated in Fig. 4-4, *A*. Note that in 4-4, *B*, on the other hand, one of the impulses reaches the depressed area at the convergence before the other and is therefore unable to propagate through alone. In Fig. 4-4, *C*, the impulse is traveling in the opposite direction through the depressed area; and because it divides instead of uniting, block results.

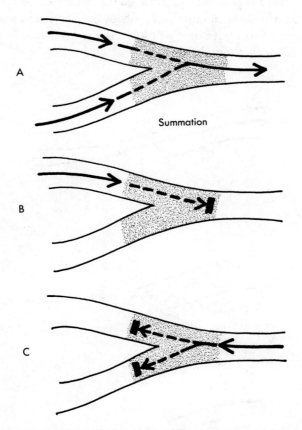

Fig. 4-4. Summation. In **A** two impulses converge within a depressed area to form a current strong enough to emerge from the depressed area, whereas only one of the impulses entering the depressed area (**B**) would be blocked. In **C** an impulse traveling in the opposite direction through the depressed area divides, instead of converging, and is blocked.

Inhibition

The term inhibition is used to describe the mechanism when one impulse, which is unable to travel through a depressed segment, reaches that segment first and leaves it refractory so a stronger impulse entering the depressed segment via another fiber is blocked.

In Fig. 4-5 impulse *1* is able to travel through the depressed segment (*A*) whereas impulse *2* is not (*B*). However, if impulse *2* reaches the depressed segment first (*C*), not only will it be blocked itself but it will leave refractory tissue in the pathway of impulse *1* and so block that impulse as well.

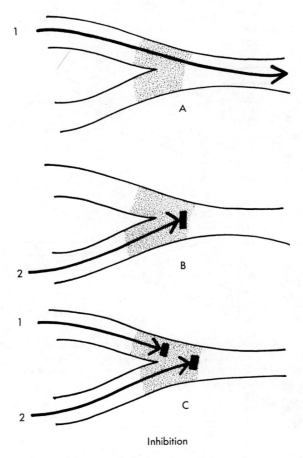

Inhibition

Fig. 4-5. Inhibition. In **A,** impulse *1* can negotiate the depressed (shaded) area; impulse *2,* on the other hand, cannot (**B**). And if this weaker impulse reaches the depressed area first (**C**), it will also block the stronger impulse (*1*).

Reflection

Another form of reentry is produced through reflection—it is possible for an impulse to turn around within a depressed segment of tissue. If the site of origin has completed its effective refractory period by the time the reflected impulse returns to it, a premature beat will result. This mechanism is diagrammatically illustrated in Fig. 4-6; two adjacent depressed fibers are shown, the upper fiber more severely depressed than the lower one.

The originating wave front (*1*) is blocked in the severely depressed fiber (*2*) but proceeds slowly in the other fiber. At *3* the wave front returns via the severely depressed fiber to the area of its origin. If the normal myocardium has completed its effective refractory period by the time the impulse reaches the interface between normal and depressed tissue, it will be propagated through the normal myocardium to produce a premature complex.

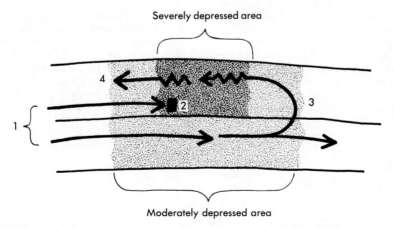

Fig. 4-6. Reflection. The impulse (*1*) is blocked in the severely depressed fiber (*2*) but proceeds slowly in the less depressed fiber to return in the opposite direction (*3*) via the severely depressed fiber to its origin (*4*).

References

1. McWilliams, J.A.: Fibrillar contraction of the heart, J. Physiol. (Lond.) **8:**296, 1887.
2. Mayer, A.G.: Rhythmical pulsation in scyphomedusae, Carnegie Institution of Washington, Publication no. 47, 1906.
3. Mayer, A.G.: Rhythmical pulsation in scyphomedusae. II. In Papers from the Tortugas Laboratory of the Carnegie Institution of Washington, Publication no. 102, Part 7, 1908.
4. Romanes, G.J.: Preliminary observations on the locomotor system of medusae, Phil. Trans. R. Soc. Lond. **166:**269, 1876.
5. Romanes, G.J.: Further observations on the locomotor system of medusae, Phil. Trans. R. Soc. Lond. **167:**659, 1877.
6. Romanes, G.J.: Concluding observations on the locomotor system of medusae, Phil. Trans. R. Soc. Lond. **171:**161, 1880.
7. Romanes, G.J.: Jelly-fish, star-fish, and sea-urchins: being a research on primitive nervous systems, London, 1885, Kegan Paul, Trench & Co.
8. Mines, G.R.: On dynamic equilibrium in the heart, J. Physiol. (Lond.) **46:**349, 1913.
9. Mines, G.R.: On circulating excitations in heart muscles and their possible relation to tachycardia and fibrillation, Trans. R. Soc. Can. **8:**43, 1914.
10. Cranefield, P.F., and Hoffman, B.F.: Reentry: slow conduction, summation, and inhibition, Circulation **44:**309, 1971.
11. Cranefield, P.F., Wit, A.L., and Hoffman, B.F.: Conduction of the cardiac impulse. III. Characteristics of very slow conduction, J. Gen. Physiol. **59:**227, 1972.
12. Gadsby, D.C., and Wit, A.L.: Normal and abnormal electrophysiology of cardiac cells. In Mandel, W.J., editor: Cardiac arrhythmias; their mechanisms, diagnosis, and management, Philadelphia, 1980, J.B. Lippincott Co.
13. Rosen, M.R., and Hordof, A.J.: Mechanisms of arrhythmias. In Roberts, N.K., and Gelband, H., editors: Cardiac arrhythmias in the neonate, infant, and child, New York, 1977, Appleton-Century-Crofts.
14. Wit, A.L., Rosen, M.R., and Hoffman, B.F.: Electrophysiology and pharmacology of cardiac arrhythmias. II. Relation of normal and abnormal electrical activity of cardiac fibers to the genesis of arrhythmias, Am. Heart J. **88:**515, 1974.
15. Cranefield, P.F.: The conduction of the cardiac impulse, Mt. Kisco, N.Y., 1975, Futura Publishing Co.
16. Carmeliet, E.E., and Vereecke, J.: Adrenaline and the plateau phase of the cardiac action potential, Pflugers Arch. **313:**303, 1969.
17. Cranefield, P.F., Wit, A.L., and Hoffman, B.F.: The genesis of cardiac arrhythmias, Circulation **47:**190, 1973.
18. Hordof, A.J., Edie, R., Malm, J.R., Hoffman, B.F., and Rosen, M.R.: Electrophysiologic properties and response to pharmacologic agents of fibers from diseased human atria, Circulation **54:**774, 1976.
19. Boyden, P.A., Tilley, L.P., Liu, S., and Wit, A.L.: Effects of atrial dilatation on atrial cellular electrophysiology: studies on cats with spontaneous cardiomyopathy [Abstract], Circulation **56** (suppl. III):48, 1977.
20. Cranefield, P.F.: Action potentials, afterpotentials, and arrhythmias, Circ. Res. **41:**415, 1977.
21. MacLeod, D.P., and Prasad, K.: Influence of glucose on the transmembrane action potential of papillary muscle, J. Gen. Physiol. **53:**792, 1969.
22. Han, J.: Ventricular ectopic activity in myocardial infarction. In Han, J., editor: Cardiac arrhythmias: a symposium, Springfield, Ill., 1972, Charles C Thomas, Publisher.

CHAPTER 5

Reentrant ventricular arrhythmias

Although from time to time there has been vociferous opposition to the claim that reentry causes ventricular extrasystoles, tachycardia, and fibrillation, there is little doubt that reentry is one of the responsible mechanisms. Moreover, since 1971 evidence has rapidly accumulated that many ventricular tachycardias—following the example of supraventricular tachycardias—also owe their existence to a circus movement.

Reentry within terminal Purkinje fibers

In 1971[1] and 1972[2,3] reentrant activity was demonstrated in vitro in canine terminal Purkinje fibers with the use of microelectrodes. This type of reentry was described as early as 1906 by Mayer[10] and later by Schmitt and Erlanger,[5] Mines,[6] and Garrey.[7]

Fig. 5-1 is a diagrammatic representation of conduction through normal terminal Purkinje fibers. The impulse travels at the same speed through all segments of the fiber, thus eliminating any possibility for reentry. It is important that conduction velocity be uniform within one locality, although conduction velocities do differ from location to location in the myocardium, ranging from 0.5 to 5 m/sec in cardiac fibers other than those of the two nodes.

Fig. 5-2 represents conduction through a severely depressed segment of the terminal Purkinje network. The shaded area has a resting membrane potential of -55 to -60 mV. Thus depolarization in this area is accomplished by Na^+/Ca^{++} currents passing through slow channels to produce a slow response action potential. The impulse *(1)* travels normally through the unaffected Purkinje twig *(2)* but is blocked at the border of the severely depressed segment *(3)*. Normal conduction, however, proceeds through the normal Purkinje network and on into the myocardium. When the propagated impulse arrives at the distal end of the severely depressed segment *(4)*, it may be blocked in this direction as well or it may enter the depressed segment and propagate slowly. When it reaches the border of normal tissue one of two things may happen: (a) It may be blocked because the normal tissue is still refractory, in which case no extrasystole occurs, or (b) it may reenter the newly repolarized normal segment and proceed on into the myocardium to produce a premature beat.

Other mechanisms for reentry within the Purkinje fibers include summation and reflection, described in the previous chapter.

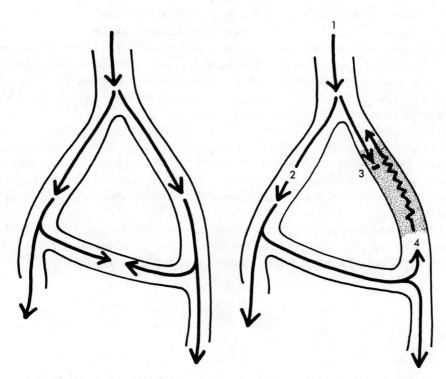

Fig. 5-1. Conduction through normal terminal Purkinje fibers. The conduction velocity is uniform.

Fig. 5-2. Conduction through a severely depressed segment of terminal Purkinje fibers. The impulse *(1)* travels normally through normal tissue *(2)*, is blocked at the severely depressed tissue *(3)*, but returns through this tissue from the opposite direction *(4)*.

Reentry through ischemic myocardial tissue

In 1977 El-Sherif and co-workers[8,9] demonstrated that the conduction disorders in ischemic myocardium closely simulated those in ischemic and depressed His-Purkinje tissue. Until this time all the models for reentry involved conductive tissue.

Fig. 5-3 is a diagrammatic representation of the conduction delays leading to reentry in the canine myocardium 3 to 7 days after myocardial infarction. It shows a web of interconnecting, depressed, slowly conducting myocardial tissue (white paths) within a bed of more severely depressed nonconducting tissue (stippled areas) surrounded by normal myocardium. This model is consistent with the known pathology of ischemic zones, in which relatively viable myocardium is interspersed with areas of infarction.[10] The depressed tissue provides "electrical avenues" as opposed to the anatomic pathways of the His-Purkinje system.

In Fig. 5-3 there are several "doors" by which the initiating impulse may gain entrance into the depressed electrical pathways. However, at some entries propagation is blocked. Note the slow devious pathway taken by the impulse until it finds an exit into nonrefractory normal tissue. Reentry then takes place; and if the strength of the activating wave front is sufficient to excite the normal tissue, a premature beat will result.

The complex interconnections in the ischemic zone would seem to invite summation and inhibition, though so far these mechanisms have been demonstrated only for depressed Purkinje fibers and not for depressed ischemic myocardium.

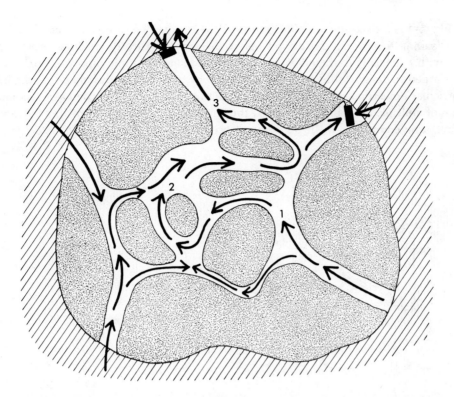

Fig. 5-3. Diagrammatic representation of conduction delays within canine myocardial tissue 3 to 7 days after an infarction. Anatomic electrical pathways are provided by a web of depressed conducting tissue (white paths) lying in a bed of severely depressed nonconducting tissue (stippled areas). The impulse travels into the depressed area via some of the paths but is blocked from doing so in others. The slowly propagating impulse may then exit through the "doors" where there was one-way block. (Modified from El-Sherif, N., Scherlag, B.J., Lazzara, R., and Hope, R.R.: Circulation **55:**686, 1977.)

Fig. 5-4 is a diagrammatic illustration of the conduction disorder in an infarcted zone leading to reentry. Displayed below this are the records obtained from that zone with a specially designed composite electrode and multiple bipolar electrodes.[8] The dashed rectangle outlines the area covered by these electrodes placed on the left ventricular epicardial surface. This combination of electrodes recorded a continuous series of multiple asynchronous spikes, thus providing evidence for the link between an initiating complex and the subsequent premature one.

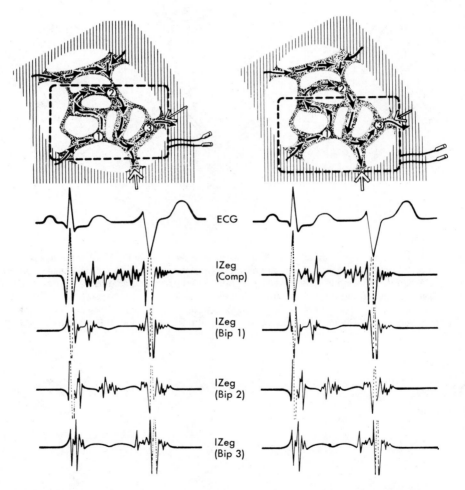

Fig. 5-4. Schematic representation of the conduction disorder in the infarction zone leading to reentry. Tracings from top to bottom represent a standard ECG lead, a composite electrode recording (*IZeg* [*Comp*]), and three close bipolar recordings (*IZeg* [*Bip, 1-3*]). (From El-Sherif, N., Scherlag, B.J., Lazzara, R., and Hope, R.R.: Circulation **55:**686, 1977. By permission of the American Heart Association, Inc.)

REENTRANT EXTRASYSTOLIC GROUPING. For the above-described reentrant beats to occur, it is necessary that the heart rate be within a critical range.[9] At rates faster than this critical rate the conduction pattern through the depressed area of tissue demonstrates a Wenckebach-like characteristic; that is, the velocity of conduction through this area will become slower and slower as the heart rate increases until it fails altogether. When conduction is slow enough to outlast the effective refractory period of the normal myocardium, a reentrant beat will result.

At rates slower than the critical rate there is less conduction delay within the depressed tissue and 1:1 conduction results with no reentrant beats. As the heart rate increases, so do the Wenckebach-like conduction characteristics of the ischemic zone.

In the experiments conducted by El-Sherif and others[9,10] trigeminal and quadrigeminal groupings were found to be the result of 3:2 and 4:3 Wenckebach-like periods, which would convert to 2:1 conduction at faster rates, resulting in a bigeminal rhythm. A higher degree of block in the reentrant pathway offers no chance for reentry, or reentry may be concealed.[10] For example, when there were 3:2 Wenckebach-like periods, the first beat of the series would experience depressed but adequate conduction through the ischemic area. The next two beats would suffer progressively deteriorating conduction through the ischemic tissue until conduction was blocked altogether by the third beat, after which the sequence would begin again. During such a sequence of three beats the second beat in the series would produce the premature beat. This is illustrated in Fig. 5-5, *A*.

Following beat 1 the normal impulse is able to enter all paths into the ischemic area and cancel out any slowly propagating abnormal currents. Following beat 2 conduction through the ischemic tissue has so deteriorated that the normal impulse cannot gain entry into every path at the perimeter of the ischemic tissue because of one-way conduction. However, the impulse may exit from the ischemic area. This is possible provided the impulse is sustained within the ischemic zone long enough for the surrounding normal tissue to repolarize. Then the wave front, trapped within the ischemic zone because of slow conduction and protected from extinction by one-way block, may find nonrefractory tissue and be propagated to produce a premature beat. Following beat 3 (the premature beat) conduction through the ischemic area will fail altogether, at which time the Wenckebach-like sequence will begin again, resulting in a pattern in which every third beat is ectopic. Fig. 5-5, *B* and *C*, illustrates 2:1 and 4:3 Wenckebach-like conduction.

Trigeminal and quadrigeminal groupings were found to be the result of 3:2 and 4:3 Wenckebach-like periods, which would convert to 2:1 conduction patterns at faster rates, resulting in a bigeminal rhythm. A higher degree of block in the reentrant pathway offers no chance for reentry, or reentry may be concealed.[10]

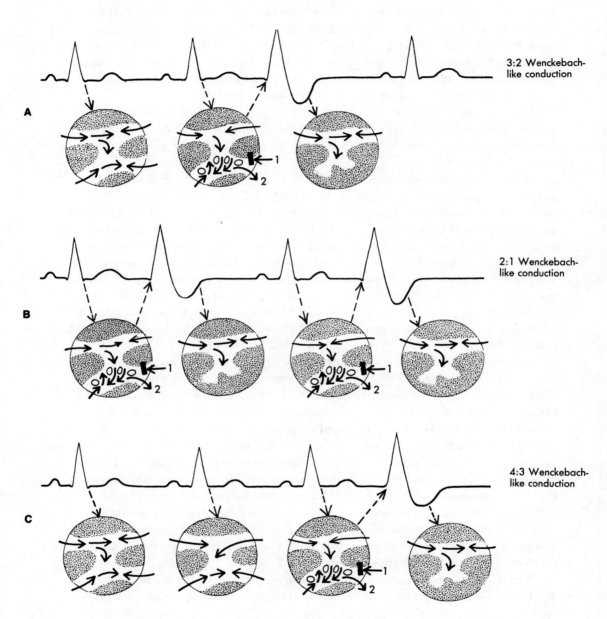

Fig. 5-5. For legend see opposite page.

Fig. 5-5. Schematic representation of conduction disorders in the infarction zone leading to 3:2, 2:1, and 4:3 Wenckebach-like periods. **A,** 3:2 Wenckebach-like conduction, producing a ventricular ectopic every third beat. Following beat no. 1 the normal impulse enters all pathways into the ischemic area to cancel out the slowly propagating impulses within. Following beat no. 2 the ischemic tissue has deteriorated and the normal impulse is prevented from entering all pathways (*1*), leaving avenues of exit available for the slowly propagating impulse, which exits (*2*) to produce a ventricular ectopic. Following beat no. 3 (the ectopic beat) conduction through the ischemic area fails completely. **B,** 2:1 Wenckebach-like conduction, producing a ventricular ectopic every other beat. Following every normal beat depressed conduction within the ischemic area produces slow conduction and the impulse is prevented from entering all pathways (*1*). This permits the reentry (*2*) of the slowly propagating impulse. Following the ventricular ectopic the impulse successfully invades all perimeters of the ischemic tissue to cancel out the slowly propagating impulse. **C,** 4:3 Wenckebach-like conduction, producing a ventricular ectopic every fourth beat. Following the first two normal beats currents enter all pathways into the ischemic tissue, although conduction within this tissue progressively deteriorates with each impulse. Following the third normal beat, conduction deterioration permits reentry as described in **A**. After the premature beat complete block through the ischemic area is present and the sequence begins again.

Concealed reentry

Concealed reentry takes place when an impulse makes a circus movement through a loop of depressed fibers but does not reenter and reexcite the heart.[2] The reentrant pathway would thus be rendered refractory without the impulse's returning to its site of origin and declaring itself on the ECG. Such an event would be noted only because of its effect on the next impulse to invade the same loop.

The term "concealed reentry" was first used in 1950[12] and again in 1955[13] by Langendorf and others, who suggested that impulse propagation could be blocked within the reentrant pathway.

Later Cranefield and associates[14] demonstrated concealed reentry in vitro using a depressed loop of canine Purkinje fiber. El-Sherif and co-workers[10] documented concealed reentry in dogs, demonstrating rate-related concealed reentry due to one of two mechanisms:

1. The reentrant impulse may be entrapped in the normal myocardial tissue bordering the ischemic zone if it leaves the reentrant pathway at the same time that the wave front from the next supraventricular beat reaches the area. This may occur when the heart rate is such that the conduction time through the reentrant pathway is about the same as or exceeds the basic cardiac cycle.
2. The reentrant wave front may never leave the depressed zone if the heart rate exceeds conduction through the reentrant pathway and the normal tissue has already been activated by the time the reentrant wave front is ready to emerge.

Concealed bigeminy

In 1961 and 1963 Schamroth and Marriott[15,16] coined the term "concealed bigeminy" as an explanation for an apparently haphazard distribution of extrasystoles that turned out not to be so.

Fig. 5-6 is an example of a ventricular bigeminy that may be intermittently latent (concealed). Although the distribution of extrasystoles at first appears to be haphazard, the number of sinus beats intervening between consecutive ectopic beats is always an odd number—1, 3, 5, 7 etc.

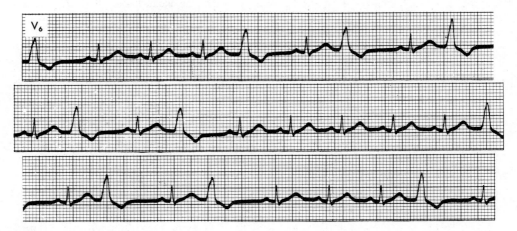

Fig. 5-6. Concealed ventricular bigeminy—a short sample from a much longer strip in which the number of sinus beats intervening between consecutive ectopics was always an odd number. The tendency to bigeminy is apparent in this sample, in which the intervening sinus beats consecutively number 3, 1, 1, 1, 1, 5, 1, 1, 3.

Reentry within the bundle branches and His bundle (macroreentry)

Macroreentry is applicable when the wave front enjoys a wider fascicular sweep (e.g., when both bundle branches and the His bundle are involved in the reentry circuit) or when, in the Wolff-Parkinson-White syndrome (Chapter 7), both the AV junction and the accessory pathway are traversed by the circulating wave.

As a rule, when ventricular tachycardia repeatedly recurs, macroreentry does not appear to be the mechanism.[17] However, when it is, it is difficult to differentiate from a supraventricular tachycardia with aberrant ventricular conduction.[17] Even with a His bundle electrogram both tachycardias may have a His bundle spike preceding the QRS complex, and both mechanisms may demonstrate a 1:1 relationship between the atrial and the ventricular deflections.

Fig. 5-7 illustrates the possible pathways of reentry involving both bundle branches, the bundle of His, and the AV node.

In *A* the coupling interval between the basic and the premature beats is long. Thus conduction proceeds at a normal velocity retrogradely up the bundle branches, bundle of His, and AV node, leaving no opportunity for reentry.

In *B* to *D* the coupling intervals are shorter and three possible mechanisms are illustrated for reentry.

In *B* retrograde conduction from the premature ventricular stimulus was initially blocked in the RBB but not in the LBB. By the time the impulse had traveled slowly up the LBB, the RBB was able to conduct that impulse anterogradely to produce a reciprocal beat.

In *C* the premature ventricular stimulus was blocked in the LBB in both directions. The impulse was still traveling slowly up the bundle of His and into the node, where it turned around and was propagated anterogradely down both bundle branches to produce a reciprocal beat. The resulting complex would, of course, be of normal configuration as long as there were no aberrancy.

In *D* the premature ventricular stimulus was blocked in the retrograde direction in the LBB. It therefore reached the LBB via its retrograde pathway up the RBB and then descended the LBB to produce a reciprocal beat.

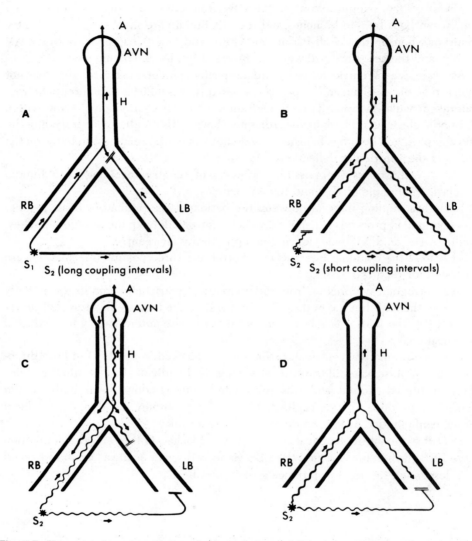

Fig. 5-7. Diagrammatic representation of events that may follow right ventricular stimulation. The possible sites of block and the circuits of reentry are depicted. *AVN*, AV node; *H*, bundle of His; *RB*, right bundle branch system; *LB*, left bundle branch system; S_1, basic ventricular drive stimulus; S_2, premature ventricular stimulus. (From Akhtar, M., et al.: Circulation **50:**1150, 1974.)

References

1. Sasyniuk, B.S., and Mendez, C.: A mechanism for re-entry in canine ventricular tissue, Circ. Res. **28**:3, 1971.
2. Wit, A.L., Hoffman, B.J., and Cranefield, P.F.: Slow conduction and re-entry in the ventricular conducting system. I. Return extrasystole in canine Purkinje fibers, Circ. Res. **30**:1, 1972.
3. Wit, A.L., Cranefield, P.F., and Hoffman, B.F.: Slow conduction and re-entry in the ventricular conducting system. II. Single and sustained circus movement in networks of canine and bovine Purkinje fibers, Circ. Res. **30**:11, 1971.
4. Mayer, A.G.: Rhythmical pulsation in scyphomedusae, Carnegie Institution of Washington, Publication no. 47, 1906.
5. Schmitt, F.O., and Erlanger, J.: Directional differences in the conduction of the impulse through heart muscle and their possible relation to extrasystolic and fibrillary contractions, Am. J. Physiol. **87**:326, 1928-1929.
6. Mines, G.R.: On dynamic equilibrium in the heart, J. Physiol. (Lond.) **46**:349, 1913.
7. Garrey, W.: Nature of fibrillary contraction of the heart. Its relation to tissue mass and form, Am. J. Physiol. **33**:397, 1914.
8. El-Sherif, N., Scherlag, B.J., Lazzara, R., and Hope, R.R.: Re-entrant ventricular arrhythmias in the late myocardial infarction period. 1. Conduction characteristics in the infarction zone, Circulation **55**:686, 1977.
9. El-Sherif, N., Hope, R.R., and Scherlag, B.J.: Re-entrant ventricular arrhythmias in the late myocardial infarction period. 2. Patterns of initiation and termination of re-entry, Circulation **55**:702, 1977.
10. El-Sherif, N., Lazzara, R., Hope, R.R., and Scherlag, B.J.: Re-entrant ventricular arrhythmias in the late myocardial infarction period. 3. Manifest and concealed extrasystolic grouping, Circulation **56**:225, 1977.
11. Cranefield, P.F.: The conduction of the cardiac impulse, Mount Kisco, N.Y., 1975 Futura Publishing Co.
12. Mack, I., and Langendorf, R.: Factors influencing the time of appearance of premature systoles (including a demonstration of cases with ventricular premature systoles due to reentry but exhibiting variable coupling, Circulation **1**:910, 1950.
13. Langendorf, R., Pick, A., and Winternitz, F.M.: Mechanisms of intermittent ventricular bigeminy. 1. Appearance of ectopic beats dependent upon length of the ventricular cycle, the "rule of bigeminy," Circulation **11**:422, 1955.
14. Cranefield, P.F., Wit, A.L., and Hoffman, B.F.: Genesis of cardiac arrhythmias, Circulation **47**:190, 1973.
15. Schamroth, L., and Marriott, H.J.L.: Intermittent ventricular parasystole with observations on its relationship to extrasystolic bigeminy, Am. J. Cardiol. **7**:799, 1961.
16. Schamroth, L., and Marriott, H.J.L.: Concealed ventricular extrasystoles, Circulation **27**:1043, 1963.
17. Akhtar, M., and others: Reentry within the His-Purkinje system. Elucidation of reentrant circuit using right bundle branch and His bundle recordings, Circulation **58**:295, 1978.

CHAPTER 6

AV nodal reentry

AV nodal reentry is the return of an impulse to activate a pathway within the AV node for the second time; when this repeatedly results, a circus movement develops. This appears to be the most common mechanism of paroxysmal supraventricular tachycardia (reciprocating tachycardia).[1-9] Knowledge of the structure of the AV node and bundle of His facilitates an understanding of the reciprocating mechanism, which in turn offers an approach to management.

Fig. 6-1 is a diagrammatic representation of the AV node and bundle of His. AV nodal tissue, with its special anatomic and electrophysiologic characteristics, lends itself to nonuniform conduction.

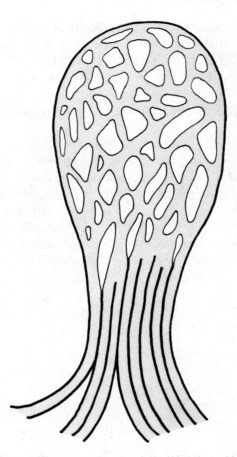

Fig. 6-1. Diagrammatic representation of the AV node and bundle of His.

Dual AV nodal pathways

The circus movement that supports the majority of paroxysmal supraventricular tachycardias is the result of functional "longitudinal dissociation"—meaning that parallel pathways are insulated from each other—within the AV node.[3-5] Since 1956 two separate pathways through the AV node have been suggested[10-16] and later demonstrated[4,17] to be the basis for this dissociation, although it is not known whether these are discrete anatomic pathways or whether the dissociation is purely functional.[18]

The two pathways, diagrammatically illustrated in Fig. 6-2, have different conduction times and different refractory periods. The pathway with slow conduction has a shorter refractory period, whereas the pathway with fast conduction has a longer refractory period.[3,10,12,17] The group of cells in the slow pathway have been called "alpha" cells,[12] and those in the fast pathway "beta" cells. If a premature impulse gains entrance to the node, it is conducted by the alpha cells whereas the beta cells block very early impulses. Thus, following an atrial premature beat, the impulse penetrates the alpha cells and then returns to the atria via the beta cells, which by this time can conduct.

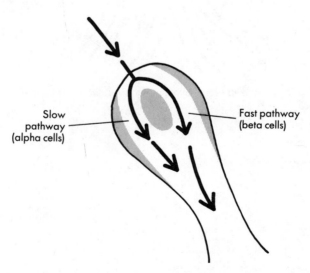

Slow
pathway
(alpha cells)

Fast pathway
(beta cells)

Fig. 6-2. Diagrammatic representation of normal conduction down the slow and the fast pathways within the AV node. The cells of the slow pathway have been designated *alpha* cells, and those of the fast pathway *beta* cells.

Mechanism of AV nodal reentry

Normally both the fast and the slow pathways are invaded by the supraventricular impulse,[3-5] which reaches the His bundle first via the fast pathway (Fig. 6-2). This is the usual sequence following a sinus beat or a relatively late atrial premature beat (APB). However, in the case of an early APB anterograde conduction may be blocked in the pathway with the longer refractory period (the fast pathway) and be conducted to the ventricles via the pathway with the shorter refractory period (the slow pathway). The PR interval will thus be prolonged due to a lengthening of the AH interval, and paroxysmal supraventricular tachycardia (PSVT) may be initiated if

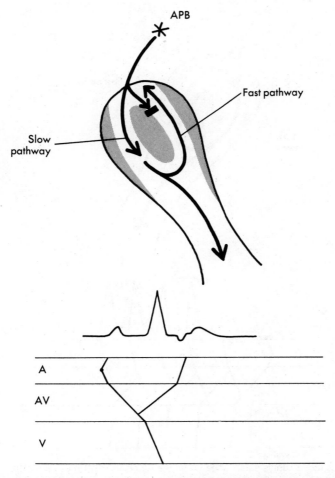

Fig. 6-3. An atrial premature beat *(APB)* may result in anterograde conduction down the slow pathway and retrograde conduction up the fast pathway to produce an atrial echo beat.

anterograde conduction down the slow pathway outlasts the refractory period of the fast pathway[2,3,5,19]; if this situation prevails, the impulse may return to the atria via the previously blocked fast pathway to produce an atrial echo (Fig. 6-3). The round trip may terminate with the atrial echo, failing anterograde transmission down the slow pathway again. However, a continuing circus movement may be established if the impulse returns again down the slow pathway and back up the fast pathway. The circus movement thus produced will result in PSVT (Fig. 6-4) and each time the distal AV node is activated, the impulse proceeds to the ventricles.

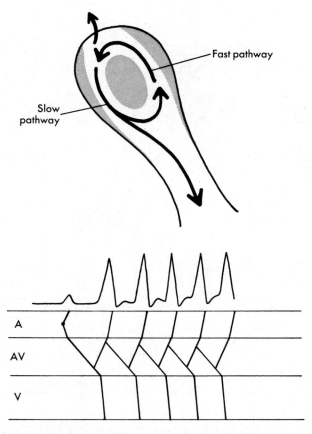

Fig. 6-4. If a circus movement is established within the AV node, PSVT may result. The most common course is anterogradely down the slow pathway and retrogradely up the fast pathway.

Studies have shown that the atria may or may not be involved in the reentry circuit.[20] Fig. 6-5 diagrammatically illustrates an AV nodal reentry circuit without atrial *or* ventricular activation (concealed conduction). Note that such a circuit, once initiated, is not dependent upon the atria or the ventricles for its perpetuation and could conceivably remain concealed to produce what appears to be complete AV block (pseudo–AV block[21]) as long as anterograde activation from the atria or retrograde activation from the ventricles does not interrupt the circuit.

AV nodal reentry may be initiated not only by an atrial premature beat but also by a junctional or even a ventricular premature beat.

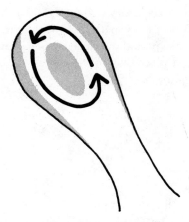

Fig. 6-5. AV nodal reentry without atrial or ventricular involvement.

Maintenance and interruption of a reentry circuit

In 1908 Mayer[22] accurately described the conditions for reentry in the following words:

> This wave will maintain itself indefinitely, provided the circuit be long enough to permit each and every point of the wave to remain at rest for a certain period of time before the return of the wave through the circuit. This single wave going constantly in one direction around the circuit may maintain itself for days traveling at a uniform rate. The circuit must, however, be long enough to allow each point to rest for an appreciable interval of time before the return of the wave. The wave is actually "trapped" in the circuit and must constantly drive onward through the tissue. The point . . . from which the . . . wave first arises is of no more importance in maintaining the rhythmical movement than is any other point on the ring.

A circus movement is interrupted if a well-timed impulse, natural or artificial, finds the gap between the head and the tail of the circulating wave and produces refractoriness. Fig. 6-6 illustrates how a circulating wave may thus be halted. A temporary pacemaker delivering rapid atrial stimulation is a tailor-made method of terminating any circus-movement supraventricular tachycardia.

A vagal maneuver will lengthen the refractory period of the AV nodal tissue and may upset the delicate balance between anterograde and retrograde conduction, thus terminating an AV nodal reentry mechanism. Pharmacologic interventions are aimed at depressing AV nodal conduction and thus interrupting the circuit. Drugs that may depress the anterograde slow pathway include digitalis, propranolol, and verapamil.[19,23-25] However, digitalis is avoided if there is any possibility that the tachycardia owes its existence to an accessory pathway. This is because digitalis shortens the refractory period of an accessory pathway[26,27] and, if atrial fibrillation should develop, a shortened refractory period in the accessory pathway may lead to a fatally rapid ventricular response. Drugs that may depress the retrograde fast pathway include procainamide and quinidine.[28]

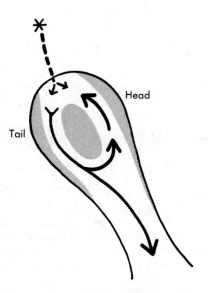

Fig. 6-6. The AV nodal reentry circuit may be interrupted by inserting an impulse and producing refractoriness between the head and the tail of the wave front.

The two types of AV nodal reciprocating tachycardia

There are two clinically distinct types of AV nodal reciprocating tachycardia: (1) the more common anterograde slow and retrograde fast ("slow-fast") mechanism, also sometimes called "the paroxysmal form," and (2) the less common mechanism using the fast pathway in the anterograde direction and the slow pathway retrogradely. This second form has been given many titles—among which are fast-slow,[29] permanent,[30] incessant,[31] chronic,[29] and persistent.[32]

SLOW-FAST (PAROXYSMAL) FORM OF SVT. This more common form of AV reciprocating tachycardia typically begins with an atrial extrasystole. It may also be initiated by a junctional extrasystole or by retrograde conduction from a ventricular extrasystole. Conduction is slow anterogradely and fast retrogradely, and the time it takes for the impulse to travel from the NH portion of the node to the atria and to the ventricles is approximately the same. Consequently this type of tachycardia is usually characterized by P' waves that are not seen because they coincide with ventricular activation.[8,30,33-35] This is illustrated in Fig. 6-7.

In Fig. 6-7 a ventricular extrasystole initiates and terminates a PSVT.

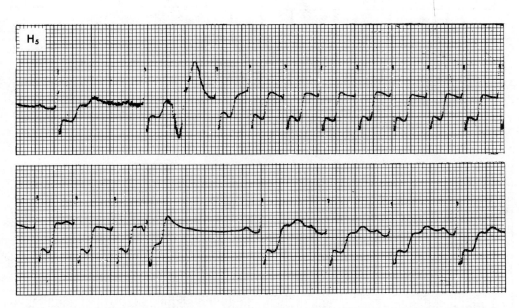

Fig. 6-7. Continuous strip from a Holter recording. After two sinus beats a ventricular extrasystole initiates a SVT. Further evidence of its reciprocating nature is that it is also terminated by a premature beat.

FAST-SLOW (PERMANENT) FORM OF SVT. The SVT that uses the fast instead of the slow pathway anterogradely is less common than the slow-fast form in adults, although it represents 50% of SVT in children.[36]

The PR interval preceding its onset is usually not prolonged. In fact, the fast-slow type of SVT may be initiated without a premature atrial beat at all.[36] It may occur spontaneously as a result of a subtle increase in sinus rate,[29] or it can be triggered, like the paroxysmal type, by atrial or ventricular premature beats.

It is claimed that, unlike the paroxysmal type, it is difficult to treat.[36] It stops from time to time, especially during rest, but starts up again after a few sinus beats. Also, unlike the paroxysmal type, the classically retrograde P′ wave (negative in leads II, III, and aVF) can easily be seen beyond the ST-T segment, preceding the next QRS complex (Fig. 6-8).

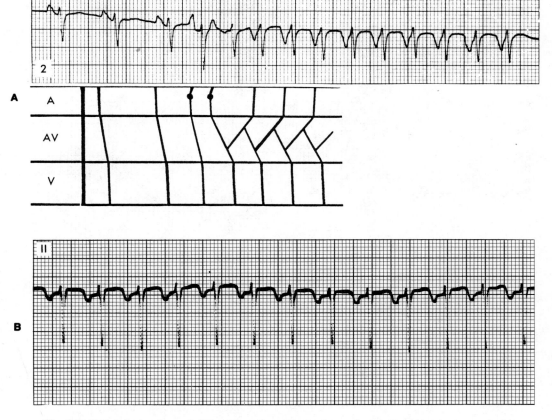

Fig. 6-8. A, A fast-slow form of AV nodal reciprocating tachycardia is initiated by the second of two APBs. **B,** Fast-slow SVT.

The tachycardia in Fig. 6-8, *A*, is initiated by the second of two atrial premature beats; the first is conducted without delay, and the second with delay. The long P'R following the second atrial extrasystole does not, as one would expect, initiate the more common type of SVT with slow anterograde and fast retrograde conduction. Since the RP' interval is so long, the slow pathway is presumably used in the retrograde direction. Fig. 6-8, *B*, is another example of the fast-slow form of SVT. Note the long RP' interval.

In Fig. 6-9 a ventricular tachycardia of 130/min initiates the fast-slow type of SVT. Note that it is not until the fifth ventricular ectopic that retrograde penetration of the AV node via the slow pathway reaches a high enough level to reenter the fast pathway without colliding with the anterograde sinus impulse. The impulse then returns to the ventricles via the fast pathway.

In Fig. 6-9 it is interesting to note the effect of the SVT, with a rate of 140/min, on the returning cycle both of the sinus node and of the ventricular ectopic focus. Both are suppressed by the overdrive of the SVT.

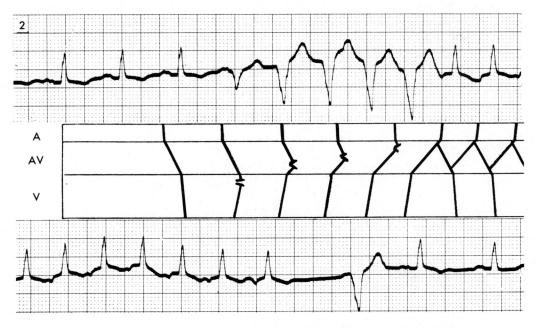

Fig. 6-9. A ventricular tachycardia initiates the less common fast-slow type of AV nodal reciprocating tachycardia. After three sinus beats a run of ventricular tachycardia begins with a fusion beat. Three subsequent ectopic ventricular impulses meet the descending sinus impulse progressively higher in the AV junction. The fifth beat of the tachycardia reaches the atria before the next sinus beat is due and returns to the ventricles to initiate a reciprocating tachycardia.

Differentiating the reciprocating supraventricular tachycardias[33]

The electrophysiologists have adduced the following clues to help in differentiating the various types of SVT:

1. The more common type of AV nodal reentry, using the slow pathway anterogradely and the fast pathway retrogradely, results in a P' wave that usually coincides with the QRS and is therefore not seen (Fig. 6-10, *A*).

2. An uncommon form of AV nodal reentry uses the fast pathway anterogradely and the slow pathway retrogradely. This usually results in a P' wave that is closer to the QRS that follows than it is to the preceding QRS (RP' > P'R) (Fig. 6-10, *A*).

3. In the reciprocating tachycardia using an accessory pathway the atria and ventricles are activated in sequence because of the relatively wide physical separation of the anterograde and retrograde pathways. Anterograde conduction is usually over the AV node and bundle of His, which takes longer than retrograde conduction over the accessory pathway. This will result in P waves that immediately follow the QRS (RP' < P'R) (Fig. 6-10, *B*).

4. In SA reentry tachycardia P waves tend to precede rather than follow QRS complexes (Fig. 6-10, *C*). Also, conduction to the ventricles is not a necessary link in the maintenance of this reentry circuit as it is with the tachycardia using an accessory pathway.

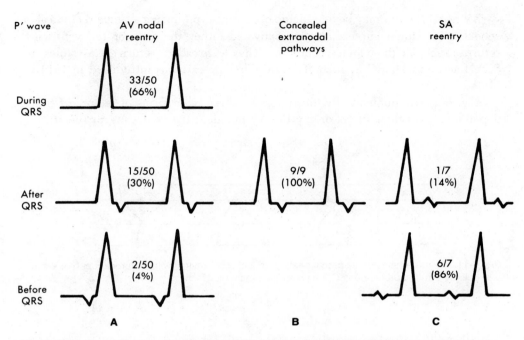

Fig. 6-10. Timing of P′ waves relative to the QRS complex during paroxysmal supraventricular tachycardia in three groups of patients. (From Wu, D., et al.: Am. J. Cardiol. **41:**1095, 1978.)

Reciprocal (echo) beats

AV nodal reentry may be an isolated occurrence, producing a single reciprocal or echo beat; a single impulse, having activated either the atria or the ventricles, returns to activate them for a second time. They were called "return extrasystoles" by Scherf and Shookhoff[37] in 1926. The term "reciprocal" was introduced in 1913 by Mines.[38]

Fig. 6-11 diagrammatically illustrates the three main forms of reciprocal beats, depending upon their site of origin: the AV junction, the ventricles, or the atria.

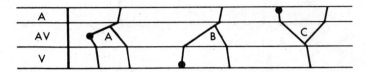

Fig. 6-11. The three forms of reciprocal beating: *A*, junctional rhythm with reciprocal beat; *B*, ventricular ectopic with reciprocal beat; *C*, reversed reciprocal beat.

AV JUNCTION (V-A-V SEQUENCE). Usually a reciprocal beat occurs when retrograde conduction to the atria from an ectopic junctional beat is long enough to permit reactivation of the ventricles. Fig. 6-12 is just such a case. The regular ectopic junctional rhythm, not preceded by a sinus P wave, is easy to spot (*A, B,* and *C*). Then what catches one's eye is a premature supraventricular beat that resets the junctional rhythm. The retrograde conduction following the junctional beats (*A, B,* and *C*) progressively lengthens (retrograde Wenckebach) until finally conduction is slow enough to permit reactivation of the ventricles.

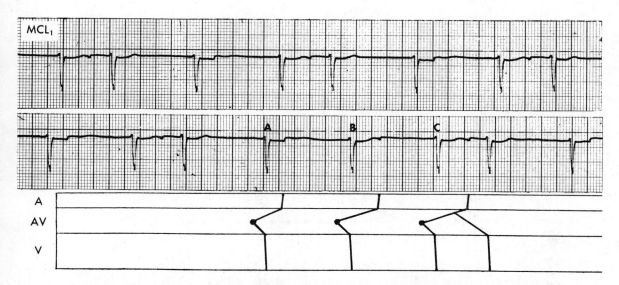

Fig. 6-12. The strips are continuous and show AV rhythm with reciprocal beating. Retrograde conduction is progressively delayed until, when the delay is sufficient, the impulse finds a responsive downward pathway and returns to reactivate the ventricles (see laddergram).

Reciprocal beating is one of the mechanisms that produce allorhythmia (i.e., a repeated arrhythmic sequence). Fig. 6-13 is an example of reciprocal beats producing an allorhythmia of three beats, each trio consisting of two junctional beats followed by a reciprocal beat.

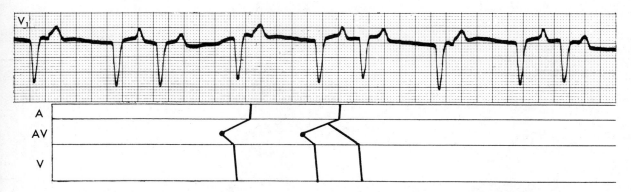

Fig. 6-13. AV rhythm with LBBB and reciprocal beating. The allorhythmia consists of two junctional beats with lengthening retrograde conduction, the second of which is followed by a reciprocal beat. The three-beat sequence then repeats itself.

VENTRICLES (V-A-V SEQUENCE). As we saw in Fig. 6-9, it is possible for a ventricular premature beat to initiate a PSVT. In Fig. 6-14 a ventricular premature beat, with slow retrograde conduction to the atria, produces a single ventricular echo or reciprocal beat.

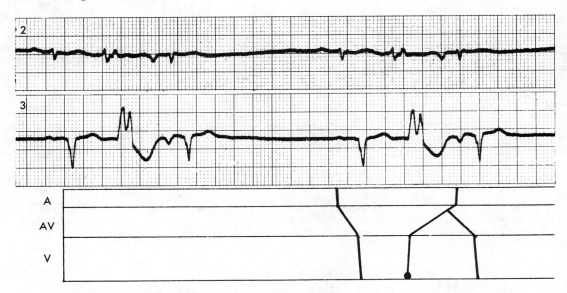

Fig. 6-14. Reciprocal beating initiated by ventricular extrasystoles with retrograde conduction.

Figs. 6-15 and 6-16 are examples of ventricular ectopic rhythms with retrograde Wenckebach conduction and ventricular echoes. In Fig. 6-15 the tracing begins with a run of ventricular tachycardia. Retrograde conduction from the first two beats lengthens until the third finally blocks (3:2 retrograde Wenckebach). There are two sinus beats before the next run of ventricular rhythm begins, to be interrupted after only two beats by a ventricular echo.

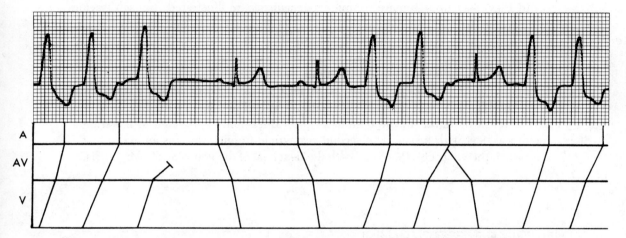

Fig. 6-15. The ventricular ectopic beats manifest retrograde Wenckebach conduction to the atria. The first group of ventricular ectopics have lengthening RP′ intervals until, after the third complex, retrograde conduction is blocked. The next group of ventricular ectopics also have retrograde Wenckebach conduction, but after the second complex the impulse returns to the ventricles to produce a ventricular echo. (From Conover, M.H.: Cardiac arrhythmias, ed. 2, St. Louis, 1978, The C.V. Mosby Co.)

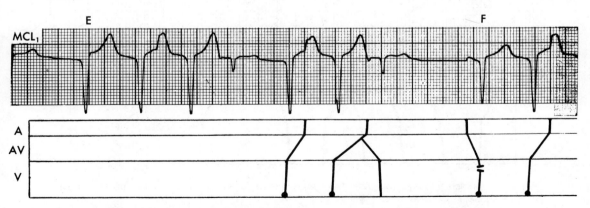

Fig. 6-16. Accelerated idioventricular rhythm with reciprocal beating. Two idioventricular beats are followed by increasingly delayed retroconduction to the atria (see laddergram). The delay following the second beat is sufficient to permit reentry and a reciprocal beat (ventricular echo). The first beats in the first and third groups (*E* and *F*) do not show retroconduction. Beat *E* does not probably because the sinus P wave is buried within it. Beat *F* is a fusion beat, with the sinus impulse therefore precluding retrograde conduction.

Fig. 6-16 is an example of accelerated idioventricular rhythm with progressively prolonging retrograde conduction culminating in a ventricular echo. If the retrograde P′ waves are elusive, follow the lines in the A tier of the laddergram—they point at the P waves.

Such reciprocal beats do not change the management of these ventricular arrhythmias. They merely alert one to the possibility that a PSVT may develop.

In Figs. 6-17 to 6-19 more complex mechanisms are illustrated. In each tracing there is a ventricular tachycardia with retrograde conduction to the atria. In the first two tracings there is retrograde Wenckebach conduction and when the R-P′ interval is long enough the impulse returns to the ventricles to produce a ventricular echo that fuses with the next expected ventricular ectopic beat.

In Fig. 6-17 (top tracing) there is ventricular tachycardia with 4:3 retrograde Wenckebach. Note that the R-P′ intervals get longer and longer until the impulse fails to reach the atria. In the bottom strip a laddergram is provided to illustrate a reciprocal beat with fusion. The second retrograde impulse spawns an anterograde impulse to the ventricles that fuses with the next beat of the ventricular tachycardia.

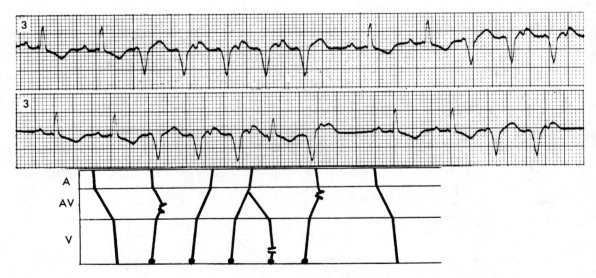

Fig. 6-17. Ventricular tachycardia (rate, 145/min) with retrograde Wenckebach in the top strip and a reciprocal beat in the lower strip.

In Fig. 6-18 there is a similar sequence. Since the lead is aVR, the retrograde P'
waves are upright. Here the third retrograde impulse turns down to reactivate the
ventricles and fuse with the next ectopic impulse of the tachycardia.

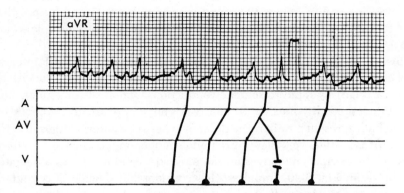

Fig. 6-18. Ventricular tachycardia (rate, 165/min) with retroconduction and reciprocal beating. Five of
the ectopic beats are diagrammed, of which the fourth represents fusion between the ectopic impulse
and reentry from the third.

In Fig. 6-19 every other beat is a fusion beat. The first ventricular ectopic on the
tracing has retrograde conduction to the atria; meanwhile the impulse turns around
in the AV node to reenter the ventricles just in time to fuse with the next ventricular
ectopic and prevent its retrograde conduction. The sequence is then repeated again
and again, masquerading as electrical alternans.

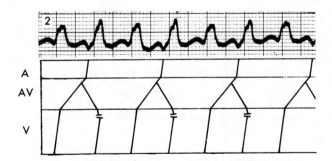

Fig. 6-19. Ventricular tachycardia at a rate of 150/min. Every other beat is a fusion beat between the
ectopic ventricular beat and a returning impulse from the preceding ectopic beat (see laddergram).

RP′ interval in V-A-V sequences. In the last eight tracings illustrating V-A-V sequences the retrograde P′ that was followed by the ventricular reciprocal beat ended a long RP′ interval. This interval is usually 0.24 second or longer and may be as long as 0.60 second or more. Occasionally the RP′ is shorter than 0.24 second, and even with an RP′ interval of only 0.12 second reciprocal beating may be possible. The shorter RPs are more often seen with junctional than with ectopic ventricular rhythms.

At first, it seems surprising that reentry can occur after a short RP interval since delayed conduction is an essential requirement for reentry and the short RP appears to speak for relatively rapid retrograde conduction. One must remember, however, that in AV junctional rhythms the RP interval is not a measure of retrograde conduction alone but represents, rather, the difference between anterograde and retrograde conduction times; thus very slow retrograde conduction, conducive to reentry, can be masked by correspondingly slow anterograde conduction, as illustrated diagrammatically in Fig. 6-20. Impulse *b* has considerable slowing of retrograde conduction, yet the masking effect of correspondingly slow anterograde conduction produces the same RP′ interval as that of the faster-conducted impulse, *a*. This masquerade is possible because the junctional discharge is a silent event, not seen on the surface ECG.

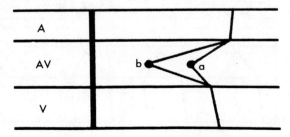

Fig. 6-20. The RP interval of junctional beats remains unchanged, provided the difference between retrograde and anterograde conduction remains the same.

ATRIA (A-V-A SEQUENCE). When an atrial impulse is conducted with some delay (prolonged PR) through the AV junction, such as occurs at the end of a Wenckebach cycle, it may return to the atria via another pathway to produce an atrial echo.[39,40]

In the top strip of Fig. 6-21 the sinus beats are conducted with PR intervals of 0.22 second and the QRS complexes are followed closely by retrograde P′ waves. In the bottom strip the same mechanism swings into a reciprocating tachycardia. Note the subtle differences between the sinus and the retrograde P waves. They are both diphasic, but as usual in V_1 the sinus diphasicity is $+-$ in contrast to the retrograde $-+$ pattern.

At times it is impossible to differentiate the atrial echo from a nonconducted atrial premature beat. Sometimes the fact that such a beat appears only after lengthening of the PR interval affords the necessary differential clue; for there is no reason why an atrial extrasystole should be dependent upon lengthening AV conduction, whereas a measure of conduction delay is clearly a promoter of reentry.[2]

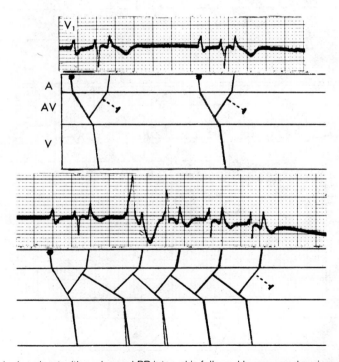

Fig. 6-21. Each sinus beat with prolonged PR interval is followed by reversed reciprocation–retroconduction to the atria, producing an atrial echo. Note that both sinus and retrograde P waves are diphasic. As is usual in V_1, the normal diphasic sinus P is $+-$ and the retrograde P′ is $-+$. In the bottom strip, instead of a single atrial echo, a run of reciprocating tachycardia is initiated. (Courtesy Dr. Leo Schamroth, Johannesburg.)

Fig. 6-22 illustrates the clue referred to above. In the top strip none of the beats with the shorter PR intervals are followed by an inverted P wave, but the one beat with a lengthened PR interval is. This establishes it as an echo rather than a nonconducted extrasystole. In each of the lower strips the third and last P wave of a 3:2 Wenckebach is followed by a retrograde P wave without an intervening QRS complex. This undoubtedly represents an atrial echo as diagrammed below the bottom strip. Just as the anterogradely reciprocal beat (ventricular echo) can complete its circuit without activating the atria,[32,41] so the reversed reciprocal beat (atrial echo) can complete its return journey without involving the ventricles.[32,40]

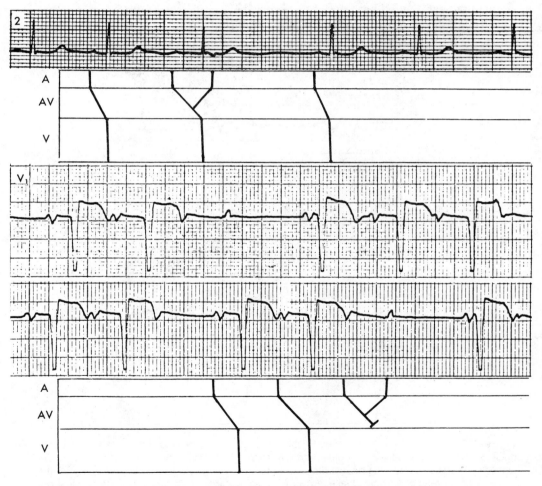

Fig. 6-22. Atrial echoes. Lead II illustrates an atrial echo resulting from lengthening of the preceding PR interval. The strips of V_1 are not continuous: each shows a 3:2 AV Wenckebach in which the third and last sinus impulse, which fails to reach the ventricles, returns to the atria to produce an echo.

References

1. Bigger, J.T., and Goldreyer, B.N.: The mechanism of supraventricular tachycardia, Circulation **42:**673, 1970.
2. Goldreyer, B.N., and Damato, A.N.: The essential role of atrioventricular conduction delay in the initiation of paroxysmal supraventricular tachycardia, Circulation **43:**679, 1971.
3. Denes, P., Wu, D., Dhingra, R.C., Chuquima, R., and Rosen, K.M.: Demonstration of dual AV nodal pathways in patients with paroxysmal supraventricular tachycardia, Circulation **48:**549, 1973.
4. Rosen, K.M., Mehta, A., and Miller, R.A.: Demonstration of dual atrioventricular nodal pathways in man, Am. J. Cardiol. **33:**291, 1974.
5. Denes, P., Wu, D., Dhingra, R., Amat-y-Leon, R., Wyndham, C., and Rosen, K.M.: Dual atrioventricular nodal pathways; a common electrophysiological response, Br. Heart J. **37:**1069, 1975.
6. Wu, D., Denes, P., Dhingra, R., Wyndham, C., and Rosen, K.M.: Determinants of fast- and slow-pathway conduction in patients with dual atrioventricular nodal pathways, Circ. Res. **36:**782, 1975.
7. Touboul, P., Huerta, R., Porte, J., and Delahaye, J.P.: Reciprocal rhythm in patients with normal electrocardiogram: evidence for dual conduction pathways, Am. Heart J. **91:**3, 1976.
8. Sung, R.J., Styperek, J.L., Myerburg, R.J., and Castellanos, A.: Initiation of two distinct forms of atrioventricular nodal reentrant tachycardia during programmed ventricular stimulation in man, Am. J. Cardiol. **42:**404, 1978.
9. Akhtar, M.: Paroxysmal atrioventricular nodal reentrant tachycardia. In Narula, O.S., editor: Cardiac arrhythmias; electrophysiology, diagnosis, and management, Baltimore, 1979, The Williams & Wilkins, Co.
10. Moe, G.K., Preston, J.B., and Burlington, H.: Physiologic evidence for a dual A-V transmission system, Circ. Res. **4:**357, 1956.
11. Mendez, C., Han, J., Garcia de Jalon, P.D., and Moe, G.K.: Some characteristics of ventricular echoes, Circ. Res. **16:**562, 1965.
12. Mendez, C., and Moe, G.K.: Demonstration of a dual A-V nodal conduction system in the isolated rabbit heart, Circ. Res. **19:**378, 1966.
13. Rosenbluth, A., and Rubio, R.: Ventricular echoes, Am. J. Physiol. **195:**53, 1958.
14. Kistin, A.D.: Multiple pathways of conduction and reciprocal rhythm with interpolated ventricular premature systoles, Am. Heart J. **65:** 162, 1963.
15. Watanabe, Y., and Dreifus, L.S.: Inhomogeneous conduction in the A-V node. A model for reentry, Am. Heart J. **70:**505, 1965.
16. Schuilenburg, R.M., and Durrer, D.: Ventricular echo beats in the human heart elicited by induced ventricular premature beats, Circulation **40:**337, 1969.
17. Wu, D., and others: Demonstration of dual atrioventricular nodal pathways utilizing a ventricular extrastimulus in patients with atrioventricular nodal re-entrant paroxysmal tachycardia, Circulation **52:**789, 1975.
18. Bharati, S., and others: Congenital abnormalities of the conduction system in two patients with recurrent tachyarrhythmias, Circulation **59:**593, 1979.
19. Wu, D., Denes, P., Dhingra, R., Khan, A., and Rosen, K.: The effects of propranolol in induction of A-V nodal reentrant paroxysmal tachycardia, Circulation **50:**665, 1974.
20. Josephson, M.E., and Kastor, J.A.: Paroxysmal supraventricular tachycardia, Circulation **54:**430, 1976.
21. Langendorf, R., and Pick, A.: Manifestations of concealed reentry in the atrioventricular junction, Eur. J. Cardiol. **1:**11, 1973.
22. Mayer, A.G.: Rhythmic pulsation in scyphomedusae. II. In Papers from the Tortugas Laboratory of the Carnegie Institution of Washington, Publication no. 102, Part 7, 1908.
23. Wu, D., Wyndham, C.R.C., Amat-y-Leon, R., Denes, P., Dhingra, R.C., and Rosen, K.M.: The effects of ouabain on induction of atrioventricular nodal reentrant paroxysmal tachycardia, Circulation **52:**201, 1975.
24. Wellens, H.J.J., Duren, D.R., Liem, K.L., and Lie, K.I.: Effect of digitalis in patients with paroxysmal atrioventricular nodal tachycardia, Circulation **52:**779, 1975.
25. Wellens, H.J.J., Tan, S.L., Bar, R.W.H., Duren, D.R., Lie, K.I., and Dohman, H.M.: Effect of verapamil studied by programmed electrical stimulation of the heart in patients with paroxysmal reentrant supraventricular tachycardia, Br. Heart J. **39:**1058, 1977.
26. Wellens, H.J.J., Farré, J., and Bar, R.W.H.: The WPW syndrome. In Mandel, W., editor: Management of difficult arrhythmias, Philadelphia, 1980, J.B. Lippincott Co.

27. Wellens, H.J.J., and Durrer, D.: Effect of digitalis on atrioventricular conduction and circus movement tachycardias in patients with Wolff-Parkinson-White syndrome, Circulation **47:**1229, 1973.

28. Wu, D., Denes, P., Bauernfeind, R., Kehoe, R., Amat-y-Leon, R., and Rosen, K.M.: Effects of procainamide on atrioventricular nodal re-entrant paroxysmal tachycardia, Circulation **57:**1171, 1978.

29. Sung, R.J., and Castellanos, A.: Supraventricular tachycardia: mechanisms and treatment, Cardiovasc. Clin. **11:**27, 1980.

30. Coumel, P., Cabrol, C., Fabiato, A., Gourgon, R., and Slama, R.: Tachycardie permanente par rythme réciproque. I. Preuves du diagnostic par stimulation auriculaire et ventriculaire. II. Traitement par l'implantation intra-corporelle d'un stimulateur cardiaque avec entrainement simultané de l'oreillette et du ventricule, Arch. Mal. Coeur **60:**1830, 1967.

31. Krikler, D., Curry, P., Attuel, P., and Coumel, P.: "Incessant" tachycardias in Wolff-Parkinson-White syndrome. I. Initiation without antecedent extrasystoles or PR lengthening. With reference to reciprocation after shortening of cycle length, Br. Heart J. **38:**885, 1976.

32. Pick, A., and Langendorf, R.: Interpretation of complex arrhythmias, Philadelphia, 1979, Lea & Febiger.

33. Wu, D., and others: Clinical electrocardiographic and electrophysiologic observations in patients with paroxysmal supraventricular tachycardia, Am. J. Cardiol. **41:**1045, 1978.

34. Wellens, H.J.J.: Value and limitations of programmed electrical stimulation of the heart in the study and treatment of tachycardias, Circulation **57:**845, 1978.

35. Wu, D., Denes, P., Amat-y-Leon, F., and others: An unusual variety of atrioventricular nodal reentry due to retrograde dual atrioventricular nodal pathways, Circulation **56:**50, 1977.

36. Coumel, P., Attuel, P., and Leclercq, J.F.: Permanent form of junctional reciprocating tachycardia: mechanism, clinical and therapeutic implications. In Narula, O.S., editor: Cardiac arrhythmias: electrophysiology, diagnosis, and management, Baltimore, 1979, The Williams & Wilkins Co.

37. Scherf, D., and Shookhoff, C.: Experimentelle Untersuchungen über die "Umkehr-Extrasystole," Wien. Arch. Inn. Med. **12:**501, 1926.

38. Mines, G.R.: On dynamic equilibrium in the heart, J. Physiol. (Lond.) **46:**349, 1913.

39. Kistin, A.D.: Atrial reciprocal rhythm, Circulation **32:**687, 1965.

40. Pick, A.: Mechanisms of cardiac arrhythmias: from hypothesis to physiologic fact, Am. Heart J. **86:**249, 1973.

41. Bix, H.H., and Marriott, H.J.L.: Reciprocal beats masquerading as ventricular captures, Am. J. Cardiol. **4:**128, 1959.

CHAPTER 7

Accessory pathways

The AV node is not the only structure that provides a reentry circuit for the support of paroxysmal supraventricular tachycardia. Congenital defects may exist in the form of extra muscular tracts or connections (accessory pathways) between the atria and the ventricles. Since these are usually extensions of atrial muscle, they conduct faster than the AV node and are often responsible for ventricular preexcitation, although, as you will see, accessory pathways may be present without or with minimal preexcitation and still provide an arrhythmogenic link.

Preexcitation may be defined as activation of part of the ventricular myocardium earlier than would be expected if the activating impulse only traveled normally via the AV junction.

A *tract* has been defined as a muscular pathway between atrium and ventricle with one end inserted into conductive tissue; as opposed to a *connection*, which is a muscular pathway between atrium and ventricle but excludes the conductive system.[1] These pathways are as follows:

1. Accessory AV connections (Kent bundles)
2. AV nodal bypass tracts (Lown-Ganong-Levine or short-PR-normal-QRS syndrome)
3. Nodoventricular and/or fasciculoventricular tracts (Mahaim fibers)

We have chosen to avoid the term "Wolff-Parkinson-White syndrome" since many patients have been shown to have Kent bundles with all of the attendant arrhythmias and yet do not exhibit the electrocardiographic signs of the originally described syndrome.

Accessory AV pathways

HISTORY. In 1915 Frank Wilson,[2] followed by Wedd[3] in 1921, Bach[4] in 1929, and Hamburger[5] in 1929, published the first examples of preexcitation, although they were not recognized as such. These investigators all thought that the broad QRS complex was an atypical bundle-branch block, as did Wolff, Parkinson, and White,[6] whose 1930 publication was entitled "Bundle branch block with short PR interval in healthy young people prone to paroxysmal tachycardia." At this time 11 cases were presented without reference to AV bypass connections.

Such muscular connections were actually described as early as 1876 by Paladino[7] and in 1893 by Kent,[8] who thought that they were the normal AV conduction pathways.

In 1914 Mines,[9] 30 years ahead of his time, suggested that these "bundles of Kent" provided a reentrant pathway for tachycardias. It was, however, not until 1932[10] and 1933[11] that the concept of AV bypass connections capable of transmitting impulses from atria to ventricles in less than the normal AV conduction time was suggested.

By 1943 and 1944 Wood and others[12] and Ohnell[13] had linked the ECG findings of short PR and broad QRS with postmortem histologic confirmation of anomalous AV connections on both sides of the heart.

CLINICAL SIGNIFICANCE OF ACCESSORY AV CONNECTIONS. ECG evidence of an accessory AV connection was nothing more than a curiosity until it became evident that some of these patients also suffered from life-threatening arrhythmias.[14] Our clinical approach to the management of these arrhythmias was given a further boost with the advent of intracardiac programmed stimulation and recordings,[15] which have also provided an understanding of anatomy and the mechanism of the associated arrhythmias.

ANATOMY. An extra anatomic connection has been documented[16-21] in patients with a short PR and a broad QRS, although such a connection may also be present with a normal ECG.[22] Its great importance is that it offers a potential reentrant pathway for the support of supraventricular tachycardia as well as ready and rapid access to the ventricles during atrial fibrillation or flutter.

Some authorities[23,24] have postulated that during the embryologic development of the heart these extramuscular connections have evaded the normal severance by the fibrous band of the AV ring of all muscle connections except the bundle of His. Others[21] have not found proof of such faulty embryologic development but have found that the accessory bundle is separate from an intact AV ring. Fig. 7-1 diagrammatically illustrates these more recent findings.

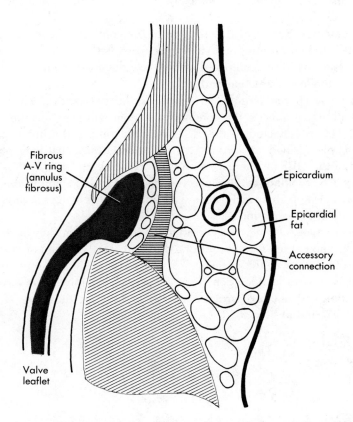

Fig. 7-1. Diagrammatic representation of a left-sided accessory atrioventricular connection. The connection skirts through the epicardial fat, being outside the AV fibrous ring. (From Becker, A.E., Anderson, R.H., Durrer, D., and Wellens, H.J.J.: Circulation **57:**870, 1978. By permission of the American Heart Association, Inc.)

ECG FEATURES. The classical ECG features of the syndrome originally described by Wolff, Parkinson, and White[6] are a short PR interval and a broad QRS. We now know the anatomic substrate of their syndrome and that this anatomy may be present without the ECG criteria.

The PR interval. If this interval is short, it is because the sinus impulse partially avoids its normal delay in the AV node by traveling rapidly down the accessory pathway.

The QRS complex. Subsequent activation of the ventricles depends upon intra-atrial conduction time from sinus node to the accessory pathway plus conduction time down the accessory pathway, compared with the conduction time from sinus node to ventricles via orthodox conduction pathways.

The delta wave. If the impulse first reaches the ventricles via the accessory pathway, it will arrive outside the conductive system and therefore be conducted more slowly. This is reflected in the ECG by a slurring of the initial part of the ventricular complex, called a *delta* wave. It is the delta wave that is responsible for the widening of the QRS (at the expense of the PR interval).

Secondary T wave changes. Because ventricular depolarization is abnormal, repolarization will also be abnormal, causing ST and T wave changes secondary to the degree and area of preexcitation.

Abnormal Q waves. Q waves are considered abnormal when they have an amplitude 25% of the succeeding R wave and/or a duration of 0.04 second or greater. Such Q waves are often seen in the presence of an accessory AV pathway and may be misdiagnosed as myocardial infarction. They are actually negative delta waves, reflecting preexcitation and not myocardial necrosis. In Fig. 7-2 there are abnormal Q waves in leads III and aVF.

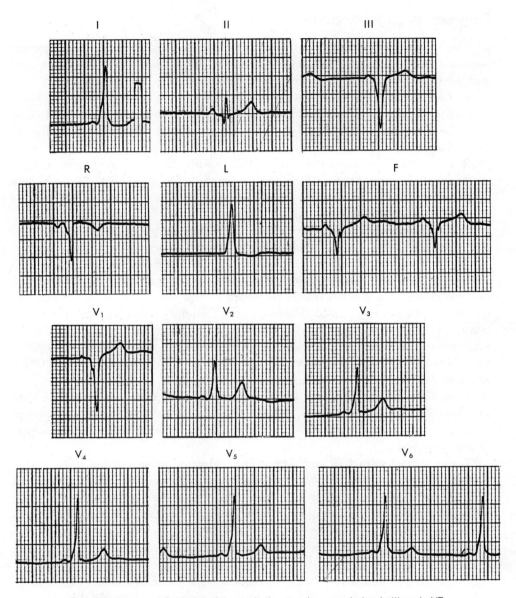

Fig. 7-2. Abnormal Q waves of preexcitation can be seen in leads III and aVF.

Degrees of preexcitation

The degree of preexcitation refers to the amount of ventricular myocardium activated via the accessory pathway. This determines the duration of the PR interval and the width of the QRS complex and is itself determined by the following[22]:

1. *Location of the accessory pathway:* The closer it is to the sinus node, the faster the impulse reaches its atrial insertion. For example, a right-sided Kent bundle provides a greater degree of preexcitation than does a left-sided one, all else being equal.

2. *Intraatrial conduction times (from sinus node to accessory pathway and from sinus node to AV node):* If the impulse generated in the sinus node reaches the atrial insertion of the Kent bundle more rapidly than it does the AV node, a greater degree of preexcitation is favored.

3. *Accessory pathway conduction time:* This is dependent upon the length of the pathway as well as the conduction velocity in the accessory pathway.

4. *AV nodal–His–Purkinje conduction time:* If intranodal conduction time is short, the degree of preexcitation may be decreased, especially if the accessory pathway is on the left side of the heart.

The degree of preexcitation determines the PR interval and the size of the delta wave, and any degree from zero to maximal is possible. The duration of the PR interval and the size of the delta wave have no bearing on the patient's vulnerability to arrhythmias. With no evidence of preexcitation at all (normal PR, normal QRS), rapid ventricular rates due to reciprocating tachycardia or atrial fibrillation may threaten life if a Kent bundle is present and open to impulse propagation in both directions. If *only* retrograde conduction is possible via the Kent bundle, the patient is protected from the life-threatening rates of atrial fibrillation but not from reciprocating tachycardia.[36]

Given normal intraatrial and intranodal conduction velocities and a short Kent bundle with rapid conduction situated close to the sinus node (i.e., right sided), the PR segment may be nonexistent (P and delta waves overlap) and the ventricles activated entirely via the accessory pathway so that the anomalous wave front blocks the entrance of the impulse through normal His-Purkinje channels. This is referred to as maximal preexcitation and is diagrammatically illustrated in Fig. 7-3, *A*. Fig. 7-3, *B* to *D*, shows progressively decreasing degrees of preexcitation.

The beats represented by Fig. 7-3, *B* and *C*, are fusion beats because the sinus impulse arrives in the ventricles via both the accessory and the normal pathway.

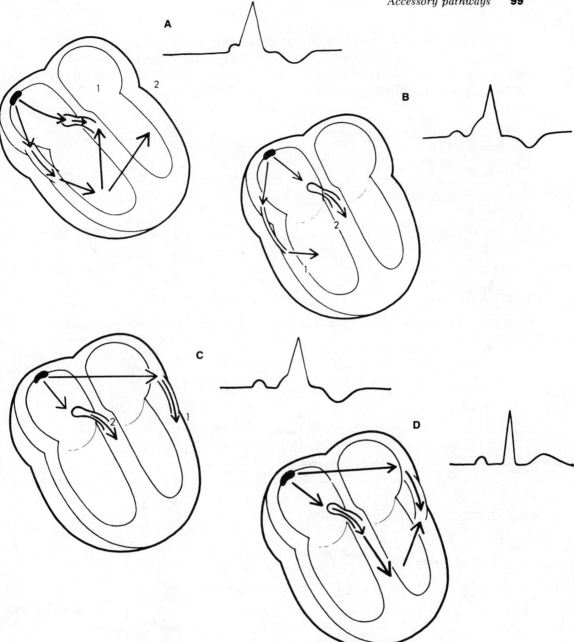

Fig. 7-3. A, Maximal preexcitation. The ventricles are activated totally by the delta force. **B,** Less than maximal preexcitation. This results in a fusion beat as long as the sinus impulse arrives in the ventricles in time to propagate. **C,** Minimal preexcitation. As the degree of preexcitation becomes less, the delta wave becomes smaller. This results in a longer PR interval and a shorter QRS duration. **D,** No preexcitation. The impulse does not conduct rapidly enough over the accessory pathway and is cancelled out by the impulse that is conducted normally through the His-Purkinje axis.

Maximal preexcitation is electrocardiographically illustrated in Figs. 7-4 and 7-5. In both cases the PR interval is only 0.09 second and the QRS complex is very broad with no well-defined ending to the delta wave. But for the short PR intervals, these ECGs could well be mistaken for LBBB.

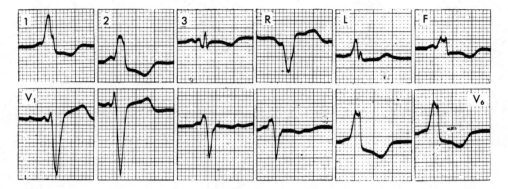

Fig. 7-4. Maximal preexcitation. The P and delta waves overlap. Note the initially positive but mainly negative QRS complex in V_1. This pattern could well be mistaken for left bundle-branch block, save for the fact that the PR interval is only 0.09 second.

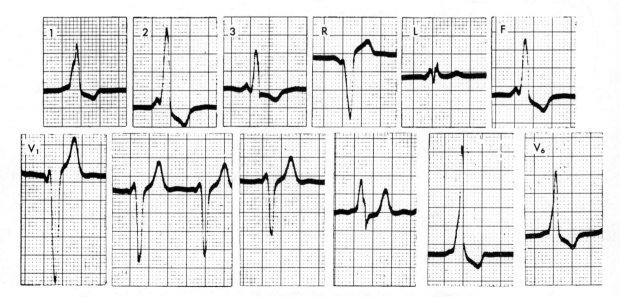

Fig. 7-5. Maximal preexcitation. The PR interval is about 0.09 second, and the widened QRS has a slow initial component well seen in several leads. The overall QRS pattern could be mistaken for left bundle-branch block.

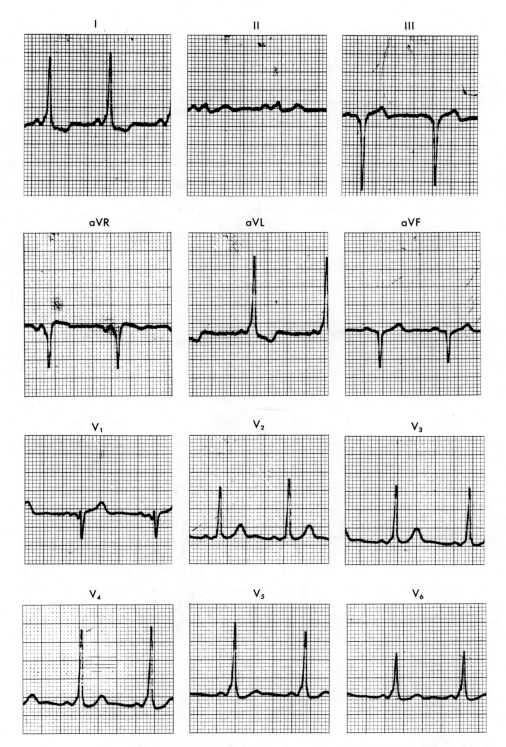

Fig. 7-6. Preexcitation with fusion. The PR interval is longer than in Fig. 7-5 and the delta wave can clearly be seen in most leads—a lesser degree of preexcitation. (From Conover, M.H.: Cardiac arrhythmias, ed. 2, St. Louis, 1978. The C.V. Mosby Co.)

In Figs. 7-6 and 7-7 the P-R intervals are 0.10 second and the delta waves can be clearly seen in most leads. The QRS in these cases is a fusion complex—a lesser degree of preexcitation than seen in Figs. 7-4 and 7-5.

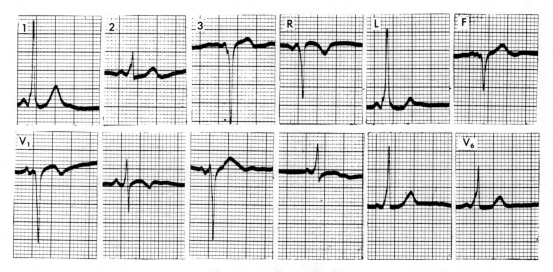

Fig. 7-7. Preexcitation with fusion. The PR interval is 0.10 second. Delta waves are well seen in several leads.

Fig. 7-8 illustrates an interesting extrasystolic phenomenon associated with preexcitation. There are several atrial premature beats each associated with shortening of the PR interval and slurring of the initial part of the QRS, clear manifestations of preexcitation. The reason for the preexcitation only with the premature atrial beat may be that the ectopic focus is located near the atrial origin of the Kent bundle and therefore the ectopic impulse gains entrance into the ventricles more rapidly.

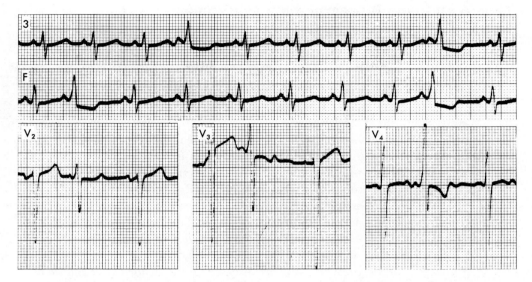

Fig. 7-8. The sinus rhythm is interrupted by numerous atrial premature beats. Each is characterized by shortening of the PR interval and widening of the QRS with slurring of its initial component—the hallmarks of preexcitation.

Mimicry by preexcitation

As indicated in Figs. 7-3, *D*, and 7-8, the existence of an accessory pathway is not always evident from the ECG. If conditions provide for a more rapid journey into the ventricles via the accessory pathway than via the normal pathway, the classical preexcitation pattern is present in the ECG: short PR, broad QRS, a delta wave, and secondary T wave changes. If, however, the sinus impulse reaches the ventricles via the normal pathways faster than via the accessory pathway, the PR and QRS will be normal.

However, when the ventricular complex is actually a fusion beat, the QRS abnormalities that result—abnormal Q waves, slurring of the ascending limb of the R wave with widening of the QRS, increased voltage of the R wave, and axis changes[22]—may beget any or all of the following misdiagnoses: myocardial infarction, intraventricular blocks, and/or ventricular hypertrophy.

Type A and type B preexcitation syndromes

The classification of preexcitation syndromes into type A and type B is simplistic. Rosenbaum and Wilson[25] originally based their subdivision into "group A" and "group B" on the QRS morphology in leads V_1, V_2, and V_E (positive electrode placed over the ensiform cartilage). Following their criteria, we call it a type A if the R wave is predominant in one or more of these leads (Fig. 7-9) and type B if there is a QS or if the S wave is dominant (Fig. 7-10).

Epicardial mapping has since shown that type B is the result of early activation of the lateral aspect of the right ventricle,[16] and that type A involves early activation of the left ventricle.[26] However, later studies[27] have shown that the accessory pathway may also insert into the IV septum and that its location is determined with confidence only when the QRS complex is the result of maximal preexcitation (activation via the accessory pathway alone), a condition that provides the best opportunity to analyze the initial forces from the accessory pathway. With minimal preexcitation this is not possible. Other handicaps in localizing the accessory pathway are (1) multiple accessory pathways, (2) the presence of heart disease, (3) the distortion of the delta wave with the P wave, and (4) the influence exerted on ventricular activation by the location (endocardial versus epicardial) of the accessory pathway.[22]

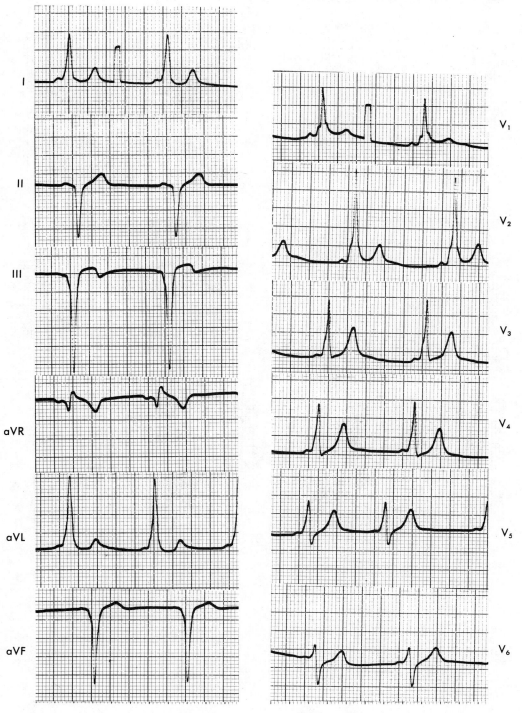

Fig. 7-9. Type A preexcitation syndrome. There is a positive delta wave in all the chest leads and a negative one in the inferior leads.

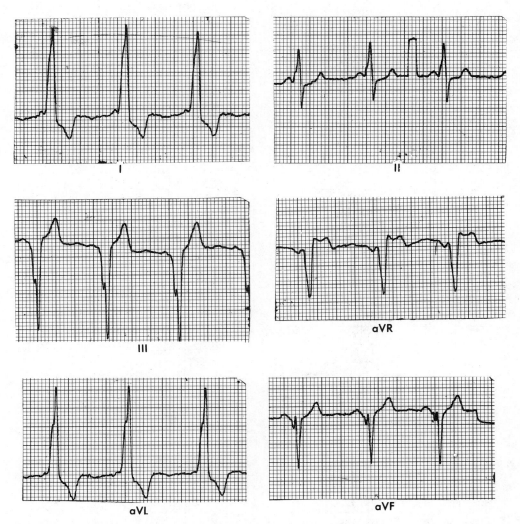

Fig. 7-10. Type B preexcitation syndrome. Note the rS pattern sometimes seen in V_1 and the QS in leads III and aVF.

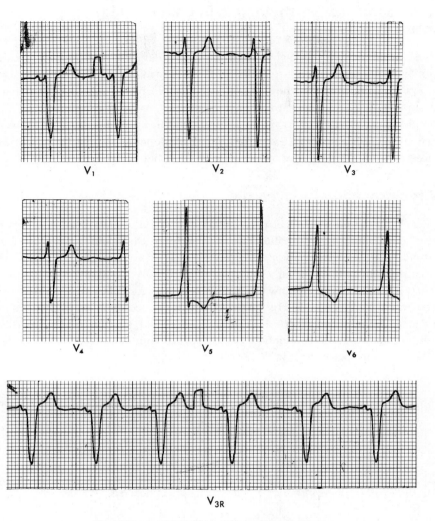

Fig. 7-10, cont'd. For legend see opposite page.

Incidence of tachyarrhythmias in patients with accessory pathways

The actual incidence of tachyarrhythmias in patients with accessory AV pathways is not known. Reported figures vary from 12% to 80%,[28,29] and Wellens and coworkers[22] consider it to be the most important underlying cause of regular paroxysmal supraventricular tachycardia, having found it to exist in as many as 57% of patients admitted with the arrhythmia. Although this figure admittedly may be influenced by patient selection, even in adults experiencing the first attack of PSVT, an accessory AV pathway was found in 36 of 75 patients (48%).[22]

AV reciprocating tachycardia

Fig. 7-11, *A* and *B*, is electrocardiograms from a 3-week-old baby. *A* was taken during sinus rhythm, and *B* illustrates AV reciprocating tachycardia (the chief arrhythmia to which these patients are prone).

Such a tachycardia is usually initiated by a critically timed atrial premature beat blocked in the accessory pathway because of its longer refractory period but conducted via the AV node and His-Purkinje axis. If the accessory pathway is no longer refractory when the impulse reaches its ventricular end, a reciprocal tachycardia may result with anterograde conduction via the normal route and retrograde conduction via the accessory pathway (Fig. 7-11, *C*).

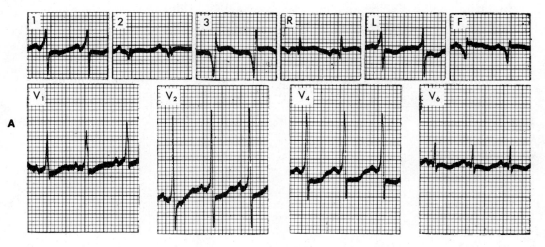

A

Fig. 7-11. A shows a type A preexcitation during sinus rhythm recorded in a 3-week-old baby.

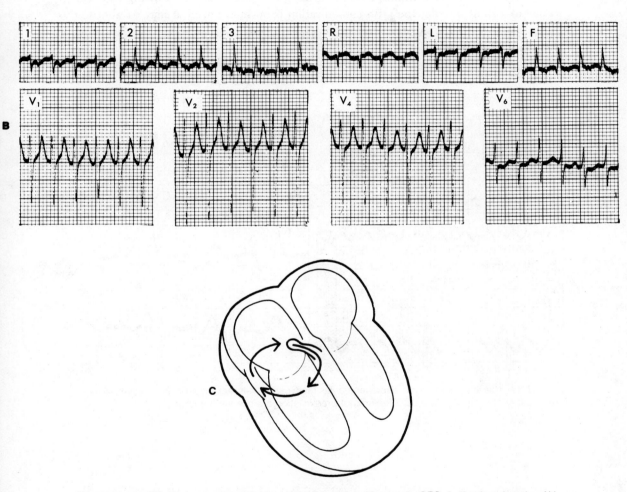

Fig. 7-11, cont'd. B shows supraventricular tachycardia with narrow QRS, indicating that the AV junction serves as the anterograde pathway and the accessory bundle as the retrograde pathway. **C** is a diagrammatic representation of the usual reentry circuit using the AV node and bundle of His in an anterograde direction and the accessory pathway in a retrograde direction.

Fig. 7-12 is another example of this more common sequence of reentry. Note the classical features of preexcitation during sinus rhythm in the right panel of Fig. 7-12 and the normal QRS in the tachycardia in the left panel.

Thus in the more common type of AV reciprocating tachycardia owing its existence to a Kent bundle, the QRS configuration is normal. Rarely it may be aberrant and then present the same differential diagnosis as any other supraventricular tachycardia with aberrancy.

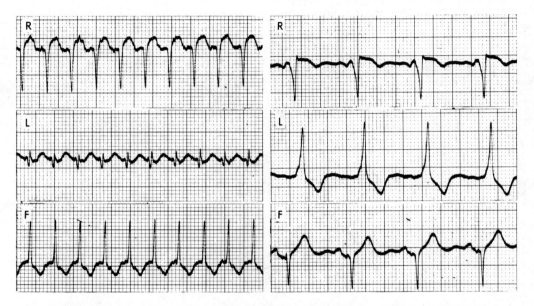

Fig. 7-12. The left panel shows supraventricular tachycardia with narrow QRS in a patient with an accessory AV pathway. The ECG features of preexcitation are seen in the right panel.

Less commonly the circulating wave front will proceed anterogradely via the accessory pathway, producing a tachycardia that is difficult to distinguish from ventricular tachycardia because of its broad QRS of maximal preexcitation (Fig. 7-13). A similar pattern may be produced when there are two accessory pathways with anterograde conduction via one pathway and retrograde conduction via the other. [27,30,31]

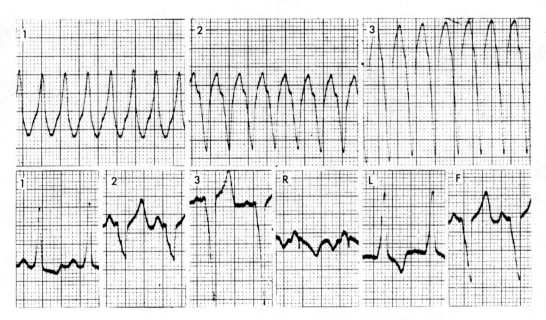

Fig. 7-13. A supraventricular tachycardia using an accessory pathway in the anterograde direction, the less common mechanism. The top panel presents standard limb leads during the tachycardia. In the bottom panel the features of preexcitation can be seen during sinus rhythm.

Fig. 7-14 illustrates an interesting potential for reentrant tachycardia due to retrograde conduction into the accessory pathway following interpolated ventricular extrasystoles. Most of the sinus beats have short PR intervals, prolonged QRS durations, and delta waves. However, the ventricular complexes following the interpolated extrasystoles are narrow and normally conducted, presumably because of concealed retrograde conduction from the extrasystole into the accessory pathway. Such retrograde penetration leaves the accessory pathway refractory and prevents it from transmitting the next sinus impulse.

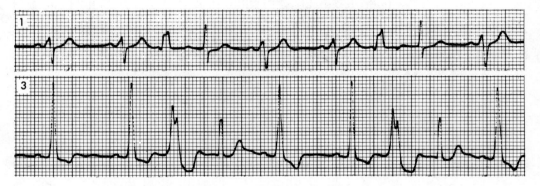

Fig. 7-14. Except for those that follow the interpolated ventricular extrasystoles, the sinus beats all have short PR intervals with delta waves. Those that follow the extrasystoles are narrow and normally conducted, presumably because of concealed retrograde conduction from the extrasystole into the accessory pathway.

Differentiating AV reciprocating tachycardia from AV nodal reentry

Sometimes the patient with a manifest accessory pathway during sinus rhythm will sustain a supraventricular tachycardia involving only the AV node (intranodal reentry). In this situation, surgical interruption of the accessory pathway is obviously futile so that this possibility must always be ruled out if surgery is under consideration.

When the P' wave can be identified during the tachycardia involving an accessory pathway, it will be close on the heels of the QRS (RP' < P'R), a fact that helps to differentiate it from the two types of AV nodal reciprocating tachycardia, in which the P' wave either is hidden in the QRS (the more common type of AV nodal reentry) or follows the QRS by a greater interval than it precedes the next (RP' > P'R). (See Fig. 6-10.)

Atrial fibrillation in the presence of an accessory pathway

Atrial extrasystoles and ventricular extrasystoles with retrograde atrial activation not only may result in a reciprocating tachycardia; they also may initiate atrial fibrillation if they invade the atrium during its vulnerable period. Less commonly atrial flutter or the tachycardia itself may deteriorate into atrial fibrillation.

If conduction during atrial fibrillation is exclusively over an accessory pathway with a short refractory period, the ventricular rates can be very high (160 to 300/min) and the rhythm may degenerate into ventricular fibrillation.[32,33] It is claimed that when RR intervals are equal to or less than 205 milliseconds the atrial fibrillation is likely to degenerate into ventricular fibrillation.[33]

Figs. 7-15 and 7-16 illustrate the tachycardia that develops as a result of atrial fibrillation and an accessory pathway. The shortest RR intervals are 0.16 and 0.18 second, prime candidates for the development of ventricular fibrillation. Note the typical irregularity of the tachycardia of atrial fibrillation as opposed to the regular reciprocating tachycardia seen in Fig. 7-12.

A

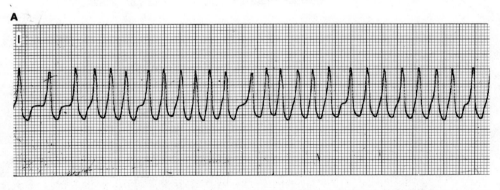

Fig. 7-15. A, Tachycardia during atrial fibrillation in the presence of an accessory pathway with a short refractory period. At times the rate is 300. Note the irregularity, typical of this arrhythmia.

Continued.

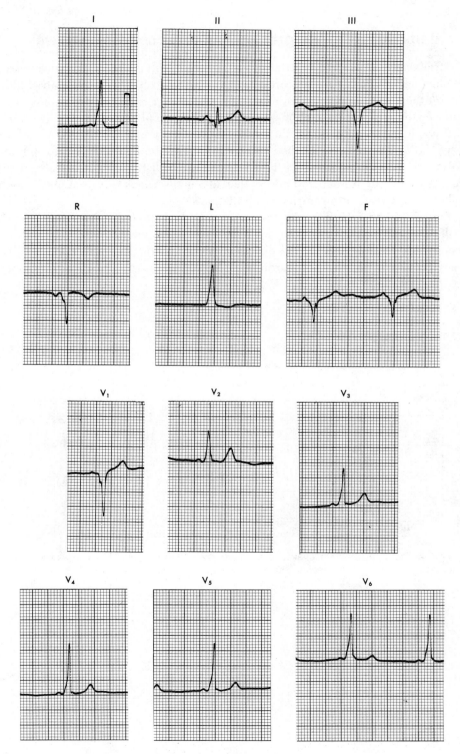

Fig. 7-15, cont'd. B, The preexcitation pattern in this patient.

Fig. 7-16, *A*, shows a typical preexcitation pattern during sinus rhythm. In panel *B* the patient is in atrial fibrillation with a ventricular response of 280/min. Several beats in the first half of lead II are evidently conducted via normal pathways at a somewhat slower rate. Note the maximal preexcitation in the remaining complexes and the irregularity of the rhythm due to the atrial fibrillation.

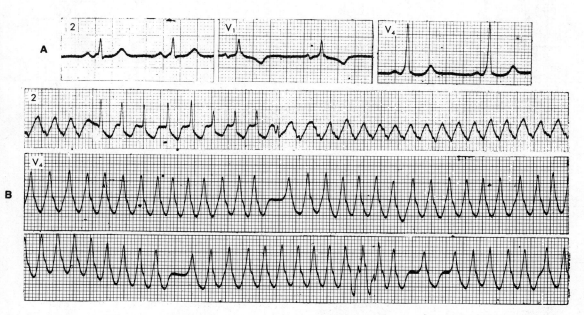

Fig. 7-16. The top panel (**A**) shows the preexcitation pattern, whereas the rhythm strips (**B**) illustrate the typical picture of atrial fibrillation during anomalous pathway conduction with a ventricular response of 280/min. Several beats in the first half of lead II are evidently conducted via normal pathways at a somewhat slower rate. Note that occasional cycles are more than twice the length of the shortest cycles.

Fig. 7-17 again illustrates atrial fibrillation and preexcitation. In *A*, note the rate of 290/min, the occasional normal conduction, and the irregularity of the rhythm. In *B*, after lidocaine, which lengthens the refractory period of accessory pathways, the rate of the ventricular response is markedly reduced.

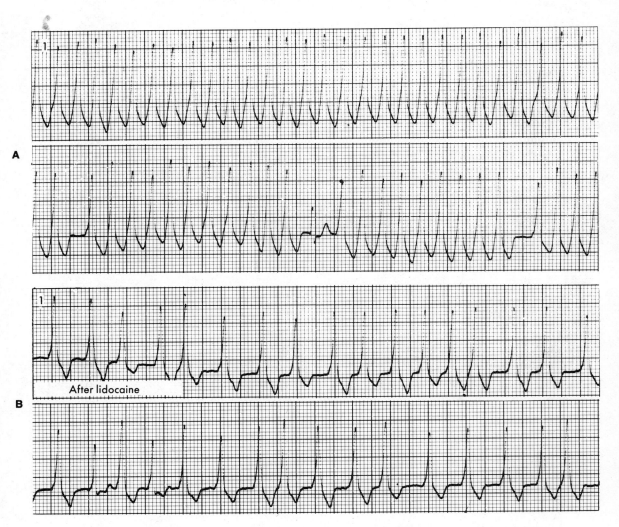

Fig. 7-17. A, The strips are continuous. From a young woman with atrial fibrillation and preexcitation. Note the rate of 290/min, the occasional normal conduction, and the occasional cycle more than twice the length of the shortest cycles. **B,** The strips are continuous and illustrate the slowing effect of lidocaine (rate, about 165/min).

Differentiating atrial fibrillation with an accessory pathway from ventricular tachycardia

Because of the maximal preexcitation during atrial fibrillation with an accessory pathway, this arrhythmia has often been mistaken for, and published as, ventricular tachycardia. Of considerable diagnostic value are the clinical setting, the regularity or irregularity of the rhythm, and the QRS morphology.

If the victim is a septuagenarian in a coronary care unit, it is probably ventricular tachycardia; on the other hand, if a 22-year-old presents in the emergency room with this arrhythmia, it is more likely preexcitation.

In the large majority of cases ventricular tachycardia is perfectly regular[34] whereas in atrial fibrillation and preexcitation the longest cycle length is often over twice the length of the shortest cycle (i.e., a greater than 100% variation).

Details of the QRS morphologic patterns that favor ventricular ectopy are described in Chapter 16, but it is important to recall that the taller left "rabbit-ear" in V_1 and the concordant precordial positivity may both be imitated by type A preexcitation; and the wide initial r wave in V_1 can be simulated by type B.

Concealed accessory pathway

When an accessory pathway is present but conducts only in the retrograde direction, it is said to be concealed since its presence is not manifest on the ECG. It is often called "concealed WPW syndrome," which is a misnomer; for without the ECG signs, there is no syndrome. The bundle of Kent conducts only retrogradely because the refractory period of the accessory pathway in the anterograde direction exceeds the sinus cycle length.[22] These patients are protected from very high ventricular rates if atrial fibrillation develops, since anterograde conduction is always through the normal route. They are, however, still vulnerable to the AV reciprocating tachycardia that often complicates the picture when an accessory pathway is present. In such cases the impulses travel retrogradely up the accessory pathway and anterogradely down the AV junction to establish a circus movement. During the tachycardia the QRS is narrow unless the rapid rate fosters aberrant conduction.

This condition should not be confused with the situation when conduction across an accessory pathway in the anterograde direction is possible but does not occur during sinus rhythm only because the impulse conducts more rapidly across the His-Purkinje axis. Distinction between the two conditions is important, because one (the concealed accessory pathway) is protected from excessively rapid ventricular rates during atrial fibrillation and the other is not.

AV nodal bypass tract (Lown-Ganong-Levine or short-PR-normal-QRS syndrome)

HISTORY. In 1952 Lown, Ganong, and Levine[35] reported the syndrome of "short P-R interval, normal QRS complex, and paroxysmal rapid heart action," that later became known as the Lown-Ganong-Levine syndrome (LGL syndrome). Many favor the abandonment of this term for the more descriptive "short-PR-normal-QRS syndrome."[36,37]

ANATOMY. Anatomic and physiologic correlations of this syndrome are controversial. The short PR and supraventricular tachycardia may be the result of an AV nodal bypass tract linking the atria directly with the penetrating bundle of His,[38] an anatomically small AV node,[39] or rapidly conducting preferential intranodal fibers.[40] Wellens and co-workers[37] and also Josephson and Kastor[40] have reported the tachycardia circuit in these patients to be completely confined to the AV node.

Of interest is the fact that the incidence of short and long PR intervals is exactly the same (1.3%) in a healthy young population, suggesting that neither is necessarily abnormal but may represent the extremities of the bell curve of normal PR intervals.[41]

Fig. 7-18 is a 12-lead tracing with a short-PR-normal-QRS pattern from a healthy individual with no history of tachycardia.

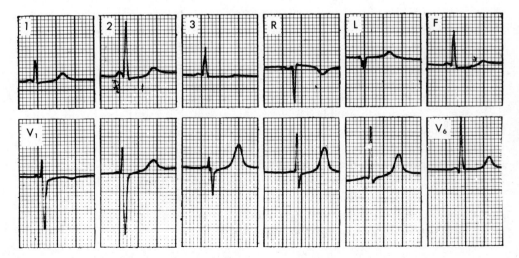

Fig. 7-18. Short-PR-normal-QRS pattern from a healthy asymptomatic individual with no history of palpitations or tachycardia. The PR interval is 0.08 second.

Nodoventricular and/or fasciculoventricular tracts (Mahaim fibers)

Nodoventricular tracts link the AV node with the ventricular myocardium. Fasciculoventricular tracts link the bundle of His (penetrating or branching portion) with the ventricular myocardium. Both types of tracts are illustrated in Fig. 7-19. They were described by Mahaim and Winston[42] in 1941 and are sometimes called Mahaim fibers.

The resulting ECG depends upon the location and length of the fiber. The expected pattern has a small delta wave that increases the QRS width less than the classical preexcitation using a Kent bundle; since the impulse emerging via a Mahaim fiber has traversed the AV node, the PR interval is within normal limits rather than foreshortened.

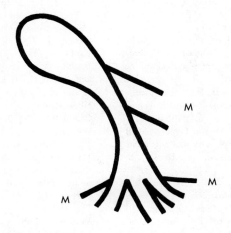

Fig. 7-19. Diagrammatic representation of several nodoventricular and fasciculoventricular tracts, sometimes called Mahaim fibers.

References

1. Anderson, R.H., Becker, A.E., and others: Ventricular preexcitation: a proposed nomenclature for its substrates, Eur. J. Cardiol. **3**:27, 1975.
2. Wilson, F.N.: A case in which the vagus influenced the form of ventricular complex of the electrocardiogram, Arch. Intern. Med. **16**: 1008, 1915.
3. Wedd, A.M.: Paroxysmal tachycardia. With reference to nomotopic tachycardia and the role of the extrinsic cardial nerves, Arch. Intern. Med. **27**:571, 1921.
4. Bach, R.: Paroxysmal tachycardia of forty-eight years duration and right bundle branch block, Proc. R. Soc. Med. **22**:412, 1929.
5. Hamburger, W.W.: Bundle branch block. Four cases of intraventricular blocks showing some interesting and unusual clinical features, Med. Clin. North Am. **13**:343, 1929.
6. Wolff, L., Parkinson, J., and White, P.D.: Bundle branch block with short P-R interval in healthy young people prone to paroxysmal tachycardia, Am. Heart J. **5**:685, 1930.
7. Paladino, G.: Contribuzione a l'anatomia, istologia e fisiologia del cuore, Moiv. Med. Chir. (Napoli) **8**:428, 1876.
8. Kent, A.F.S.: Researches on structure and function of mammalian heart, J. Physiol. **14**: 233, 1893.
9. Mines, G.R.: On circulating excitations in heart muscles and their possible relation to tachycardia and fibrillation, Trans. R. Soc. Can., ser. 3, sec. 4, **8**:43, 1914.
10. Holzmann, M., and Scherf, D.: Ueber Elektrokardiogramme mit verkürzter Vorhof-Kammer-Distanz und positiven P-Zacken, Z. Klin. Med. **121**:404, 1932.
11. Wolferth, C.C., and Wood, F.C.: The mechanism of production of short P-R intervals and prolonged QRS complexes in patients with presumably undamaged hearts. Hypothesis of an accessory pathway of auriculoventricular conduction (bundle of Kent), Am. Heart J. **8**: 297, 1933.
12. Wood, F.C., Wolferth, C.C., and Geckeler, G.D.: Histological demonstration of accessory muscular connections between auricle and ventricle in a case of short P-R interval and prolonged QRS complex, Am. Heart J. **252**: 454, 1943.
13. Ohnell, R.F.: Preexcitation, a cardiac abnormality, Acta Med. Scand. **152** (suppl.):74, 1944.
14. Dreifus, L.S., and others: Ventricular fibrillation, a possible mechanism of sudden death in patients with the Wolff-Parkinson-White syndrome, Circulation **43**:520, 1971.
15. Wellens, H.J.J.: Contribution of cardiac pacing to our understanding of the Wolff-Parkinson-White syndrome, Circulation **43**:520, 1971.
16. Durrer, D., and Roos, J.P.: Epicardial excitation of the ventricles in a patient with Wolff-Parkinson-White syndrome (type B), Circulation **35**:15, 1967.
17. Durrer, D., Shoo, L., Schuilenburg, R.M., and Wellens, H.J.J.: The role of premature beats in the initiation and termination of supraventricular tachycardia in the Wolff-Parkinson-White syndrome, Circulation **36**:644, 1967.
18. Castellanos, A., Jr., and others: His bundle electrograms in two cases of Wolff-Parkinson-White (pre-excitation) syndrome, Circulation **41**:399, 1970.
19. Gallagher, J.J., Sealy, W.C., Wallace, A.G., and Kasell, J.: Correlation between catheter electrophysiological studies and findings on mapping of ventricular excitation in the WPW syndrome. In Wellens, H.J.J., Lie, K.I., and Janse, M.J., editors: The conduction system of the heart, Philadelphia, 1976, Lea & Febiger.
20. Sealy, W.C., and Wallace, A.G.: Surgical treatment of the Wolff-Parkinson-White syndrome, J. Thor. Cardiovasc. Surg. **68**:757, 1974.
21. Becker, A.E., Anderson, R.H., Durrer, D., and Wellens, H.J.J.: The anatomical substrates of Wolff-Parkinson-White syndrome: a clinicopathologic correlation in seven patients, Circulation **57**:870, 1978.
22. Wellens, H.J.J., Farré, J., and Bar, W.H.M.: The Wolff-Parkinson-White Syndrome. In Mandel, W.J., editor: Cardiac arrhythmias: their mechanisms, diagnosis, and management, Philadelphia, 1980, J.B. Lippincott Co.
23. Ferrer, M.I.: Preexcitation, Am. J. Med. **62**: 715, 1977.
24. Verduyn-Lunel, A.A.: Significance of annulus fibrosus of heart in relation to AV conduction and ventricular activation in cases of Wolff-

Parkinson-White syndrome, Br. Heart J. **34:** 1263, 1972.

25. Rosenbaum, F.F., Hecht, H.H., Wilson, F.N., and Johnston, F.D.: Potential variations of the thorax and the esophagus in anomalous atrioventricular excitation (Wolff-Parkinson-White syndrome), Am. Heart J. **29:**281, 1945.

26. Wallace, A.G., Sealy, W.C., Gallagher, J.J., Svenson, R.H., Strauss, H.C., and Kasell, J.: Surgical correction of anomalous left ventricular preexcitation: Wolff-Parkinson-White (type A), Circulation **49:**206, 1974.

27. Gallagher, J.J., Pritchett, E.L.C., Sealy, W.C., Kasell, J., and Wallace, A.G.: The preexcitation syndromes, Prog. Cardiovasc. Dis. **20:**285, 1978.

28. Bellet, S.: Clinical disorders of the heart beat, ed. 3, Philadelphia, 1971, Lea & Febiger.

29. Averill, K.M., Fosmoe, R.J., and Lamb, L.E.: Electrocardiographic findings in 67,375 asymptomatic subjects. IV. Wolff-Parkinson-White syndrome, Am. J. Cardiol. **6:**108, 1960.

30. Gallagher, J.J., Sealy, W.C., Kasell, J., and Wallace, A.G.: Multiple accessory pathways in patients with the preexcitation syndrome, Circulation **54:**571, 1976.

31. Wellens, H.J.J., Farré, J., Bar, R.W.: Stimulation studies in the Wolff-Parkinson-White syndrome. In Narula, O., editor: Clinical electrophysiology, Philadelphia, 1979, F.A. Davis Co.

32. Dreifus, L.S., Haiat, R., Watanabe, Y., Arriaga, J., and Reitman, N.C.: Ventricular fibrillation, a possible mechanism of sudden death in patients with the Wolff-Parkinson-White syndrome, Circulation **43:**520, 1971.

33. Bashore, T.M., Sellers, T.D., Gallagher, J.J.,

and Wallace, A.G.: Ventricular fibrillation in the Wolff-Parkinson-White syndrome [Abstract], Circulation **54** (suppl. II):187, 1976.

34. Wellens, H.J.J., and others: The value of the electrocardiogram in the differential diagnosis of a tachycardia with a widened QRS complex, Am. J. Med. **64:**27, 1978.

35. Lown, B., Ganong, W.F., and Levine, S.A.: The syndrome of short P-R interval, normal QRS complex and paroxysmal rapid heart action, Circulation **5:**696, 1952.

36. Sherf, L., and Neufeld, H.N.: The pre-excitation syndrome: facts and theories, New York, 1978, Yorke Medical Books.

37. Wellens, H.J.J., Lubbers, W.J., and Losekoot, T.G.: Preexcitation. In Roberts, N.K., and Gelband, H., editors: Cardiac arrhythmias in the neonate, infant, and child, New York, 1977, Appleton-Century-Crofts.

38. Sherf, L.: The atrial conduction system: clinical implications, Am. J. Cardiol. **37:**814, 1976.

39. Caracta, A.R., Damato, A.N., Gallagher, J.J., and others: Electrophysiological studies in the syndrome short P-R interval, normal QRS complex, Am. J. Cardiol. **31:**245, 1973.

40. Josephson, M.E., and Kastor, J.A.: Supraventricular tachycardia in Lown-Ganong-Levine syndrome: atrionodal versus intranodal reentry, Am. J. Cardiol. **40:**521, 1977.

41. Marriott, H.J.L.: Preexcitation "syndromes." In Contemporary electrocardiography, vol. 2., no. 7, Baltimore, 1980, The Williams & Wilkins Co.

42. Mahaim, I., and Winston, R.M.: Recherches d'anatomie comparée et de pathologie expérimentale sur les connexions hautes du faisceau de His-Tawara, Cardiologia **5:**189, 1941.

CHAPTER 8

Concealed conduction

So long as it is traveling in the specialized conduction system, the cardiac impulse writes nothing in the surface tracing because of the small amount of tissue involved. However, if an impulse travels a limited distance within the system, even though it leaves no trace of its own on the record, it can interfere with the formation or propagation of another impulse. When such interference can be recognized in the tracing because of an unexpected conduction delay or postponement of an impulse, it is known as *concealed conduction*. One may therefore define concealed conduction as the propagation of an impulse within the specialized conduction system of the heart, which can be recognized only from its effect on the subsequent beat or cycle.

Historical background

The first indirect electrocardiographic evidence of concealed AV conduction came in 1925 when Lewis and Master[1] demonstrated in the canine heart the effect of blocked impulses on subsequent conduction. During the same period Ashman[2] was performing like experiments on the turtle heart. Twenty years before this time Erlanger[3] had noted concealed conduction in his studies on complete heart block and had postulated with Engelmann that delayed conduction was caused by incomplete penetration of the junctional tissues causing partial refractoriness.

In 1927 Kaufmann and Rothberger[4] were the first to clinically apply the concept of concealed conduction. These authors proposed that the alternation of ventricular cycle length seen in a case of atrial flutter with 2:1 ventricular response was secondary to concealed deeper penetration into the AV junction by every other blocked flutter wave (diagrammatically illustrated in Fig. 8-1).

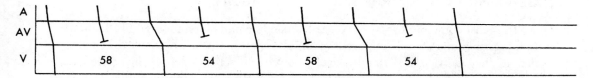

Fig. 8-1. Diagram of atrial flutter with 2:1 AV conduction and alternation of the ventricular cycle length secondary to concealed deeper penetration of alternate blocked impulses (the first clinical invocation of concealed conduction, Kaufmann and Rothberger, 1927).

The term *concealed conduction* was not introduced until 1948, when Langendorf[2] succinctly defined it in the title of his published paper: "Concealed A-V Conduction: the Effect of Blocked Impulses on the Formation and Conduction of Subsequent Impulses."

In 1950 Soderstrom[6] and later Moe and co-workers[7] showed that the irregular ventricular response in atrial fibrillation was a function of concealed conduction.

The mechanism of concealed conduction was outlined in detail in 1956 by Katz and Pick[8] and was demonstrated experimentally as a possibility in any part of the conduction system in 1961 by Hoffman, Cranefield, and Stuckey.[9] Finally, in 1969, direct evidence of concealed AV conduction was obtained in His bundle recordings performed by Lau, Damato, and co-workers.[10]

An understanding of this mechanism has proved to be most useful in interpreting arrhythmias that would otherwise be unexplainable in the surface ECG.

Concealed conduction in atrial fibrillation

The most common display of concealed conduction is seen in atrial fibrillation.[11] In this arrhythmia literally hundreds of impulses per minute are available for conduction to the ventricles. If hundreds of impulses are crowded into the space of 1 minute, it stands to reason that there can be little measurable variation in their spacing. You would then expect the AV node to conduct whenever it became nonrefractory, which would be at regular intervals. This, however, is not what happens. The ventricular response to atrial fibrillation is chaotically irregular because numerous impulses are competing for pathways in the AV junction. Some penetrate incompletely, leaving the AV junction refractory yet not producing a QRS complex (concealed conduction); others are blocked; and a few get through, resulting in (a) haphazard activation of the ventricles and (b) reduction in the number of impulses that pass the AV barrier. In fact, the more rapid the bombardment of the AV node by vagrant impulses from the fibrillating atria, the more the concealed conduction and the slower the ventricular response.

Fig. 8-2, *A*, is a regular supraventricular tachycardia at a rate of 148/min. In *B* atrial fibrillation has developed in the same patient, with the ventricular rate reduced to less than 100/min. In this patient it is evident that the AV junction is able to conduct 148/min *(A)*; yet when atrial fibrillation ensues, the AV junction can conduct only 100 beats/min because of concealed conduction.

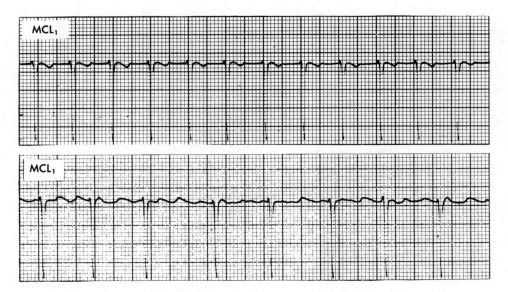

Fig. 8-2. The top strip shows a regular supraventricular tachycardia at a rate of 148/min. When atrial fibrillation develops (bottom strip), AV conduction to the ventricles is reduced to less than 100/min.

Interpolated ventricular extrasystoles with concealed retrograde conduction

Ventricular extrasystoles often conduct retrogradely all the way to the atria. In fact, Kistin and Landowne[12] showed that this happened nearly half the time. It is therefore likely that a majority of ectopic ventricular impulses are conducted at least as far as the AV junction. Such conduction is evident only if it has an effect on the next cycle; and this is most likely if the next beat is soon due, like the beat following an *interpolated* ventricular premature beat (VPB) sandwiched, as it is, between two consecutive sinus beats. If the VPB penetrates retrogradely into the AV junction, it leaves the junction refractory so that the imminent descending impulse may be delayed in its passage through the AV junction to the ventricles. Thus the PR interval of the sinus beat following the VPB is prolonged.

Fig. 8-3 graphically illustates such a case. In fact, the PR interval following the VPB is so long that it creates the impression of supraventricular prematurity in the following beat. When the ventricular rhythm is irregular, the atrial rhythm often seems to be also irregular. The laddergram indicates the regularity of the sinus rhythm and the concealed retrograde conduction from the VPB.

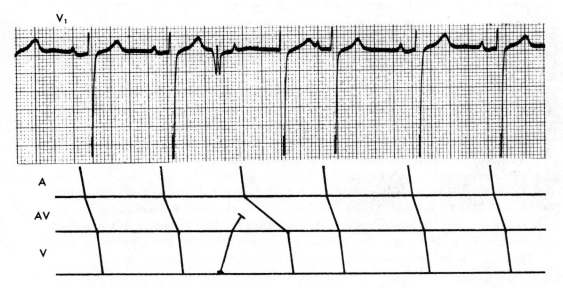

Fig. 8-3. The third beat is an interpolated ventricular extrasystole, which, thanks to retrograde concealed conduction, prolongs the next PR interval to about 0.50 second.

In Fig. 8-4 there are three interpolated VPBs, all of which are followed by concealed retrograde conduction. Note in the laddergram that the sinus P waves are right on time, a fact not immediately perceived in the tracing. The PR prolongation following each VPB varies depending upon how soon the P wave follows on the heels of the VPB. The closer it is, the longer the PR interval (a shorter RP results in a longer PR); and the later the P, the shorter the PR.

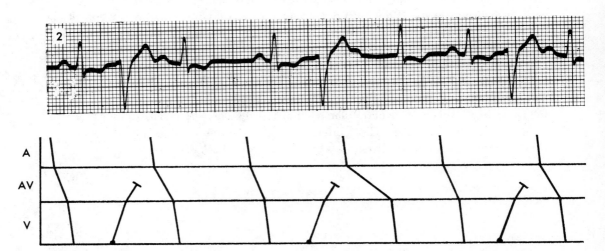

Fig. 8-4. The second, fifth, and eighth beats are interpolated ventricular extrasystoles that prolong the ensuing PR intervals by concealed retrograde conduction.

Fig. 8-5 shows the progressive effect of interpolated ventricular bigeminy on the PR interval, producing a Wenckebach-like effect. Three of the P waves in this tracing are detectable only because of the way they distort the T waves, especially since this distortion is at a time when a sinus P wave is expected (see laddergram). The first VPB is interpolated, and its retrograde concealed conduction lengthens the following PR interval. Since the sinus rhythm is regular and the VPBs are precisely coupled, the next sinus P wave falls earlier on the downslope of the ectopic T—resulting in an even longer PR interval. This sequence continues, the sinus P waves falling progressively closer to the preceding ectopic beat. Thus the fifth P wave of the series ends such a short RP interval that it is not conducted. The first three VPBs are interpolated; the fourth is not and the Wenckebach-like cycle begins again.

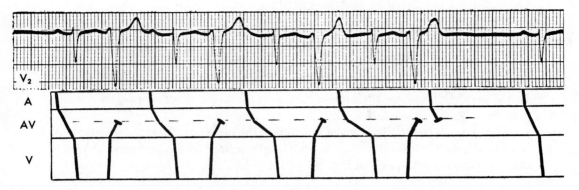

Fig. 8-5. Interpolated ventricular bigeminy produces a Wenckebach-like effect because of retrograde concealed conduction. The first VPB lengthens the next PR, which automatically "pushes" the next couplet (sinus beat + VPB) to the right, bringing the ectopic beat nearer to the next P wave (shorter RP). Thus the next retrograde conduction is closer to the next descending impulse and the PR is prolonged still further. This sequence is repeated until finally, after the fourth extrasystole, the descending impulse fails to get through.

Fig. 8-6 is another example of the same mechanism. In this case, however, because of the slower sinus rate, the P waves are quite evident and the PR lengthening is easily appreciated. The sequence consists of two VPBs that are interpolated and a third that is not. The third VPB is followed by a ventricular escape beat.

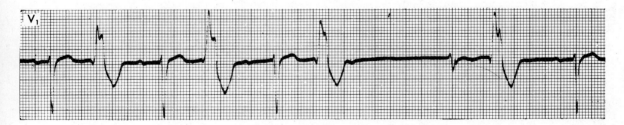

Fig. 8-6. Another example of ventricular bigeminy with concealed retrograde conduction producing progressive lengthening of the PR interval until the fourth sinus impulse fails to get through. Following the "dropped" beat the cycle ends with a ventricular escape beat.

Concealed junctional extrasystoles

Concealed junctional extrasystoles discharge the AV junction while both antero-grade and retrograde conduction is blocked. Such an event is totally silent on the surface ECG; and yet its diagnosis may be extremely important in the management of the patient, for concealed junctional beats can imitate type I (Wenckebach) and type II AV block[5,13-15] and are themselves thought to indicate significant junctional disease.[16]

Wenckebach periodicity may be imitated in the presence of concealed junctional bigeminy since the PR may progressively lengthen until a beat is dropped.[5] This is diagrammatically illustrated in Fig. 8-7.

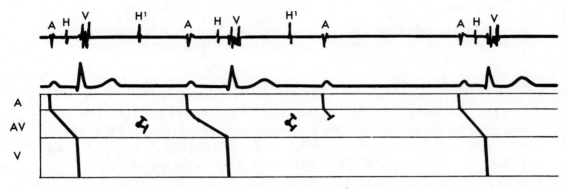

Fig. 8-7. Diagrammatic representation of how concealed junctional extrasystoles can imitate Wencke-bach conduction. The His-bundle recording, ECG, and laddergram are shown depicting concealed junctional bigeminy mimicking the Wenckebach phenomenon. Note that the first junctional extra-systole lengthens the following AH and PR intervals; the next extrasystole then prevents conduction altogether and simulates the dropped beat of a Wenckebach period. Key to His-bundle records: *A,* atrial activation; *H,* His-bundle activation; *V,* ventricular activation; *H',* junctional extrasystole.

Type II AV block may be imitated if a single concealed junctional extrasystole suddenly prevents conduction of a sinus impulse (Fig. 8-8) or if concealed penetration involves the proximal His-Purkinje system as well.[17,18] Since the development of type II AV block is a widely accepted indication for a permanent implanted pacemaker, one has a serious responsibility to rule out concealed junctional extrasystoles.

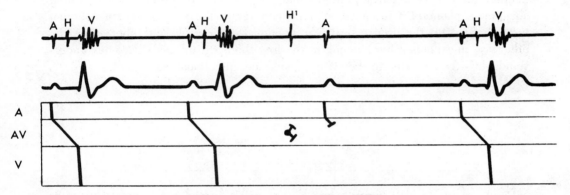

Fig. 8-8. Diagrammatic representation of how concealed junctional extrasystoles can mimic type II AV block. Without prior lengthening of the PR interval, the junctional extrasystole prevents conduction of the next sinus impulse. Key to abbreviations as in Fig. 8-7.

ECG CLUES TO CONCEALED JUNCTIONAL EXTRASYSTOLES. Although such extrasystoles can be documented only with the aid of His bundle electrograms, which may indeed be necessary if there is a question of pacing the patient, they can be strongly suspected from the following clues[19]:

1. Abrupt, unexplained lengthening of the PR interval
2. The presence of apparent types I and II AV block in the same tracing
3. Apparent type II block in the presence of a normal QRS
4. The presence of manifest junctional extrasystoles elsewhere in the tracing

In the top tracing of Fig. 8-9 there is an abrupt and unexplained lengthening of the PR interval. This lengthening is certainly not due to the Wenckebach phenomenon, since the next sinus impulse is conducted with a shorter PR interval and there are no nonconducted beats. In the bottom tracing there is the same, abrupt, unexplained lengthening of the PR interval followed by two normally conducted beats and then what looks like an interpolated VPB with concealed retrograde conduction to the atria, manifested by the long PR interval. Herein lies the clue to the abrupt unexplained PR prolongations. The laddergram illustrates their explanation: if instead of a VPB the bizarre beat is a junctional extrasystole with aberration, the otherwise unexplained lengthening of the first three PR intervals becomes understandable—they are due to the effect of concealed junctional extrasystoles.

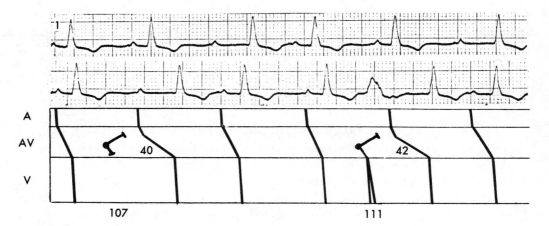

Fig. 8-9. The strips are not continuous. In the top strip the two longer PR intervals and ventricular cycles are caused by concealed junctional extrasystoles (as diagrammed under the beginning of the bottom strip). Further along in the bottom strip there is a junctional extrasystole, conducted to the ventricles with LBBB aberration, producing the same effect on the next PR interval. (Courtesy Dr. Leo Schamroth, Johannesburg.)

Concealed conduction affecting impulse formation

In the bottom tracing of Fig. 8-10 there is a sudden unexpected interruption of an accelerated junctional rhythm. The junctional rate averages 64/min and is dissociated from the slightly slower sinus rhythm. In the top tracing the junctional rhythm is interrupted when a sinus impulse (P wave in the T of the third junctional beat) is conducted to the ventricles (ventricular capture); then after two normal sinus beats the accelerated junctional rhythm takes over again. Toward the end of the bottom tracing the same thing almost occurs a second time but now the sinus impulse fails to reach the ventricles. It does, however, discharge the AV pacemaker and interrupt the junctional rhythm. Thus, concealed conduction is recognized because an expected beat fails to appear.

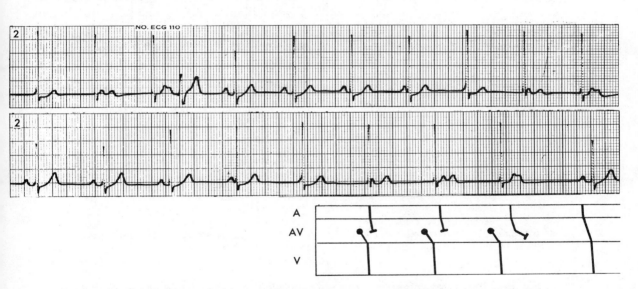

Fig. 8-10. AV dissociation between an accelerated junctional rhythm at a rate of 74/min and a slightly slower sinus rhythm. In the top strip the fourth beat is a ventricular capture conducted with aberration. At the end of the bottom strip there is another attempted capture, but the sinus impulse fails to reach the ventricle. It does, however, reach and discharge the junctional pacemaker (see laddergram).

In Fig. 8-11 another junctional rhythm has a sudden unexpected interruption. Each junctional beat is followed by a retrograde P′ wave and the RP′ interval lengthens with each beat. It is only when the RP′ interval has lengthened critically that the junctional rhythm is abruptly interrupted. The readiest explanation is illustrated in the laddergram. Delayed retrograde conduction has permitted reentry with a resulting abortive reciprocal beat. The retrograde impulse with the longest RP′ interval turns down toward the ventricles but fails to reach its destination. It does, however, succeed in discharging and thus resetting the junctional focus, leaving in its tracks an unexpected pause.

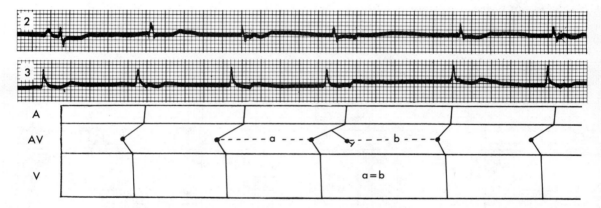

Fig. 8-11. In lead 2 the first beat is a sinus beat. Then a mildly accelerated junctional rhythm takes over at a rate of 62/min with retrograde conduction to the atria. The RP lengthens progressively (potential retrograde Wenckebach), and after the fourth beat a longer ventricular cycle develops. The same sequence is repeated twice in lead 3, where the mechanism is diagrammed. A critical degree of retrograde conduction delay enables the retrograde impulse to reenter a downward path and discharge and reset the junctional pacemaker, though it fails to reach the ventricles.

Fig. 8-12 illustrates yet another form of concealed retrograde conduction. In this tracing there is a junctional escape rhythm of 36/min resulting from an underlying sinus bradycardia and arrhythmia. Three VPBs can be seen in the two strips. In the top strip these VPBs do not disturb the basic junctional cycle length, which varies between 161 and 166. However, the VPB in the second strip postpones the junctional beat. We can infer from this that the ventricular ectopic impulse has traveled retrogradely into the AV junction, discharged the junctional pacemaker, and reset its rhythm.

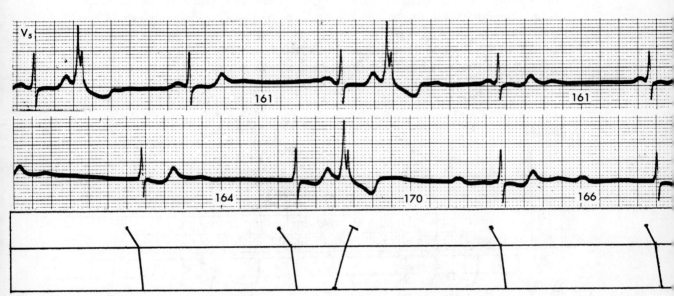

Fig. 8-12. An idiojunctional pacemaker at a rate of 36/min is dissociated from an irregular but even slower sinus rhythm. The two VPBs in the top strip do not interfere with the regularity of the junctional firing, but the one in the bottom strip does. The mechanism is diagrammed below the second strip. This VPB, by concealed retrograde conduction to the AV junction, resets the idiojunctional pacemaker.

Fig. 8-13 is an interesting example of how consecutive atrial premature beats can suggest some degree of AV block. Note in the top tracing that there is an APB in the second and fourth T waves. On each occasion it is immediately followed by a second one, which is late enough in the cycle to conduct normally to the ventricles; yet it is not conducted, suggesting AV block, and the pause ends with a junctional escape beat. Compare this to the bottom tracing from the same patient, in which on two occasions a single APB with the same coupling interval as in the top tracing is conducted. One would think that if some APBs premature enough to land on the T wave can be conducted certainly the second of each pair of APBs in the top strip, which land well beyond the T wave, could be easily conducted. The explanation for this failure of conduction is that the first of each pair of APBs in the top strip has penetrated the AV junction and left it refractory so that the second of the pair is blocked.

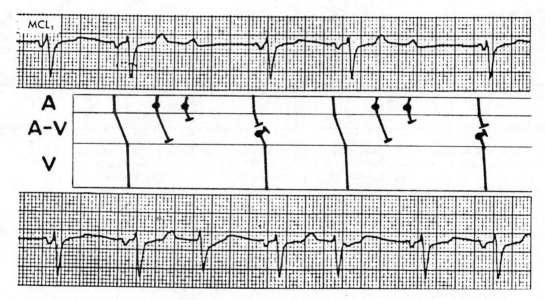

Fig. 8-13. The strips are not continuous. On two occasions in the top strip there are pairs of APBs neither of which is conducted. The first is not conducted because of refractoriness due to the preceding sinus conducted beat. The second is not conducted because of incomplete penetration of the junction by the preceding APB.

In Fig. 8-14 the same mechanism explains the failure of the second of a pair of APBs to be conducted when the first of the pair is conducted with RBBB aberration at the end of the tracing. The underlying rhythm is sinus with nonconducted atrial bigeminy.

For a more exhaustive listing of complex manifestations of concealed conduction see Chan and Pick.[19]

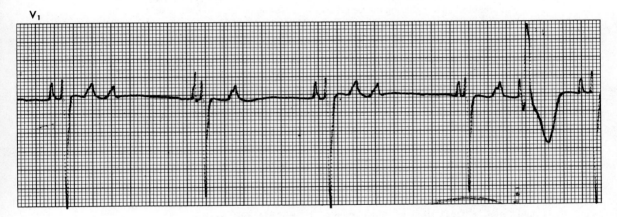

Fig. 8-14. Bigeminal nonconducted APBs. Following the first and third ventricular complexes there are two APBs in a row; the second of these is not conducted probably because of incomplete penetration into the AV junction by the preceding APB. At the end of the strip an APB is conducted with RBBB aberration. There is an artifact in the second sinus P wave.

References

1. Lewis, T., and Master, A.M.: Observations upon conduction in the mammalian heart. A-V conduction, Heart 12:209, 1925.
2. Ashman, K.: Conductivity in compressed cardiac muscle; supernormal phase in conductivity in compressed auricular muscle in the turtle heart, Am. J. Physiol. 74:140, 1925.
3. Erlanger, J.: On the physiology of heart block in mammals, with especial reference to the causation of Stokes-Adams disease, J. Exp. Med. 7:676, 1905.
4. Kaufmann, R., and Rothberger, C.J.: Der-Uebergang von Kammerallorhythmien in Kammer-Arrhythmie in klinischen Fällen von Vorhofflattern, Alternans der Reisleitung, Z. Ges. Exp. Med. 57:600, 1927.
5. Langendorf, R.: Concealed A-V conduction: the effect of blocked impulses on the formation and conduction of subsequent impulses, Am. Heart J. 35:542, 1948.
6. Sodorstrom, N.: What is the reason for the ventricular arrhythmia in cases of atrial fibrillation? Am. Heart J. 40:212, 1970.
7. Moe, G.K., Abildskov, J.A., and Mendez, C.: An experimental study of concealed conduction, Am. Heart J. 67:338, 1964.
8. Katz, L.N., and Pick, A.: Clinical electrocardiography. I. Arrhythmias, Philadelphia, 1956, Lea & Febiger.
9. Hoffman, B.F., Cranefield, P.F., and Stuckey, J.H.: Concealed conduction, Circ. Res. 9:194, 1961.
10. Lau, S.H., Damato, A.N., Berkowitz, W.D., and Patton, R.D.: A study of atrioventricular conduction in atrial fibrillation and flutter in man using His bundle recordings, Circulation 40:69, 1965.
11. Langendorf, R., and others: Ventricular response in atrial fibrillation: role of concealed conduction in the AV junction, Circulation 32:69, 1965.
12. Kistin, A.D., and Landowne, M.: Retrograde conduction from premature ventricular contractions, a common occurrence in the human heart, Circulation 3:738, 1951.
13. Langendorf, R., and Mehlman, J.S.: Blocked (non-conducted) A-V nodal premature systoles imitating first and second degree heart block, Am. Heart J. 34:500, 1947.
14. Rosen, K.M., Rahimtoola, S.H., and Gunnar, R.M.: Psuedo A-V block secondary to premature nonpropagated His bundle depolarization. Documentation by His bundle electrocardiography, Circulation 42:367, 1970.
15. Pick, A.: Mechanisms of cardiac arrhythmias: from hypothesis to physiologic fact, Am. Heart J. 86:249, 1973.
16. Narula, O.S.: His bundle electrocardiography and clinical electrophysiology, Philadelphia, 1975, F.A. Davis Co.
17. Cohen, A.C., Langendorf, R., and Pick, A.: Intermittent parasystole; mechanism of protection, Circulation 48:761, 1973.
18. Castellanos, A., and others: Pseudo AV block produced by concealed extrasystoles arising below the bifurcation of the His bundle, Br. Heart J. 36:457, 1974.
19. Chan, A.Q., and Pick, A.: Reentrant arrhythmias and concealed conduction, Am. Heart J. 97:644, 1979.

CHAPTER 9

Abnormal automaticity and triggered activity

There are two ways in which an impulse may be spontaneously initiated: (1) phase 4 automaticity or (2) triggered activity. Cells in many regions of the normal heart are capable of spontaneous impulse initiation by one or the other of these two mechanisms.

Until Mines[1] demonstrated reentry in cardiac muscle, it was widely held that all arrhythmias were caused by enhanced automaticity. In 1973 and 1974 Cranefield[2] and Cranefield and Aronson[3] described yet another arrhythmogenic mechanism: the initiation of delayed afterdepolarizations which, if they attain threshold potential, may cause rapid nondriven impulses called "triggered activity." Before Cranefield, Segers[4] and then Bozler[5] recorded afterdepolarizations in atrial fibers of normal hearts. Thus there are three known arrhythmogenic mechanisms: reentry, abnormal automaticity, and triggered activity. Reentry has been discussed in detail in the preceding chapters.

Abnormal automaticity

Automaticity is the capability of a cell to depolarize spontaneously, reach threshold, and initiate an action potential. In normal hearts only the SA node does this. Cells in other regions of the heart that possess the property of automaticity are called latent pacemakers; they are found in the distal AV node, bundle of His, bundle branches, Purkinje fibers, and some cells of the AV valves.[6-8]

Normally automaticity is not a property of working myocardial cells. However, it has been shown that if the membrane potential of these cells is reduced to −60 mV[9-11] or if the heart is diseased,[12] abnormal automaticity may develop even in working atrial and ventricular muscle in the form of slow response action potentials (p. 51).

SPONTANEOUS IMPULSE INITIATION RATE. Two things affect the intrinsic rate of spontaneous impulse initiation:

1. The rate of slow diastolic depolarization (phase 4)
2. The proximity of the maximum diastolic potential to the threshold potential

The rate of slow diastolic depolarization is primarily determined by a gradual decrease in outward potassium current, resulting in a decrease in the resting membrane potential (it becomes less and less negative) until the threshold potential is reached and an action potential is initiated (Chapter 3). The SA node dominates the heart because it reaches threshold potential faster than the latent pacemaker cells and is also under the control of the vagus nerve and sympathetic system. It thus adjusts its rate of slow diastolic depolarization to the needs of the body, at the same time exerting overdrive suppression (p. 44) on all other pacemaker cells to keep them latent. An increase in vagal activity will result in suppression of SA node automaticity, as will a decrease in sympathetic activity. Enhanced and depressed automaticity are illustrated in Fig. 9-1.

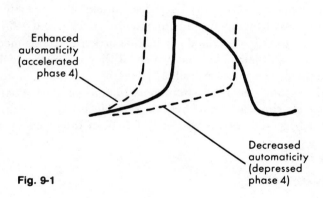

Fig. 9-1

The proximity of the maximal diastolic potential to the threshold potential is illustrated in Figs. 9-2 and 9-3. *Maximal diastolic potential* is attained after full repolarization. It is the most negative level of transmembrane potential achieved by the cell. *Threshold potential* is the transmembrane potential that must be achieved before the gates to the fast sodium channels open and an action potential can be initiated. The normal relationship of these two features to each other is illustrated in Fig. 9-2, *A*.

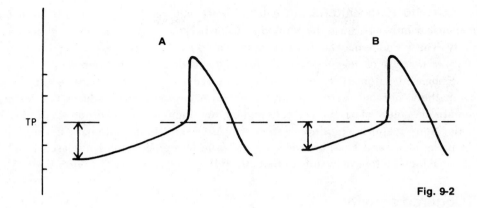

Fig. 9-2

A decrease in maximal diastolic potential, that is, a less negative resting membrane potential, causes automaticity to be enhanced because the membrane is then closer to threshold potential (Fig. 9-2, *B*) and it takes less time for threshold to be reached. This increases the rate of impulse formation.

A decrease in threshold potential, that is, a threshold potential at a more negative level, enhances automaticity for the same reason (Fig. 9-3, *B*).

An increase in threshold potential (a more positive level) depresses automaticity in that it takes longer for the membrane to depolarize to this more positive level; this decreases the rate of impulse formation.

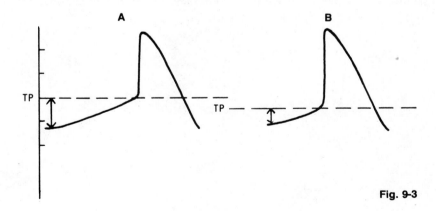

Fig. 9-3

ECTOPIC PACEMAKERS. An ectopic focus will assume the role of dominant pacemaker either because the SA node fails or because of its own enhanced automaticity. The SA node may fail because of increased vagal or decreased sympathetic activity or because of degeneration of SA node cells due to sinus disease.

Enhanced automaticity of a latent pacemaker may be secondary to increased sympathetic nervous system activity or to cardiac disease that reduces the resting membrane potential of involved cells and endows them with a faster rate than the SA node. Norepinephrine produces a steeper phase 4 slope in the automatic fibers of the SA node, atria, and His-Purkinje system. If the norepinephrine is released locally, pacemaking function may shift to that site.[13,14]

Triggered activity

The second means by which rhythmic impulses can be initiated in cardiac cells is delayed afterdepolarization. Cranefield[2] and Cranefield and Aronson[3] described a slow depolarization occurring after an action potential, which Cranefield termed "delayed afterdepolarization" (Fig. 9-4, *A*, open arrow).

This afterdepolarization is somehow dependent upon the preceding action potential. It is never self-initiated and is often preceded by an after-hyperpolarization (solid arrow in Fig. 9-4, *A*). If the afterdepolarization reaches threshold potential, it will produce a premature action potential called a triggered impulse[3,4,15] because it arises as a result of the preceding beat. It is thus distinguished from automatic activity, which needs no preceding event for its initiation.

A triggered impulse may itself be followed by a series of afterdepolarizations and action potentials (Fig. 9-4, *B*), each being generated by the preceding one,[16] to produce a run of accelerated rhythm or tachycardia.

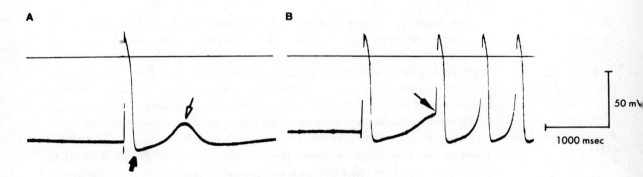

Fig. 9-4. A, Driven action potential followed by a delayed hyperpolarization (solid arrow) and a delayed afterdepolarization (open arrow). **B,** A driven action potential followed by a delayed afterdepolarization that reaches threshold and a nondriven action potential (arrow) that arises from the peak of the afterdepolarization. (From Wit, A.L., Boyden, P.A., Gadsby, D.C., and Cranefield, P.F.: In Narula, O.S., editor: Cardiac arrhythmias: electrophysiology, diagnosis, and management, Baltimore, 1979, The Williams & Wilkins Co.)

CONDITIONS INCREASING THE AMPLITUDE OF AFTERDEPOLARIZATIONS.
Afterdepolarizations can be present without producing an action potential, since an action potential is produced only when threshold is reached. Some conditions that may increase the amplitude of the afterdepolarization so that it may reach threshold are

1. *An increase in the drive rate of the fiber*[2,3]: Even if only a single cycle shortens, as with an atrial or ventricular premature beat, there will be an increase in the amplitude of the afterdepolarization. If this increase reaches threshold, it will initiate triggered activity,[17] which perpetuates itself, in that the short coupling interval of the VPB causes a still greater increase in amplitude of the next afterdepolarization.[16]

2. *Catecholamines:* Norepinephrine has been found to increase the amplitude of the afterdepolarization in the fibers of the coronary sinus, mitral valve, and diseased atrial tissue.[18-20] Low concentrations of catecholamines still permit triggering as long as there is an increase in the drive rate. Conversely, in the presence of low drive rates, triggering is still possible if the level of catecholamines is high.[9] As one might expect, acetylcholine lowers the amplitude of the afterdepolarization, decreases the rate, and often stops triggered activity.[19]

3. *Digitalis:* In vitro digitalis causes the action potentials of Purkinje fibers to develop delayed afterdepolarizations; the amplitude of these is enhanced when the fiber is driven more rapidly.[21-24]

DELAYED AFTERDEPOLARIZATIONS AS A CAUSE OF ARRHYTHMIAS. No one has yet established that triggered activity resulting from delayed afterdepolarizations is arrhythmogenic in the living human heart. However, it is postulated that APBs or simply an increase in the atrial rate may initiate triggered activity in the atria and that such arrhythmias will be electrocardiographically indistinguishable from those caused by reentry.[16]

Cranefield[17] has suggested that the exactly coupled extrasystoles often seen secondary to digitalis toxicity may be the result of delayed afterdepolarization, since digitalis has been shown in vitro to produce afterdepolarizations and to enhance their amplitude by increasing the driving rate of the fiber.

MECHANISM OF AFTERDEPOLARIZATIONS. The electrophysiologic mechanism causing afterdepolarizations and the enhancement of their amplitude is not known. However, it is known that drugs which impair current flow through the slow Na^+/Ca^{++} channel will also reduce the amplitude of afterdepolarizations and prevent the appearance of triggered activity.[17-19]

References

1. Mines, G.R.: On circulating excitations in heart muscles and their possible relation to tachycardia and fibrillation, Trans. R. Soc. Can., ser 3, sec. 4, **8:**43, 1914.
2. Cranefield, P.F.: Ventricular fibrillation, N. Engl. J. Med. **289:**732, 1973.
3. Cranefield, P.F., and Aronson, R.S.: Initiation of sustained rhythmic activity by single propagated action potentials in canine Purkinje fibers exposed to sodium-free solution or to ouabain, Circ. Res. **34:**477, 1974.
4. Segers, M.: Le rôle des potentiels tardifs du coeur, Mem. Acad. R. Med. Beig. Ser. II **1:**1, 1941.
5. Bozler, E.: The initiation of impulses in cardiac muscle, Am. J. Physiol. **138:**273, 1943.
6. Wit, A.L., Fenoglio, J.J., Wagner, B.M., and Bassett, A.L.: Electrophysiological properties of cardiac muscle in the anterior mitral valve leaflet and the adjacent atrium in the dog. Possible implications for the genesis of atrial dysrhythmias, Circ. Res. **32:**731, 1973.
7. Bassett, A.L., Wit, A.L., and others: Ectopic impulses originating in the tricuspid valve and contiguous atrium, Fed. Proc. **33:**445, 1974.
8. Fenoglio, J., Jr., and others: Canine mitral complex; ultrastructural and electromechanical properties, Circ. Res. **31:**417, 1972.
9. Katzung, B.: Effects of extracellular calcium and sodium on depolarization-induced automaticity in ginea pig papillary muscle, Circ. Res. **37:**118, 1975.
10. Brown, H.F., and Noble, S.J.: Membrane currents underlying delayed rectification and pacemaker activity in frog atrial muscle, J. Physiol. (Lond.) **204:**717, 1969.
11. Imanishi, S., and Surawicz, B.: Automatic activity in depolarized guinea pig ventricular myocardium: characteristics and mechanisms, Circ. Res. **39:**751, 1976.
12. Gadsby, D.C., and Wit, A.L.: Normal and abnormal electrophysiology of cardiac cells. In Mandel, W.J., editor: Cardiac arrhythmias: their mechanisms, diagnosis, and management, Philadelphia, 1980, J.B. Lippincott Co.
13. Armour, J.A., Hageman, G.R., and Randall, W.C.: Arrhythmias induced by local cardiac nerve stimulation, Am. J. Physiol. **223:**1068, 1972.
14. Geesbreght, J.M., and Randall, W.C.: Area localization of shifting cardiac pacemakers during sympathetic stimulation, Am. J. Physiol. **220:**1522, 1971.
15. Cranefield, P.F.: The conduction of the cardiac impulse: the slow response and cardiac arrhythmias, Mount Kisco, N.Y., 1975, Futura Publishing Co.
16. Wit, A.L., Boyden, P.A., Gadsby, D.C., and Cranefield, P.F.: Triggered activity as a cause of atrial arrhythmias. In Narula, O.S., editor: Cardiac arrhythmias: electrophysiology, diagnosis, and management, Baltimore, 1979, The Williams & Wilkins Co.
17. Cranefield, P.F.: Action potentials, afterpotentials, and arrhythmias, Circ. Res. **41:**415, 1977.
18. Wit, A.L., and Cranefield, P.F.: Triggered activity in cardiac muscle fibers of the simian mitral valve, Circ. Res. **38:**85, 1976.
19. Wit, A.L., and Cranefield, P.F.: Triggered and automatic activity in the canine coronary sinus, Circ. Res. **41:**435, 1977.
20. Boyden, P.A., Tilley, L.P., Lie, S., and Wit, A.L.: Effects of atrial dilatation on atrial cellular electrophysiology: studies on cats with spontaneous cardiomyopathy [Abstract], Circulation **56** (suppl. III): 48, 1977.

CHAPTER 10

Supernormality

Supernormal excitability was first described in 1912 for nerve[1] and in 1938 for heart muscle.[2] With the advent of the microelectrode, supernormal excitability was first demonstrated in 1953[3] in isolated Purkinje fibers from sheep and calves. Since that time intracellular stimulation methods have demonstrated supernormal excitability in the bundle branch–Purkinje system[4] and in Bachmann's bundle[5] but not in the AV node,[6] bundle of His,[4] or working myocardium.[5]

The supernormal period

The supernormal period occurs at the end of phase 3. It is that period during which a stimulus of less than the normally required intensity can initiate a propagatable action potential.

Supernormal excitability is diagnosed when the myocardium responds to a stimulus that is ineffective when applied earlier or later in the cycle. During the supernormal period the cell has recovered enough to respond to a stimulus; and since the membrane potential is still reduced, it requires only a little additional depolarization to bring the fiber to threshold. Thus a smaller stimulus than is normally required elicits an action potential during the supernormal phase of excitability.

The shaded areas in Fig. 10-1 illustrate the supernormal period and its relationship to the total refractory period. There is a point within this time that the current requirement for excitation is at its minimum. This is indicated by x within the shaded areas. Spear and Moore[7] have found that the duration of the supernormal phase remains the same in spite of changes in the action potential duration. Thus, as the action potential shortens, the supernormal period occupies more of it.

Fig. 10-2 is an example of supernormal excitability. In this tracing a failing pacemaker is ineffective except when the pacing stimulus lands between the nadir and the end of the T wave.

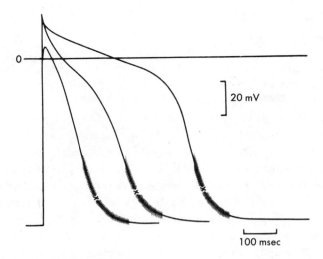

Fig. 10-1. Relationship between the supernormal period and the total refractory period. (X indicates moment of maximal supernormality.) Above are shown superimposed action potentials. The longest-duration action potential was evoked at a basic cycle length of 800 milliseconds. The shorter action potentials were successively evoked premature beats at cycle lengths of 460 and 251 milliseconds. The shaded areas delineate the boundaries of the period of supernormal excitability. The Xs within the shaded area indicate the point of minimum current requirements. (From Spear, J.F., and Moore E.N.: Circulation **50:**1144, 1974. By permission of the American Heart Association, Inc.)

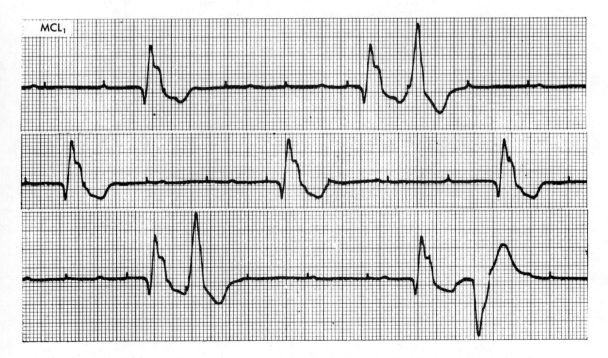

Fig. 10-2. The strips are continuous. Complete AV block with very slow left idioventricular rhythm. The implanted pacemaker is ineffective except on two occasions when the stimulus lands in the "supernormal" phase of excitability—toward the end of the T wave.

Supernormal conduction

Supernormal conduction is not better than normal, only better than expected. Conduction is better earlier in the cycle than later and occurs when block is expected.

Spear and Moore[7] have demonstrated the relationship between supernormal excitability and supernormal conduction; the mechanism is as follows: A conduction wave relies for its propagation on local currents flowing across the membranes just in front of the propagating action potential. If the downstream cells can be brought to threshold faster because of reduced current requirement for excitation during late repolarization, then conduction velocity is improved over that expected at a later time in diastole, when current requirements to reach threshold are greater.

Supernormal conduction can be seen in Fig. 10-3. Most of the sinus impulses are conducted with RBBB. However, there are two early beats that are conducted normally, suggesting supernormal conduction in the RBB. This is also an example of critical rate RBBB, since the sinus impulses following the APB end a longer cycle (overdrive suppression) and are conducted normally.

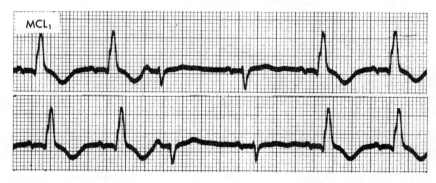

Fig. 10-3. The strips are not continuous. Supernormal conduction in the RBB. The third beats in the two tracings are APBs with normal conduction in the face of an underlying RBBB with much longer cycles.

Concealed supernormal conduction

In Fig. 10-4 there are two instances of manifest supernormal conduction (fifth beat in each tracing) and two instances of concealed supernormal conduction (after the first beat in each tracing). Supernormal conduction is evident just beyond the middle of each strip. The sinus P waves deforming the ST segment in the top strip and the T wave in the bottom represent impulses that are conducted whereas later sinus impulses, with an expected better chance of conduction, are blocked.

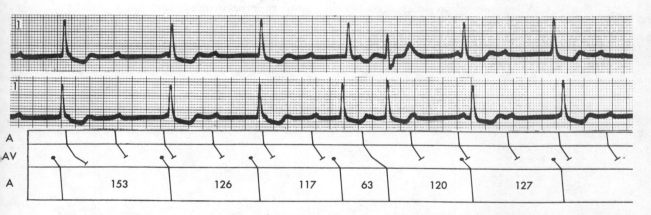

Fig. 10-4. The strips show a significant degree of AV block with a junctional escape rhythm at a rate of 48/min. The first cycle in each strip is longer than the other cycles because the atrial impulse immediately following the first QRS is conducted into the AV junction and resets the junctional pacemaker (see laddergram). The fifth beat in each strip is conducted from the somewhat later atrial impulses deforming the ST segment or T wave of the preceding beat. Since these atrial impulses are much earlier in the cycle than many that are not conducted at all, they may be considered examples of supernormal conduction; and since the impulses after the first QRS do not reach the ventricles and their conduction is only inferred, they are examples of concealed supernormal conduction.

Concealed supernormal conduction is not quite so easy to recognize. Apart from the two instances of capture due to manifest supernormal conduction, notice the irregularity of the junctional escape rhythm in the face of a significant degree of AV block. The following principle often facilitates a diagnosis: When an independent rhythm (in this case junctional) manifests two cycle lengths, subtract the shorter from the longer, *starting from the end of the long cycle*. At that point look for possible clues which may explain what has lengthened this cycle beyond its shorter fellows. Applying this principle to the tracing at hand, note that just preceding the spot to which you have measured in the longer cycle there is a sinus P wave. Clearly this is causally related to the lengthened cycle and implies penetration of that sinus impulse into the AV junction, thus discharging and resetting the junctional pacemaker. The postponement of the next expected junctional beat earmarks this as concealed conduction.

Mimics of supernormal conduction

When conduction is better earlier than later, supernormality is certainly a possibility. However, other mechanisms[8-10] should also be considered, some of which are listed below. Keep in mind that you may not always be able to prove your point conclusively.

1. Concealed junctional extrasystoles
2. Phase 4 (paradoxical critical rate)
3. Reentry with ventricular echo
4. The gap phenomenon

CONCEALED JUNCTIONAL EXTRASYSTOLES. In Fig. 10-5 the underlying sinus rhythm is regular at 68/min. Note that each time there is a shorter RP interval it is complemented by a shorter PR interval, suggesting supernormal conduction of these alternate beats. A much more likely explanation, postulated by Langendorf[11] in 1948, is that the longer PRs are the result of concealed junctional extrasystoles, as illustrated in the laddergram.

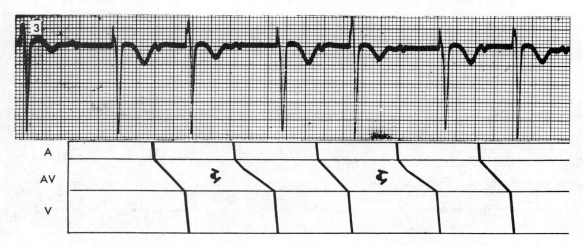

Fig. 10-5. Concealed junctional extrasystoles mimicking supernormal conduction.

PHASE 4 (PARADOXICAL CRITICAL RATE).[12-15] Enhanced phase 4 depolarization within the bundle branch system may result in BBB (phase 4 block, p. 164). In such a case the maximum diastolic potential immediately follows repolarization, from which point the membrane potential is steadily reduced. Thus an action potential initiated early in the cycle (immediately following repolarization) would have a steeper and higher phase 0 and consequently better conduction than would an action potential initiated later in the cycle.

In Fig. 10-6 the underlying rhythm is a sinus bradycardia at 50/min with a faster junctional escape rate of 56/min producing AV dissociation. If the fibers of the RBB have enhanced automaticity, late-arriving impulses due to the bradycardia find a reduced membrane potential and conduction is blocked. Since diastolic depolarization begins immediately after repolarization, the membrane potential is maximum early in the cycle; in fact, the earlier the better. Note that all the beats except two early ones are conducted with RBBB. When ventricular capture occurs (fifth beat), there is much less evidence of BBB, suggesting that conduction occurred either before the membrane potential could be reduced or because the impulse arrived during the phase of supernormal excitability in the RBB.

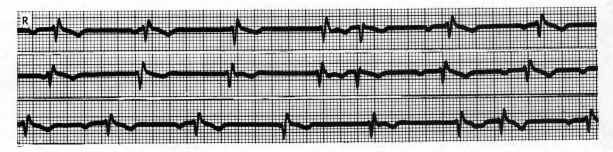

Fig. 10-6. The strips are continuous. A junctional rhythm with RBBB aberration is dissociated from a slightly slower sinus rhythm. The three early beats are ventricular captures; and the first two are conducted with much less evidence of RBBB, suggesting conduction during the "supernormal" phase of the RBB or conduction prior to reduction of the membrane potential.

CONCEALED REENTRY. Fig. 10-7 is another example of simulated supernormal conduction. A shorter PR interval (fourth beat) unexpectedly interrupts what starts out to be a Wenckebach sequence. Since the P wave of this impulse is close to the preceding T wave, one might suspect supernormal conduction. A more likely explanation is that after the lengthened PR interval of the third beat there is reentry with retrograde conduction (see laddergram). The descent of the next atrial impulse thwarts this attempt at an atrial echo. However, further (anterograde) reentry produces a ventricular echo as the impulse returns to the ventricles, making it appear that the atrial impulse was conducted during a period of supernormality.

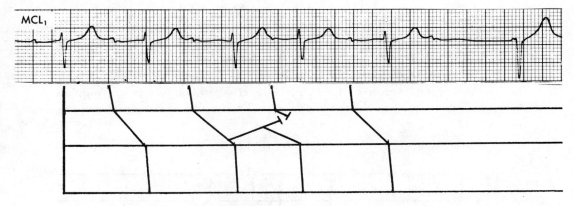

Fig. 10-7. Concealed reentry as a mimic of supernormal conduction.

THE GAP PHENOMENON. The gap phenomenon was originally described by Moe and his associates[16] in 1965 as a zone in which premature atrial stimuli encountered AV block whereas if the stimulus were earlier or later AV conduction was accomplished. Since that time as many as six types of gaps have been described for anterograde conduction.[17]

The more commonly encountered gaps, thought to be functional in nature, are dependent upon a difference in refractoriness between the cells at two different levels in the AV conduction system so that a premature atrial beat is blocked in the His-Purkinje system but not in the AV node. This is because the shortest time between two atrial impulses needed for the AV node to conduct (functional refractory period) is less than the effective refractory period of the His-Purkinje system.

Fig. 10-8 diagrammatically illustrates the mechanism of the gap phenomenon. In A a premature atrial beat is not conducted to the ventricles because the impulse traverses the AV node rapidly enough to arrive while the His-Purkinje system is still in its effective refractory period. In B, with a shorter coupling interval the impulse travels more slowly through the AV node, which is in its relative refractory period. By the time this impulse traverses the AV node the His-Purkinje system has completed its effective refractory period and conduction is possible. Ventricular activation results.

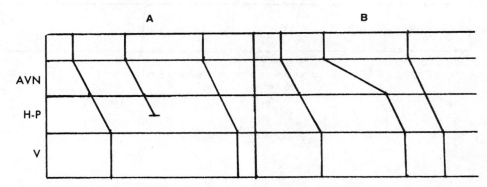

Fig. 10-8. Diagrammatic representation of the mechanism of the gap phenomenon. The initial block is in the His-Purkinje system (**A**). The required conduction delay is in the AV node (**B**).

Fig. 10-9 diagrammatically illustrates another level for the gap phenomenon, in which the effective refractory period of the His-Purkinje system exceeds both the functional and the effective refractory period of the AV node. This means that the His-Purkinje system and not the AV node is the site of conduction delay. In *A* a premature atrial beat is blocked within the His-Purkinje system. In *B*, at a shorter coupling interval, a premature atrial beat is delayed in the proximal His-Purkinje system, probably the bundle branches,[15] giving the distal portion time to recover. Ventricular activation results.

From these two examples you can see that the gap phenomenon depends on conduction delay in fibers activated during their relative refractory period when conduction velocity is slower than it would have been if activation had occurred later in the cycle. Other types of gap phenomenon are described in which the required conduction delay is in the bundle of His,[18] proximal AV node,[17] or the atria.[18]

The gap phenomenon has also been described in a retrograde direction[19]; and, in fact, this is thought to occur more frequently than during anterograde conduction. The site of retrograde block is the AV node or upper reaches of the His-Purkinje system whereas the gap-produced retrograde delay in conduction is lower in the His-Purkinje system.

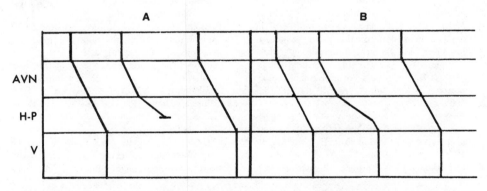

Fig. 10-9. Diagrammatic representation of the mechanism of another type of gap phenomenon. The initial block is low in the His-Purkinje system (**A**). The required conduction delay is in the bundle branches (**B**).

References

1. Adrian, E.D., and Lucas, K.: On the summation of propagated disturbances in nerve and muscle, J. Physiol. **44**:68, 1912.
2. Cranefield, P.E., Hoffman, B.E., and Siebens, A.A.: Anodal excitation of cardiac muscle, Am. J. Physiol. **190**:383, 1957.
3. Weidmann, S.: Effects of calcium ions and local anesthetics on electrical properties of Purkinje fibers, J. Physiol. **129**:568, 1955.
4. Spear, J.F., and Moore, E.N.: The effect of changes in rate and rhythm on supernormal excitability in the isolated Purkinje system of the dog. A possible role in re-entrant arrhythmias, Circulation **50**:1144, 1974.
5. Childers, R.W., Merideth, J., and Moe, G.J.: Supernormality in Bachmann's bundle: an in vivo and in vitro study, Circ. Res. **22**:363, 1968.
6. Puech, P., Guimond, C., and ohers: Supernormal conduction in the intact heart. In Narula, O.S., editor: Cardiac arrhythmias: electrophysiology, diagnosis, and management, Baltimore, 1979, The Williams & Wilkins Co.
7. Spear, J.F., and Moore, E.N.: Supernormal excitability and conduction. In Wellens, H.J.J., Lie, K.I., Janse, M.J., editors: The conduction system of the heart: structure, function, and clinical implications, Philadelphia, 1976, Lea & Febiger.
8. Moe, G.K., and others: An appraisal of "supernormal" A-V conduction, Circulation **38**:5, 1968.
9. Damato, A.N., and others: Observations on the mechanism of one type of so-called supernormal A-V conduction, Am. Heart J. **82**:725, 1971.
10. Gallagher, J.J., and others: Alternative mechanisms of apparent supernormal atrioventricular conduction, Am. J. Cardiol. **31**:362, 1973.
11. Langendorf, R.: Concealed A-V conduction: the effect of blocked impulses on the formation and conduction of subsequent impulses, Am. Heart J. **35**:542, 1948.
12. Singer, D.H., Lazzara, R., and Hoffman, B.F.: Interrelationships between automaticity and conduction in Purkinje fibers, Circ. Res. **21**:537, 1967.
13. Rosenbaum, M.B., Elizari, M.V., Lazzari, J.O., and others: The mechanisms of intermittent bundle branch block: relationship to prolonged recovery, hypopolarization, and spontaneous diastolic depolarization, Chest **63**: 666, 1973.
14. Pick, A., and Fishman, A.P.: Observations in heart block. Supernormality of A-V and intraventricular conduction and ventricular parasystole under the influence of epinephrine, Acta Cardiol. **5**:270, 1950.
15. Hoffman, B.F.: Physiology of A-V transmission, Circulation **24**:506, 1961.
16. Moe, G.K., Mendez, C., and Han, J.: Aberrant A-V impulse propagation in the dog heart. A study of functional bundle branch block, Circ. Res. **16**:261, 1965.
17. Damato, A.N., Akhtar, M., and others: Gap phenomena: antegrade and retrograde. In Wellens, H.J.J., Lie, K.I., Janse, M.J., editors: The conduction system of the heart: structure, function, and clinical implications, Philadelphia, 1976, Lea & Febiger.
18. Wu, D., Denes, P., Dhingra, R., and Rosen, K.: Nature of gap phenomenon in man, Circ. Res. **34**:682, 1974.
19. Akhtar, M., Damato, A.N., and others: The gap phenomenon during retrograde conduction in man, Circulation **49**:811, 1974.

CHAPTER 11

Phase 3 and phase 4 block

Determinants of conduction velocity reviewed

Conduction velocity depends upon, among other things, the rate of rise of phase 0 of the action potential (dV/dt) and the height to which it rises (V_{max}), which are in turn voltage dependent; that is, the more negative the membrane potential at the time of stimulation, the greater will be the amplitude and the faster the rise of phase 0 and the greater will be the conduction velocity. The resting membrane potential, in its turn, is dependent upon the concentration gradient of potassium, which we discussed in detail in Chapter 3.

Fig. 11-1 illustrates that, if a stimulus occurs either during phase 3 or during phase 4 of the action potential, the membrane potential at the time of stimulation is reduced and conduction is compromised; hence the term "phase 3" and "phase 4" block.

In Fig. 11-1, *A*, the ECG shows an APB conducted with aberration. The action potential of the RBB is shown above the ECG tracing and indicates that aberration occurs because the stimulus reaches the RBB during phase 3 when the membrane potential is only −65 mV. At this time only about half of the fast sodium channels are available for activation. The resulting action potential is a slow channel response and conduction fails.

In Fig. 11-1, *B*, the ECG shows a bradycardia with RBBB. The action potential of the RBB indicates enhanced automaticity so that by the time the impulse arrives in the RBB the membrane potential has been reduced. The resulting action potential is a slow channel response and conduction fails.

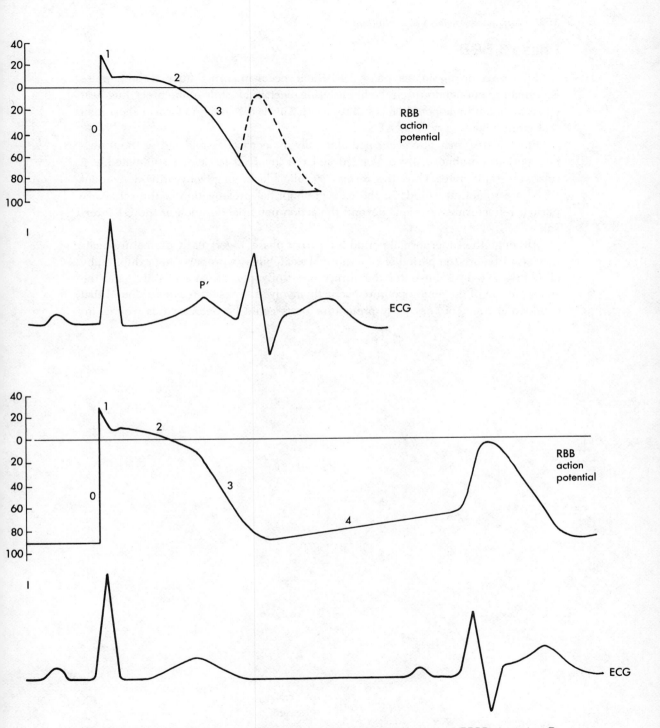

Fig. 11-1. Phase 3 and phase 4 block. **A,** An APB is conducted with phase 3 RBBB aberration. **B,** Phase 4 RBBB.

Phase 3 BBB

Functional or physiologic phase 3 BBB may occur in normal fibers if the impulse is premature enough to reach the fiber during electrical systole of the preceding beat when the membrane potential is still reduced. This is the common form of aberration that often follows very early APBs.

Phase 3 BBB may also occur pathologically if electrical systole and/or the refractory period are abnormally prolonged and the involved fascicle is stimulated at a relatively rapid rate. Thus the terms "systolic block" or "tachycardia-dependent BBB" are sometimes used. In the case of abnormal prolongation of the refractory period, refractoriness extends beyond the action potential duration or the QT interval.

Although the supernormal period is a part of phase 3, very early premature beats may occur before the period of supernormal excitability, a property not exhibited by all fibers. Fig. 11-2 illustrates the abrupt onset of supernormal excitability and the small portion of the action potential actually involved. Spear and Moore[1] found that conduction times of very early premature beats could be decreased as well as increased.

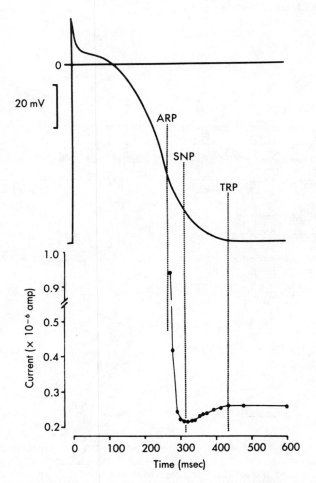

Fig. 11-2. Excitability determination in a canine Purkinje fiber. The excitability curve is displayed beneath the action potential and represents the minimum depolarizing current necessary to evoke a · response at the time indicated. *TRP,* Total refractory period; *ARP,* absolute refractory period; *SNP,* minimum current requirements to excite the fiber during the supernormal period. (From Spear, J.F., and Moore, N.: In Wellens, H.J.J., Lie, K.I., and Janse, M.J., editors: The conduction system of the heart, Hingham, Mass., 1976, Martinus Nijhoff, Publishers.)

Fig. 11-3 illustrates examples of right bundle-branch block aberration due to phase 3 block, following an APB. In such cases it is often difficult or impossible to make the distinction between a physiologic phase 3 BBB and a pathologic one involving lengthening of the refractory period.

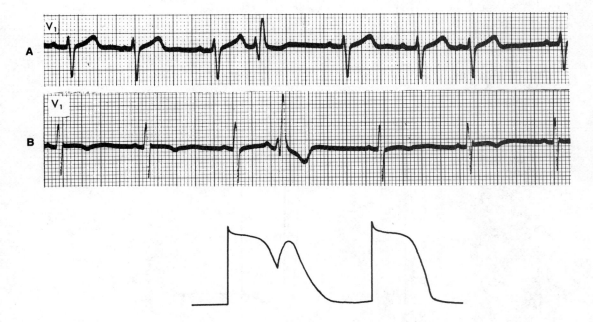

Fig. 11-3. Phase 3 BBB. In both **A** and **B,** after three normally conducted beats, an atrial extrasystole arises and its impulse arrives at the RBB, which is still refractory; it is therefore conducted with RBBB aberration. In **A** the second and seventh beats are also extrasystoles, but they are less premature and are therefore conducted normally. The action potentials illustrate the mechanism.

Fig. 11-4 gives two more examples of phase 3 BBB. In *A* there is RBBB, and in *B*, LBBB. Both develop in response to a gradual shortening of the cycle length until it becomes shorter than the refractory period of one of the bundle branches, whereupon aberrant conduction develops and persists until the cycle lengthens enough for normal conduction to recur. The BBBs seen in these two tracings are secondary to a pathologic prolongation of the action potential and/or refractory period in the respective bundle branches.

Rate-dependent BBB is the term used when such a block comes and goes with changes in heart rate.

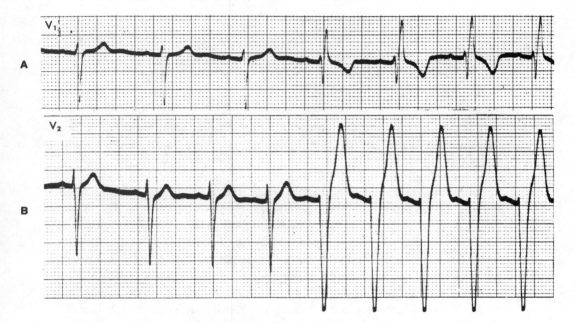

Fig. 11-4. Phase 3 BBB. **A,** From a 19-year-old student nurse. As her sinus rate accelerates and the cycle shortens in response to gentle exercise, progressively increasing degrees of RBBB develop ("critical-rate" or "rate-dependent" RBBB). **B,** From a 64-year-old man with severe coronary disease. As his sinus rate accelerates, the cycles shorten; LBBB develops at a critical rate of just over 100/min.

Critical rate is the term given to the rate at which the bundle-branch block develops during acceleration or disappears on slowing. It is of interest that rate-dependent BBB develops at a faster critical rate than at which it disappears. Note in Fig. 11-5 that although rate-dependent BBB develops when the rate reaches 66/min (cycle = 91) normal conduction is not restored until the rate falls to 56/min (cycle = 108).

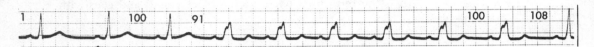

Fig. 11-5. Rate-dependent LBBB. As the sinus rhythm accelerates, LBBB develops when the rate exceeds 60/min (cycle length <100); but for normal conduction to resume, the rate must fall below 60/min (cycle length >100).

There are two reasons for this phenomenon:
1. As the heart rate accelerates, the refractory period shortens; because of this, normal conduction tends to be preserved. Conversely, as the heart rate slows, the refractory period lengthens. It is thus necessary for the heart rate to slow down more than one would expect in order to reestablish normal intraventricular conduction.
2. Perhaps more important is the fact that once BBB is established the depressed BB will be activated late transseptally via the still conducting BB; it will therefore recover later than the conducting BB. The operative sequence is illustrated in Fig. 11-6. It is obvious then that once BBB is established the actual cycle for the blocked branch does not begin until about halfway through the QRS complex. For example, in the case of the rate-dependent LBBB (Fig. 11-5) it takes approximately 0.06 second for the impulse to negotiate the unaffected right bundle and the septum and reach the depressed left branch. Therefore the left branch actually *begins* its cycle 0.06 second after the right branch. It follows that for normal conduction to resume, the cycle during deceleration—as measured from the *beginning* of one QRS to the beginning of the next QRS—must be longer than the "critical" cycle during acceleration by at least 0.06 second.

Two more examples of phase 3 BBB can be seen in Fig. 11-7. This time the fact that the BBB is rate dependent is revealed only because of the pause following VPBs in *A* and a nonconducted APB in *B*. In each case the complex ending the pause achieves normal intraventricular conduction.

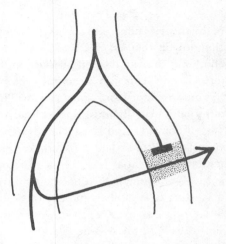

Fig. 11-6. Diagram to illustrate one of the two mechanisms responsible for the fact that the "critical rate" is different (faster) during acceleration from what it is during deceleration (see text).

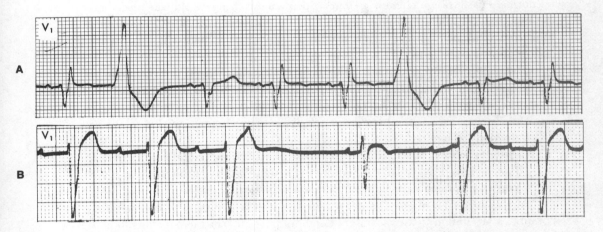

Fig. 11-7. Examples of postextrasystolic revelation of rate-dependent BBB. **A,** After each of the ventricular extrasystoles, the returning sinus beat manifests a lesser degree of RBBB than do the sinus beats ending the normal (shorter) sinus cycles. **B,** After three sinus beats conducted with first-degree AV block and LBBB, a nonconducted atrial extrasystole results in a prolonged ventricular cycle, at the end of which the returning sinus beat is conducted with normal PR and normal intraventricular conduction, demonstrating that both the AV delay and the LBBB are rate dependent.

Phase 4 BBB

Phase 4 block is one of the theories offered to explain the development of abnormal intraventricular conduction only at the end of a lengthened cycle. Since one would expect conduction to be better at the end of a longer diastole, this form of aberration is known as paradoxical critical rate. It is also sometimes referred to as bradycardia-dependent BBB; but this is unsatisfactory as an inclusive term because it is not always necessary to achieve a rate that merits the designation bradycardia.

Phase 4 block occurs late in diastole and is associated with the cyclical reduction in resting membrane potential typical of latent pacemaker cells. If these cells are activated when their membrane potential is so reduced, conduction disturbances may result like those that develop when activation occurs during phase 3.[2-4]

One would expect to see this type of aberration in the setting of bradycardia or enhanced automaticity of latent pacemaker cells. However, in spite of the fact that bradycardia is common and cells with phase 4 depolarization are abundant, phase 4 block is not frequently seen and most reported cases are associated with organic heart disease. Singer and Cohen[4] offer this explanation: In normal fibers conduction is well maintained at membrane potentials above −70 to −75 mV. Significant conduction disturbances are first manifested when the membrane is below −70 mV at the time of stimulation, and local block appears at −65 to −60 mV. Since the threshold potential for normal His-Purkinje fibers is −70 mV, spontaneous firing would take place before the membrane could actually be reduced to the potential necessary for conduction impairment or block. Therefore phase 4 block is always pathologic when it does occur and requires one or more of the following:

1. The presence of slow diastolic depolarization, which need not be enhanced.
2. A decrease in excitability (shift in threshold potential toward zero) so that, in the presence of significant bradycardia, enough time elapses before the arrival of the impulse for the bundle-branch fibers to reach a potential at which conduction is impaired.
3. A deterioration in membrane responsiveness so that significant conduction impairment develops at −75 instead of −65 mV. This would also negate the necessity for such a long cycle before conduction falters.

Membrane responsiveness is determined by the relationship of the membrane potential at excitation to the maximum height of phase 0. Thus hypopolarization (the loss of maximal diastolic potential) is an important factor in phase 4 block, since it itself causes both a decrease in excitability and enhanced automaticity.[5]

Two examples of phase 4 BBB can be seen in Fig. 11-8. In *A* the longer sinus cycles end with LBBB; in *B* the lengthened postextrasystolic cycles end with RBBB conduction.

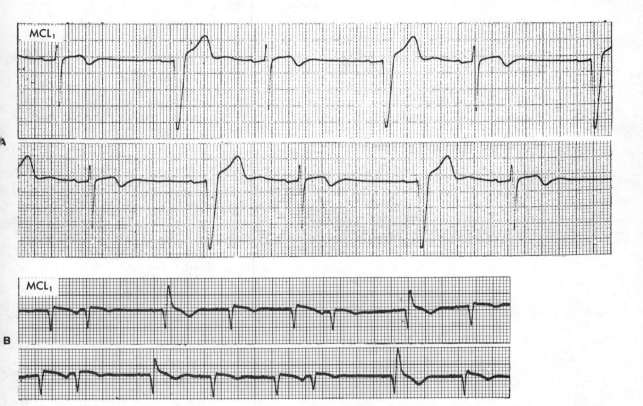

Fig. 11-8. Paradoxical critical rate. **A,** All the longer cycles (range, 138 to 142) end with LBBB whereas the shorter cycles (range, 107 to 110) end with improved, virtually normal, intraventricular conduction. The alternately longer and shorter sinus cycles are presumably due to a 3:2 sinus Wenckebach. **B,** The sinus rhythm is repeatedly interrupted by atrial extrasystoles. The conducted beats ending the lengthened postextrasystolic cycles all show RBBB, whereas the shorter sinus cycles and the even shorter extrasystolic cycles show more normal intraventricular conduction.

Phase 3 and phase 4 AV block

Phase 3 and phase 4 block may also be the cause of intermittent AV block whenever the necessary conditions exist in the only available AV connection. For example, in a patient with complete LBBB and hypopolarization of the right bundle, complete heart block could conceivably be precipitated by a critical slow rate (phase 4 block). On the other hand, if this same patient had an abnormal lengthening of the refractory period in the right bundle, complete heart block could result from a critical increase in heart rate (phase 3 block).

References

1. Spear, J.F., and Moore, E.N.: Supernormal excitability and conduction. In Wellens, H.J.J., Lie, K.I., and Janse, M.J., editors: The conduction system of the heart; structure, function, and clinical implications, Philadelphia, 1976, Lea & Febiger.
2. Singer, D.H., Lazzara, R., and Hoffman, B.F.: Interrelationships between automaticilty and conduction in Purkinje fibers, Circ. Res. **21:** 537, 1967.
3. Singer, D.H., Yeh, B.K., and Hoffman, B.F.: Aberration of supraventricular escape beats [Abstract], Fed. Proc. **23:**158, 1967.
4. Singer, D.H., and Cohen, H.C.: Aberrancy: electrophysiologic aspects and clinical correlations. In Mandel, W.J., editor: Cardiac arrhythmias, Philadelphia, 1980, J.B. Lippincott Co.
5. Rosenbaum, M.B., Elizari, M.V., et al.: Relevance of phase 3 and phase 4 block in clinical electrophysiology. In Befeler, B., editor: Selected topics in cardiac arrhythmias, Mt. Kisco, N.Y., 1980, Futura Publishing Co.

CHAPTER 12

Laddergrams

Laddergrams are simple line drawings in tiers that represent different levels of the heart (SA node, atria, AV junction, and ventricles). The lines from tier to tier reflect the conduction sequence within the heart and are best drawn with a slant to represent the progress of the impulse. The lines are precisely aligned with the corresponding ECG events (P waves and QRS complexes) so that AV conduction, in particular, can be accurately extrapolated. The number of tiers used depends upon what is being illustrated; three will serve most purposes: one for atrial activation (A), one for AV conduction (AV), and the third for ventricular activation (V), as in Fig. 12-1. Other tiers can be added when necessary. For example, if you wish to illustrate type I or II SA block, a narrow tier is added to the atrial tier for SA nodal activation; if you want to, you can even use another tier between the ones for SA nodal and atrial activation to illustrate conduction through the perinodal fibers. If necessary, several divisions can be made of the AV tier (node, His bundle, and Purkinje fibers) and an extra tier can be tacked on below the ventricular tier to permit illustration of ventricular ectopic activity and microreentry mechanisms. In short, *the laddergram can be tailored to fit your need*.

Fig. 12-1 shows the simplest of laddergrams using the three basic tiers. A gentle slope is used to indicate the passage of time as the impulse spreads through the atrium (complex *a*); this sloping line should begin in the atrial tier at a spot directly under the beginning of the P wave. Some authorities do not slant the atrial line at all but draw it straight down from the onset of the P wave, especially when it is apparent that the SA node is pacing the heart (complex *b*). Others make a dot at the top of the atrial tier to indicate the point of origin of the impulse (complex *c*). Sometimes, as a visual aid when the mechanism is more complicated, an arrowhead is used (complex *d*) to indicate the direction of impulse spread. It doesn't really matter which method you use, as long as it illustrates what you want it to.

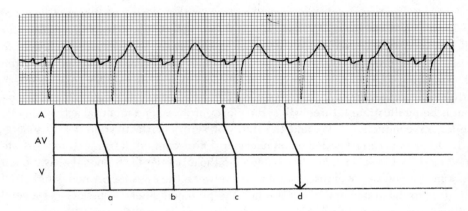

Fig. 12-1. Four methods used to illustrate the same complex. *A*, Atria; *AV*, AV junction; *V*, ventricles.

When constructing a laddergram, first mark in what you can see and then draw in what is inferred. For example, using a straightedge, draw the atrial lines right under the beginning of the P waves so that the sinus rhythm is accurately reflected in the laddergram. Then draw in ventricular activity. If you have determined that the ventricular complexes are the result of conduction from the atria, indicate this by beginning the slope at the top of the ventricular tier right under the beginning of the QRS complex and ending at the bottom of the V tier at a point corresponding to the end of the QRS complex. Then join up the two lines to reflect what is inferred, that is, AV conduction.

Illustrating supraventricular ectopic mechanisms

APBs. In Fig. 12-2 a laddergram illustrates atrial premature beats. The leading point is placed midway down the atrial tier to indicate an ectopic focus.

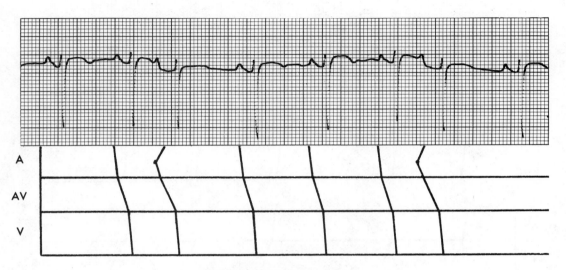

Fig. 12-2. Atrial premature beats.

NONCONDUCTED APBs. In Fig. 12-3, *A*, there is one nonconducted APB. Block is represented as being in the AV junction, although the impulse may never have penetrated the node at all. The level of the block cannot be known without His bundle electrograms; but since the point of this particular laddergram is to illustrate a nonconducted APB, the block can be indicated anywhere after the atrial and before the ventricular tier. If however, you wish to illustrate that the block is in the AV node as opposed to the His-Purkinje system, the laddergram may look like Fig. 12-3, *B*, with the divisions of the AV conduction system delineated. The beat following the pause is a junctional escape (note the shorter PR interval).

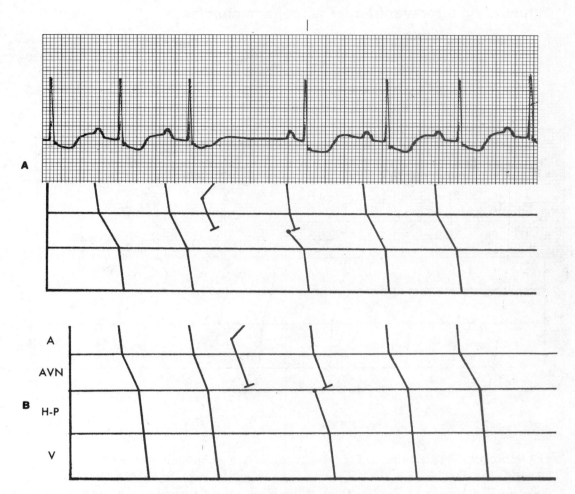

Fig. 12-3. *AVN*, AV node, *H-P*, His-Purkinje system.

AV NODAL REENTRY. Laddergrams are particularly helpful in illustrating this mechanism. Reflecting lines are drawn in the AV tier, as seen in Figs. 12-4 and 12-5. The lines proceeding anterogradely conduct to the ventricles and meet the V tier directly under the onset of the QRS. The lines proceeding retrogradely show conduction to the A tier. Often the P′ wave is not seen in paroxysmal supraventricular tachycardia because it is buried within the QRS. It is drawn on the laddergram whether it is seen or not—sometimes with a dashed line if it is invisible. If the mechanism involves an accessory pathway, the P′ wave occurs midway between the QRS complexes.

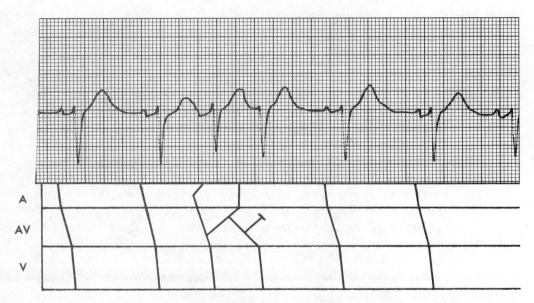

Fig. 12-4. AV nodal reentry.

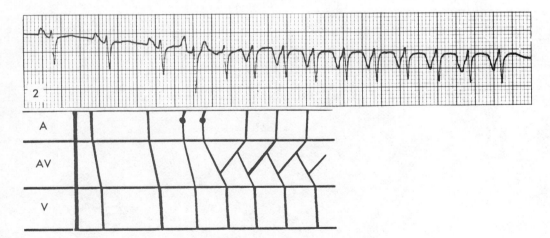

Fig. 12-5. AV nodal reentry.

When constructing this laddergram, first draw in all the P waves that can be seen, varying their slopes according to whether they are sinus, ectopic, or retrograde. Then draw in the ventricular complexes, slanting them slightly anterogradely to indicate a supraventricular mechanism. Now you are ready to illustrate the AV nodal reentry mechanism. Draw a straight line from the end of the APB to the top of the V tier where the first QRS of the tachycardia begins. Now, a short distance up this line, illustrate retrograde conduction by drawing a line from this point to the beginning of the first retrograde line in the A tier. The next anterograde line will begin a short distance down the retrograde line in the AV tier and end at the top of the V tier where the next QRS begins; and so on, until the tachycardia terminates.

ATRIAL FLUTTER. Fig. 12-6 shows atrial flutter at a rate of 306/min. The normal response of the AV node to a rapidly firing atrial ectopic focus is Wenckebach conduction, which is reflected in this tracing by the group beating (pairs) and the alternating relationship of the F′ wave to the following QRS. When drawing the laddergram for atrial tachycardia or flutter, it is important to remember that the P′ immediately preceding the QRS is not necessarily the one to have conducted. Pick and Langendorf[1] long ago pointed out that the AV conduction time in atrial flutter is considerably prolonged owing to the effect of concealed conduction of the numerous atrial impulses. They calculated that the usual "FR" interval during 2:1 conduction probably measured between 0.26 and 0.46 second. (The "FR" interval in atrial flutter is measured in the inferior leads from the lowest point—nadir—of the negative component of the flutter wave to the beginning of the QRS.)

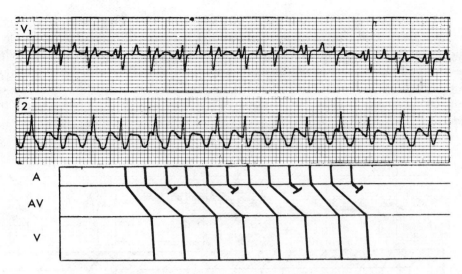

Fig. 12-6. Atrial flutter with 3:2 Wenckebach periods.

ATRIAL FLUTTER WITH WENCKEBACH CONDUCTION. In Fig. 12-6 there is a Wenckebach sequence of 3:2. Note the paired ventricular complexes and the alternating F-R relationship. In constructing the laddergram, proceed as above by first drawing in the atrial impulses, then the ventricular, and finally AV conduction. Remember that the FR interval in atrial flutter will usually be greater than 0.26 second. In this case the shortest one is 0.30 second.

ATRIAL FLUTTER WITH EXIT BLOCK OUT OF THE FLUTTER FOCUS. To graph the tracing in Fig. 12-7, you need an additional tier because pairing of the flutter waves themselves must be accounted for (in V_1 the flutter wave is a positive peak). When beats are grouped in pairs, one should always think of 3:2 Wenckebach conduction. Although in atrial flutter it is undecided whether the mechanism is reentry or enhanced automaticity, either mechanism could exhibit an exit block out of the flutter focus.

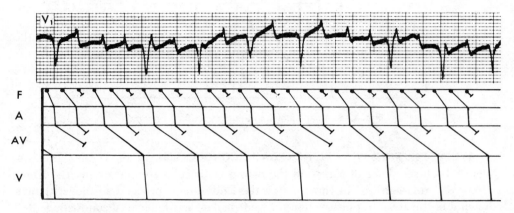

Fig. 12-7. Atrial flutter with 3:2 Wenckebach conduction out of the flutter focus; in the AV junction there is 2:1 conduction at a higher level and 5:4 Wenckebach conduction at a lower level.

To construct such a laddergram, draw an extra tier above the atrial tier to accommodate the ectopic focus. Then draw the atrial waves in the A tier and measure the length of the Wenckebach period (the distance between the two F waves beginning the short cycle); in this case it is 0.56 second. Since a 3:2 Wenckebach is assumed, the 0.56 second is divided by 3 (0.19 sec). Now plot the discharge of the ectopic focus at 0.19-second intervals beginning at a spot in the F tier immediately preceding the Wenckebach period (just before the F wave ending the long cycle). The first two ectopic discharges are conducted with lengthening conduction time and the third is blocked, creating the atrial bigeminy. Now the ventricular beats can be drawn in the V tier and AV conduction established, revealing in addition a 5:4 AV Wenckebach.

Illustrating SA block

SA conduction problems are illustrated by drawing an extra tier at the top of the laddergram. This segment represents the SA node and the perinodal fibers, silent zones on the surface ECG.

SA WENCKEBACH. Fig. 12-8 has all the classical signs of Wenckebach conduction: group beating, shortening RR intervals, and pauses less than twice the shortest cycle (see Chapter 16). However, since the PR intervals are short and all equal, the Wenckebach must be higher in the conduction system between the sinus node and the atrial musculature.

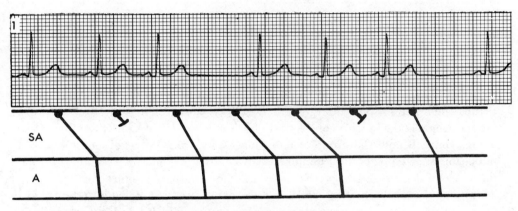

Fig. 12-8. 4:3 sinus Wenckebach.

In constructing this laddergram you may wish to illustrate only SA conduction, as we have, since there is no AV or ventricular problem. After drawing a tier for sinus and atrial activity, fill in what you can see—the P waves. The events in the SA node and perinodal fibers are concealed and must be extrapolated from the pattern of their activity, the PP intervals. Now measure the distance between the P waves ending the long cycles and divide that number by 4, which represents the number of P waves seen plus the one assumed to be lost ($240 \div 4 = 60$). This number (0.60 sec) represents the sinus cycle. Begin shortly before the P wave ending the pause and walk out the sinus cycle at the top of the SA tier. Now you can indicate conduction between sinus firing and atrial activation and clearly show a Wenckebach sequence.

SA WENCKEBACH WITH JUNCTIONAL ESCAPE. Fig. 12-9 is another SA Wenckebach. This time the pauses are interrupted by junctional escape beats, so the AV and V tiers are used in addition to the SA and A segments.

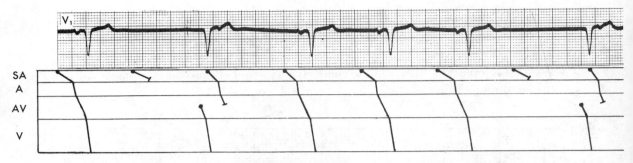

Fig. 12-9. 5:4 sinus Wenckebach with junctional escape beats.

It could be that you would begin this laddergram without spotting the mechanism; constructing the laddergram, however, is an excellent way to arrive in a logical fashion at the mechanism. You will first draw the P waves into the A tier. In so doing, you will note the group of four, suggesting a 5:4 Wenckebach. There is a noticeable shortening of the PP interval between the first and the second cycle, and the longest PP intervals are less than twice the shortest; therefore this must indeed be a 5:4 sinus Wenckebach. The ventricular complexes are now drawn into the laddergram. All of them are of supraventricular origin, so begin your line at the top of the V tier directly under the beginning of the QRS and slant it anterogradely. The two junctional escape beats are illustrated by placing dots in the AV tier just ahead of the junctional complexes and connecting the dots to the ventricular complex in the V tier. Now calculate the whole Wenckebach period as before by measuring the distance between the P waves ending the pauses. Count the number of P waves between pauses, add one for the missing P wave, and divide this number (5) into the total Wenckebach cycle (525 ÷ 5 = 105). The sinus cycle is 105, which is walked out in the SA tier beginning just before a P wave ending the longest atrial cycle (located immediately after the junctional escape beat). Now connect these dots with the lines in the A tier, and the illustration of a 5:4 SA Wenckebach with junctional escape beats is complete.

Fig. 12-10 is another SA Wenckebach. Why not cover our laddergram and try plotting this one on your own?

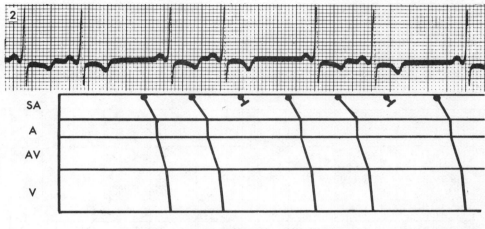

Fig. 12-10

Illustrating junctional ectopic mechanisms

The junctional ectopic focus is represented within the AV tier by a dot or simply by making that point the leading edge of conduction. However, the time of the junctional discharge is not known from the surface ECG. The location of the retrograde P′ with respect to the QRS is not even helpful, because whether or not and where the retrograde P′ wave appears are determined by the speed of retrograde conduction as compared to anterograde conduction (Fig. 12-11). The RP′ interval is not a measure of retrograde conduction per se but represents the difference between anterograde and retrograde conduction (Fig. 12-12).

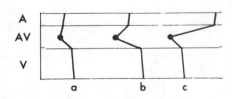

Fig. 12-11. The relationship of atrial to ventricular activation depends on the rate of conduction in each direction.

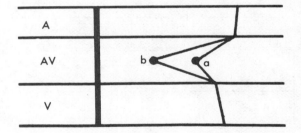

Fig. 12-12. The RP interval of junctional beats remains unchanged provided the difference between retrograde and anterograde conduction remains the same.

JUNCTIONAL RHYTHM WITH RECIPROCAL BEATS. Figs. 12-13 and 12-14 are examples of a junctional rhythm with progressively lengthening retrograde conduction culminating in reciprocal beats. In both cases retrograde conduction is slower than anterograde conduction.

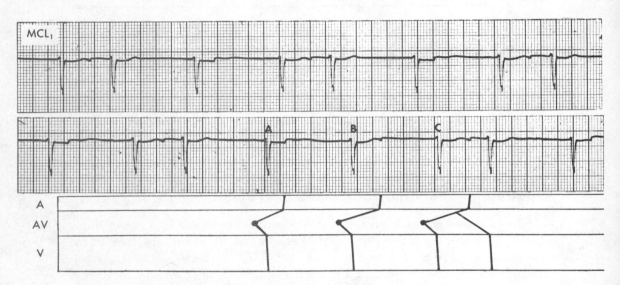

Fig. 12-13. Junctional rhythm with reciprocal beats.

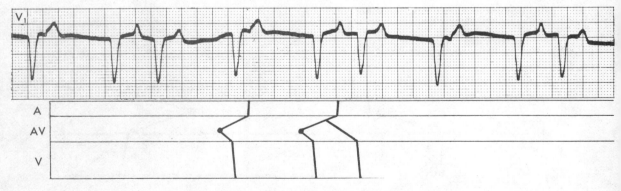

Fig. 12-14. Junctional rhythm with reciprocal beats.

To construct the laddergram, first draw in the P waves, showing their retrograde pathway by starting the slant up and forward from the bottom of the A tier. Then draw in the ventricular lines, reflecting their supraventricular origin by slanting them from the top of the V tier down. Now pick a reasonable spot in the AV tier preceding the ventricular lines to indicate the junctional discharge. The exact location of this position in the AV tier is not important, since this information is not known without a His bundle electrogram; but just keep the distance between the junctional impulse and its propagation through the ventricles consistent. Now you can establish anterograde and retrograde conduction, and note that retrograde conduction is lengthening until there is sufficient delay to permit the impulse to find a responsive downward pathway and return to the ventricles.

JUNCTIONAL ESCAPE. Fig. 12-15 illustrates a sinus bradycardia that results in a junctional escape rhythm. First mark off the sinus impulses and then the retrograde P' waves, noting that the first negative P' is not as deep as the ones that follow. This is obviously a fusion beat, since the sinus impulse was expected at that same time. Fusion is illustrated by the two lines opposing each other in the same tier. Now mark off the ventricular complexes and establish AV conduction. Note that the PR interval of the third complex is shorter by 0.04 second than the preceding ones and therefore is not conducted to the ventricles. The third beat and those following it are junctional. This is illustrated by placing the dot in the AV tier just preceding the ventricular lines. Now anterograde and retrograde conduction from the junctional focus is drawn, as is the sinus conducted beat.

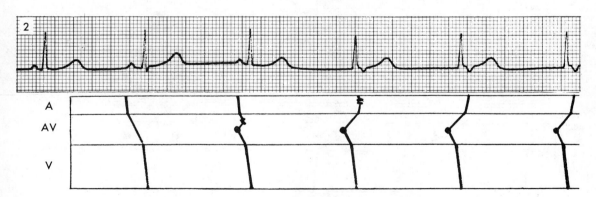

Fig. 12-15. Sinus bradycardia resulting in a junctional escape rhythm. There is one atrial fusion beat.

ACCELERATED IDIOJUNCTIONAL RHYTHM WITH WENCKEBACH EXIT BLOCK.

One of the manifestations of digitalis toxicity in atrial fibrillation is an accelerated idiojunctional rhythm with Wenckebach block (out of or below the junctional pace-maker). Fig. 12-16 is such a case, and the laddergram is useful in illustrating this mechanism. In lead V_2 there is group beating and shortening RR intervals, two of the footprints of Wenckebach. Paired beats are noted in lead V_4, and the absolute regu-larity of the independent junctional pacemaker is seen in V_3.

In constructing this laddergram for V_4, begin by drawing in the ventricular lines; the atrial tier can be left empty in atrial fibrillation. Since pairs usually reflect a 3:2 Wenckebach, you will divide by 3 once you determine the length of the full Wencke-bach period (the distance between two Rs ending the long cycle). This is 184, and the distance between junctional impulses is 63. Begin to plot these intervals at the center of the AV tier just preceding the first beat of one of the Wenckebach cycles (the QRS ending the pause) and then establish AV conduction. Conduction time length-ens, the third junctional impulse is finally blocked, and the sequence begins again (3:2 Wenckebach).

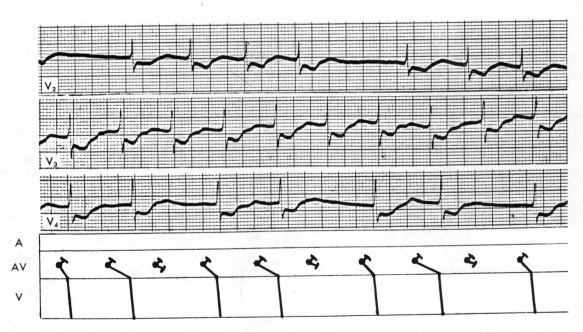

Fig. 12-16. Atrial fibrillation with an accelerated junctional rhythm (rate, 98/min) and 3:2 Wenckebach below or exit block from the junctional pacemaker.

CONCEALED JUNCTIONAL BEATS. Useful applications of the laddergram are for concealed junctional extrasystoles and for the blocked beat of the junctional tachycardia with Wenckebach exit block. Figs. 12-17 to 12-19 are examples of how nicely these mechanisms can be illustrated with the laddergram. The concealed junctional beat is drawn as a dot with both retrograde and anterograde block.

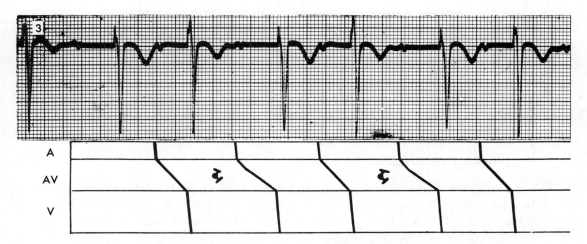

Fig. 12-17. Concealed junctional extrasystoles produce alternating PR and RR intervals.

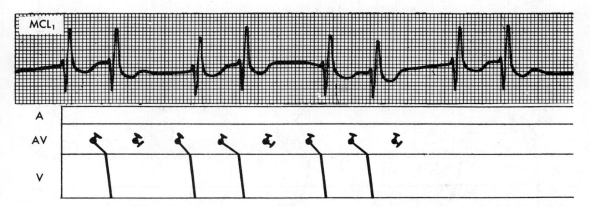

Fig. 12-18. Junctional tachycardia with 3:2 Wenckebach conduction below or exit block from the junctional pacemaker and RBBB.

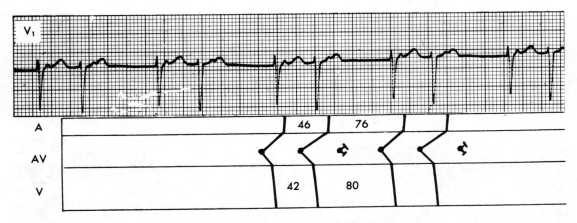

Fig. 12-19. Junctional tachycardia with simultaneous bidirectional (anterograde and retrograde) 3:2 Wenckebachs producing bigeminal grouping.

Illustrating ventricular ectopics

A ventricular ectopic beat is reflected in the laddergram by drawing the line beginning at the bottom of the V tier at a spot directly under the beginning of the ectopic QRS. Then draw the line forward and upward to clearly indicate the ventricular origin of the impulse (Fig. 12-20).

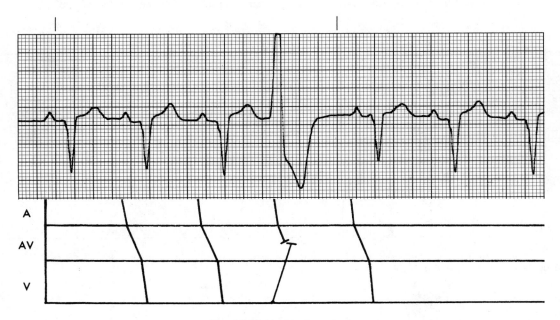

Fig. 12-20. Ventricular ectopic.

VENTRICULAR FUSION. These complexes are illustrated in the laddergram by showing two lines meeting within the V tier; one line begins at the bottom of the V tier (ventricular ectopic beat) and the other enters the V tier from the AV tier (a supraventricular impulse). You can usually tell by the PR interval and the shape of the complex how much of the line in the V tier should be ventricular in origin and how much should be supraventricular (Fig. 12-21).

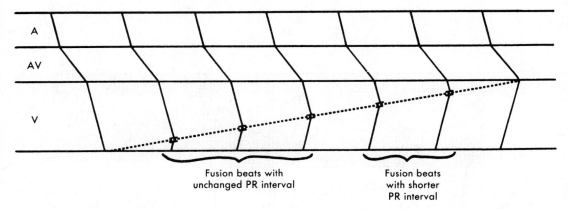

Fusion beats with unchanged PR interval

Fusion beats with shorter PR interval

Fig. 12-21. Laddergram illustrating progressively "higher" levels of fusion within the ventricles. The first beat represents a pure sinus beat; the last beat, a pure ventricular ectopic. Note that at first the PR interval remains the same as that of the sinus beat (as long as the sinus impulse invades the ventricles before or no later than the ectopic center fires); but when the ectopic center fires before the sinus impulse arrives, the PR becomes shorter than that of the sinus beat.

In Fig. 12-22 four fusion beats are indicated (*1* to *4*) in which the PR intervals progressively lengthen. It is evident that the QRS complexes become more and more normal in contour as the supraventricular impulse captures more and more of the ventricular myocardium.

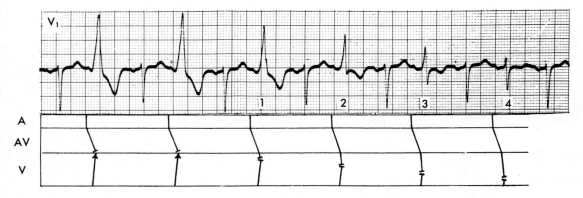

Fig. 12-22. Ventricular fusion.

In Fig. 12-23 there is an atrial fusion beat because of an underlying atrial parasystole (longer strip in 14-5, *B*). Fusion is always illustrated on the laddergram by two opposing lines in the same tier. You can use your imagination to illustrate the atrial parasystolic focus; we have chosen to represent it by a dot within a circle in the atrial (*A*) tier. Note that the parasystolic focus fired once without capturing the atria because of refractoriness due to the previous sinus beat.

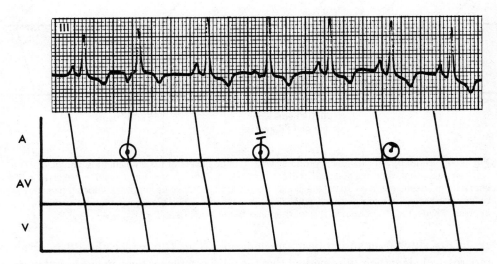

Fig. 12-23. Atrial fusion because of atrial parasystole. For a longer tracing see Fig. 14-5, *B*. (Courtesy Alan Lindsay, M.D., Salt Lake City.)

VENTRICULAR MICROREENTRY. If you wish to illustrate the mechanism for ectopic impulse formation within the ventricles, an extra ectopic (E) tier can be added at the bottom of the V tier. In Fig. 12-24 two possible microreentry mechanisms are illustrated in the E tier.

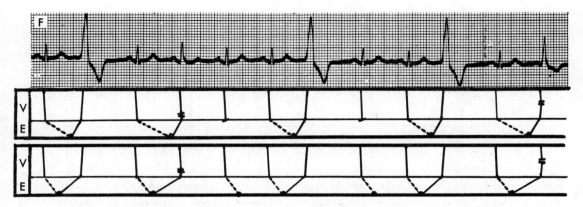

Fig. 12-24. If reentry is the mechanism for these ventricular extrasystoles, the laddergrams depict two possible explanations for the lengthening coupling intervals: Wenckebach-like conduction occurring in the afferent (upper diagram) and the efferent (lower diagram) limb of the reentry circuit.

Now it's your turn

We have outlined the principles necessary for constructing laddergrams. Now try your hand at drawing the rather intricate diagrams needed to illustrate the mechanisms of the next four figures. After putting your best hand forward, turn the page and see if you have illustrated the mechanisms correctly. Fig. 12-25 reviews the three mechanisms for reciprocal beating.

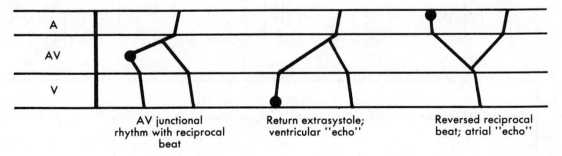

Fig. 12-25. The three forms of reciprocal beating ("echo" beats).

Interpretation to Figs. 12-26 to 12-28

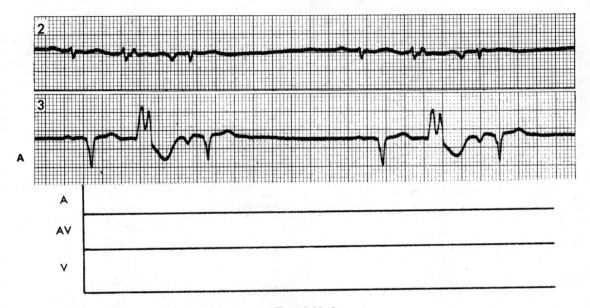

Fig. 12-26, A

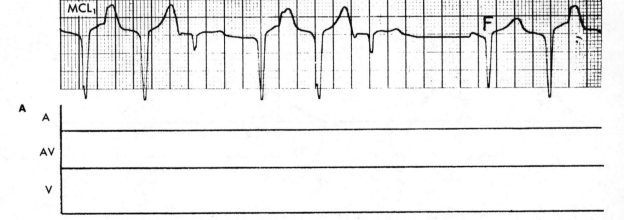

Fig. 12-27, A

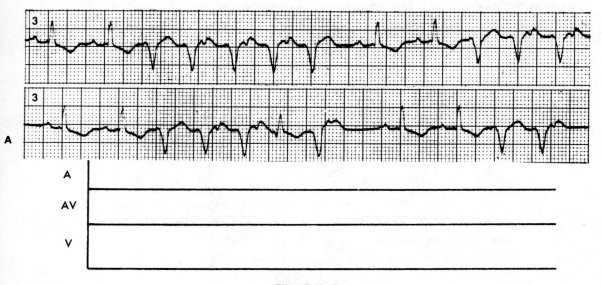

Fig. 12-28, A

Fig. 12-26: Reciprocal beating initiated by ventricular extrasystoles. Each trio of beats consists of a sinus beat, a ventricular extrasystole with retrograde conduction, and a reciprocal beat.

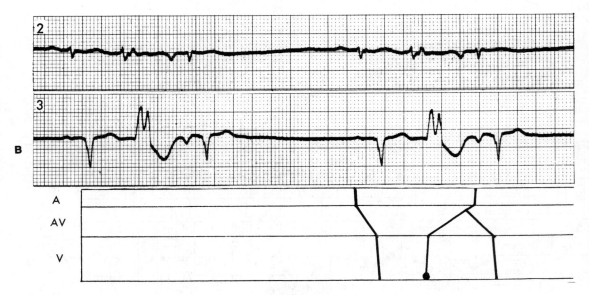

Fig. 12-26, B

Fig. 12-27: Accelerated idioventricular rhythm with reciprocal beating. Two idioventricular beats are followed by increasingly delayed retroconduction to the atria, delay after the second being sufficient to permit reentry and a reciprocal beat. The second-to-last beat is a fusion beat.

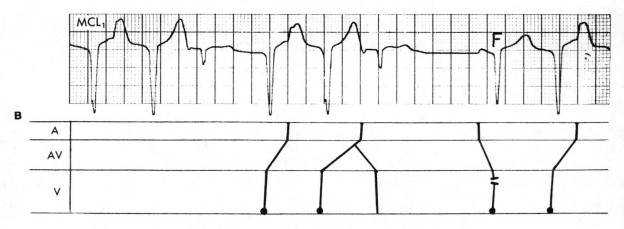

Fig. 12-27, B

Fig. 12-28: Ventricular tachycardia with retrograde conduction to the atria, a reciprocal beat, and ventricular fusion.

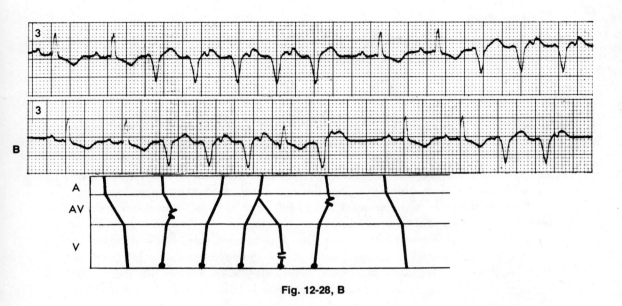

Fig. 12-28, B

Reference

1. Besoain-Santander, M., Pick, A., and Langendorf, R.: A-V conduction in auricular flutter, Circulation 2:604, 1950.

CHAPTER 13

Fusion

A fusion beat is the complex (ventricular or atrial) that results when two impulses simultaneously activate parts of the same myocardial territory (ventricular or atrial myocardium). The simultaneous spreading impulses produce a hybrid complex usually possessing recognizable features of the patterns produced by each alone. The fusion beat is unrecognizable clinically and is a purely electrocardiographic diagnosis.

Three of the more common mechanisms for fusion are diagrammatically represented in Fig. 13-1. They are as follows:

A: Ventricular fusion resulting from the simultaneous spread of a descending sinus impulse and an ectopic ventricular one in any of the following forms— ventricular extrasystole or escape, ventricular tachycardia in the absence of retrograde conduction to the atria, accelerated idioventricular rhythm (AIVR), parasystole, or a paced ventricular beat. Ventricular fusion involving a sinus impulse is obviously likely to occur only with end-diastolic ectopic beats.

B: Ventricular fusion resulting from the simultaneous spread of two supraventricular impulses, one of them via an accessory pathway and the other via the normal route (preexcitation syndrome).

C: Atrial fusion resulting from the simultaneous spread of a sinus impulse and a retrograde one from either the AV junction or the ventricles.

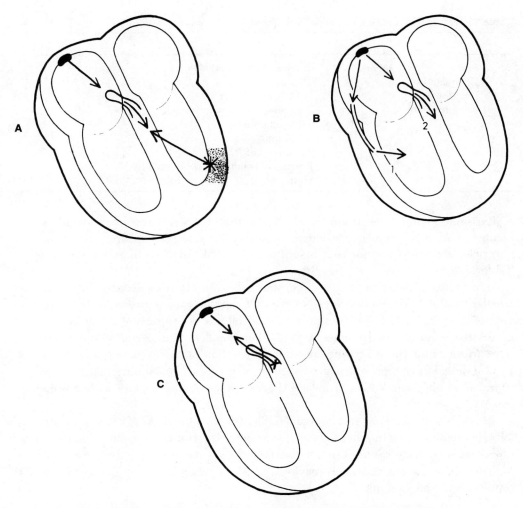

Fig. 13-1. A, Ventricular fusion because of ventricular ectopic activity. **B,** Ventricular fusion because of preexcitation. **C,** Atrial fusion.

Table 13-1. *Potential partners in fusion (any impulse in **A** can fuse with any in **B**)*

A	B
Sinus	Ectopic ventricular
Ectopic atrial	Extrasystole
Junctional	Tachycardia
Ectopic ventricular	Accelerated idioventricular
	Parasystole
	Escape
	Pacemaker
	Junctional conducted preferentially
	Sinus or ectopic atrial conducted by Kent bundle

Less often ventricular fusion can also result from the simultaneous spread of two ectopic ventricular impulses, as when two idioventricular pacemakers, one in each ventricle, are competing for control. All the potential fusion partners are shown in Table 13-1.

The ventricular fusion beat is of considerable value in recognizing ectopic ventricular rhythms. Most authorities believe that the presence of fusion favors ectopy with 85% to 90% odds. The argument runs as follows: if a supraventricular impulse enters the ventricles and merges with another impulse, that second impulse must have arisen within the ventricles since the AV junction would be rendered refractory by one descending supraventricular impulse, negating the possibility that a second supraventricular impulse could invade the ventricles in time to fuse with the first one.

Most of the time this is probably true; but Kistin[1] demonstrated that it was possible for a descending sinus impulse to fuse in the ventricles with an aberrantly conducted junctional beat. One explanation for this is that the junctional impulse spreads via Mahaim fibers to the ventricle, leaving the AV junction clear for passage of the simultaneous sinus impulse.

Ventricular fusion

CLINICAL SIGNIFICANCE. The clinical significanc of ventricular fusion is simply that of the ventricular ectopic beat that contributes to it. Evaluation is in the light of the total clinical picture, and its significance is not altered because the ectopic happens to collide with a supraventricular impulse. The fact that there is fusion is purely circumstantial and relevant only to the extent that the ventricular ectopic itself is relevant.

There is some evidence that end-diastolic ectopics can be the result of excessive stretch of the conductive fibers within the ventricles, such as would occur with an elevated left ventricular end-diastolic pressure secondary to congestive heart failure.

DIAGNOSIS. There are three main principles in the diagnosis of ventricular fusion[2]:

1. It should be diagnosed only if you have cogent reason to believe that two impulses were due at that moment. This is so self-evident that it seems unnecessary to say it; but there is an observed tendency for interpreters to hastily invoke fusion when an offbeat complex is not readily explained—and there is no doubt that "fusion beats" are plucked out of insubstantial air more than any other electrocardiographic phenomenon.
2. Ventricular fusion beats generally show a contour and a duration that are intermediate between the contour and duration of complexes of the fusing impulses (see *Exception* below).
3. The PR interval of a ventricular fusion beat may be the same as that of the sinus rhythm, or it may be shorter; but if it is shorter, it is not more than about 0.06 second shorter than the sinus PR. This is because virtually any ectopic impulse can reach the AV junction within 0.06 second and, once it has reached the junction, the way is barred for a descending impulse to enter the ventricles and fuse.

Exception to rule 2 above. When fusion occurs between a supraventricular impulse in the presence of BBB and an ectopic impulse arising in the ventricle on the same side as the BBB, the resulting fusion complex may be narrower than either the ectopic or the BBB pattern (see p. 215); similarly, if fusion develops between two ectopic ventricular impulses simultaneously arising from each ventricle, the resulting complex may be narrower than either ectopic.

In Fig. 13-2, *A*, the end-diastolic VPB is preceded by a PR interval of only 0.06 second; clearly the sinus impulse has not been conducted to the ventricles and there is therefore no chance of fusion. In the same patient Fig. 13-2, *B*, shows another end-diastolic VPB. This time the PR interval is 0.16 second instead of the underlying 0.22 and the complex is a fusion beat. If a similar ventricular ectopic occurred following an even longer PR interval, say 0.18 second, it is easy to visualize that the morphology of the ventricular complex would be quite different again from the fusion beat seen in *B*, looking more like the sinus and less like the ectopic. Going one step further, if the ectopic ventricular focus did not discharge until after the sinus impulse actually entered the ventricles, the complex would be different still and would now

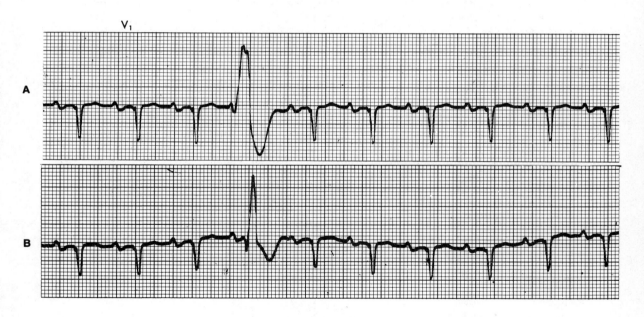

Fig. 13-2. End-diastolic ventricular extrasystoles. In **A** there is no chance for fusion because the PR interval is only 0.06 second. In **B** the ventricular extrasystole begins 0.14 second after onset of the P wave; thus fusion is possible.

have the same PR interval as the conducted sinus beats (0.22 sec). Even if the ventricular ectopic focus were discharging with the same PR interval each time, the morphology of the fusion complexes might vary because of slight variation in the amount of myocardial tissue activated each time by the two fusing impulses, and because the ectopic focus could discharge at any time fom the beginning of the normal QRS until it was itself activated by the normal impulse, thus producing the same PR each time but varying shapes to the fusion beat. Likewise, even with the same coupling interval (normal QRS to ectopic), each time the sinus cycle may vary slightly resulting in different fusion complexes.

Fig. 13-3 shows ventricular bigeminy in which the coupling intervals are long enough to deposit the extrasystoles after every other sinus P wave. Ventricular fusion beats (labeled *1*, *2*, *3*, and *4*) result from the gradually lengthening coupling interval. The first two extrasystoles capture the whole ventricular myocardium; but beginning with the third extrasystole, there is time for the sinus impulse to enter the ventricles before they have been completely activated from the ectopic center. As the coupling interval and with it the PR interval lengthens, the sinus contribution to the ventricular fusion complex increases (see laddergram).

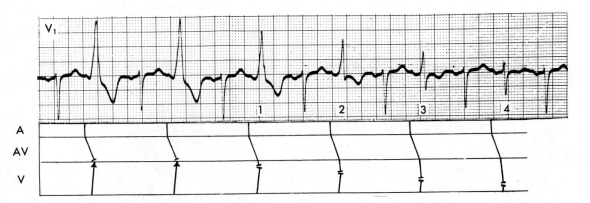

Fig. 13-3. End-diastolic ventricular extrasystoles landing after every other P wave. After the first two extrasystoles their coupling intervals progressively lengthen so that fusion occurs (beats 1, 2, 3, and 4) at progressively "lower" levels in the ventricles with more and more contribution from the sinus impulse. The PR interval of beat 4 is as long as that of the sinus beats.

Occasionally the coincidence of a more or less simultaneous atrial and ventricular extrasystole produces ventricular fusion, which may simulate an APB with aberration. An example of this coincidence is illustrated in Fig. 13-4. The third beat (*A*) is an APB, the fifth and last beats (*V*) are VPBs, and the eighth beat (*F*) is a fusion beat between atrial and ventricular extrasystoles. If the fusion beat is taken out of context without the evidence of the surrounding beats, it is seen as a bizarre QRS-T preceded by a premature P wave and is therefore diagnosed as an APB with aberration. Since a fusion beat is partly an ectopic ventricular beat, it carries clinical and therapeutic implications different from those of an APB.

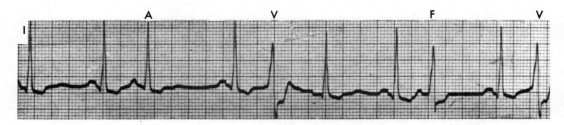

Fig. 13-4. *A*, Atrial extrasystole; *V*, ventricular extrasystole; *F*, fusion between simultaneous atrial and ventricular extrasystoles.

Fig. 13-5 is an accelerated idioventricular rhythm with a rate almost the same as the sinus rhythm. Thus when the sinus rhythm slows just a little, the ventricular ectopic focus discharges. In such a situation ventricular fusion is common (the second to sixth beats). The last three are pure ventricular ectopic beats, but they are somewhat distorted by the simultaneous occurrence of sinus P waves.

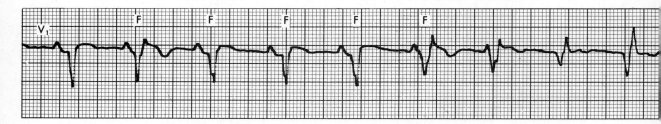

Fig. 13-5. Ventricular fusion beats due to an accelerated idioventricular rhythm.

In Fig. 13-6 note the changing shapes of the fusion beats, a phenomenon that contributes to diagnostic confusion when the mechanism is poorly understood. This patient's PR interval is 0.18 second; with the VPBs the PR shortens by 0.2 to 0.6 second, resulting in varying degrees of fusion. The shorter the PR, the greater is the contribution from the ectopic impulse to the fusion beat.

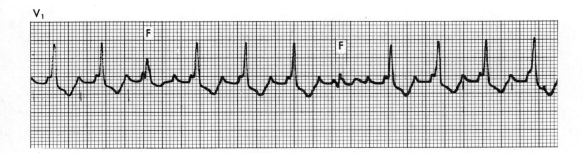

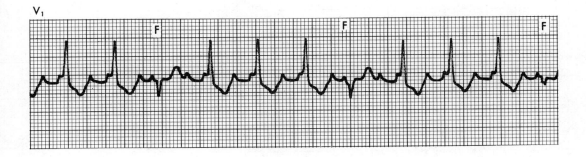

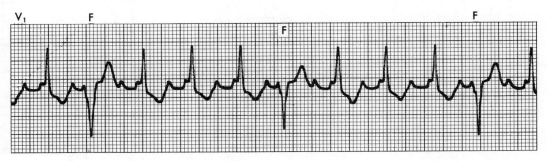

Fig. 13-6. Varying degrees of ventricular fusion resulting in changing QRS shapes.

Fig. 13-7 again shows the confusing face of bigeminal end-diastolic ventricular ectopy. The sinus beats are conducted with RBBB. In the top tracing *(A)* one might even suspect supernormal AV and intraventricular conduction since P waves with shorter PR intervals precede the narrower normal-looking beats. However, a second tracing *(B)* clearly indicates that *the narrower complexes are really fusion beats* and that the shortening of the PR interval is the result of the premature ventricular ectopic and not a true reflection of AV conduction time. Since the *right* BBB complex is normalized by fusion with a ventricular beat, the ectopic focus must be in the *right* ventricle.

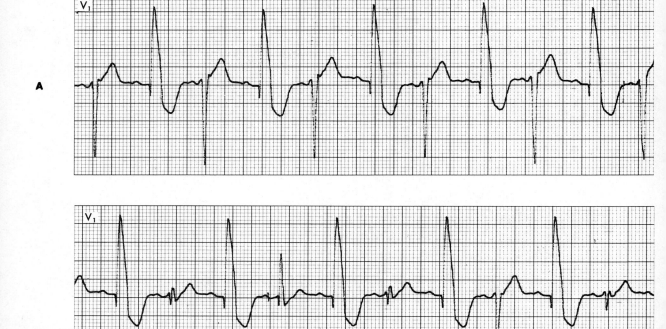

Fig. 13-7. Ventricular fusion every other beat. In **A** fusion normalizes the QRS when the underlying mechanism is RBBB, simulating supernormal conduction. In **B** it is evident that the narrower complexes are really fusion beats.

Fig. 13-8 shows the same arrhythmia, bigeminal end-diastolic VPBs, all of which produce multiform fusion beats.

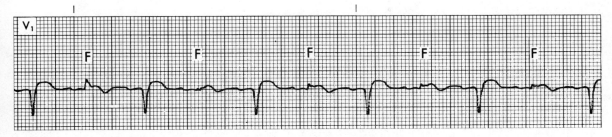

Fig. 13-8. Bigeminal end-diastolic ventricular extrasystoles producing multiform fusion beats.

Fusion in parasystole

Fig. 13-9 is a parasystolic rhythm with one fusion beat. Note that even though the first ventricular ectopic is end-diastolic it is not a fusion beat. This is because the underlying PR interval is 0.14 second and the ventricular complex begins only 0.04 second after the onset of the P wave, giving the ectopic impulse 0.10 second to activate the ventricles before the sinus impulse is expected.

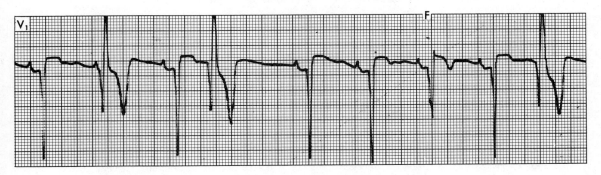

Fig. 13-9. Ventricular parasystole with fusion *(F)*.

Take a good look at Fig. 13-10 and use your calipers before you read on! The intervals between the negative deflections are approximately the same, but we hope you didn't mistake the artifact for ventricular parasystole with fusion. Note that the deep negative deflections do not interrupt or disturb the cardiac cycle. They are therefore clearly artifacts.

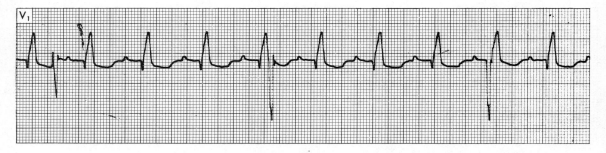

Fig. 13-10

Fusion during accelerated idioventricular rhythm (AIVR)

AIVR is a common source of fusion. This is because its rate is often closely similar to the competing sinus rate. The ectopic focus therefore asserts itself just as soon as the sinus rate slows slightly. This is nicely illustrated in Fig. 13-11. When the sinus cycle lengthens by as little as 0.04 second, a fusion beat occurs. The ectopic ventricular focus is firing at a rate of 88/min; as long as the sinus rhythm remains at 90/min or faster, as at the beginning of the strip, the enhanced ventricular automaticity is not manifest. In this tracing the sinus rhythm slows slightly, after the third beat permitting fusion until, at the seventh beat, the ectopic focus assumes complete control of the ventricles with no contribution from the sinus impulse.

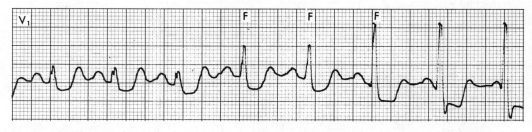

Fig. 13-11. Ventricular fusion *(F)* between the sinus impulses and an accelerated idioventricular rhythm.

Fig. 13-12 is a champion tracing, boasting no less than 37 consecutive fusion beats! At the beginning of the tracing are pure ectopic beats, at the end pure sinus beats. Between the two Xs all are fusion beats with the varying contributions from the isorhythmic sinus and ventricular impulses producing a kaleidoscope of configurations.

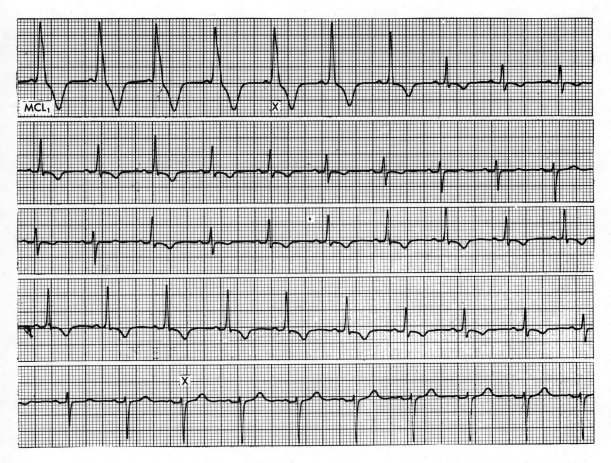

Fig. 13-12. Fusion in profusion! In these five continuous strips, between the complexes marked X, there are 37 consecutive fusion beats between the sinus impulses and a competing accelerated idioventricular rhythm.

Fig. 13-13 illustrates a similar mechanism but looks completely different because of the underlying LBBB. Note the three fusion beats in the middle of the tracing, the last of which actually normalizes the complex, presumably because the ectopic focus is in the left ventricle. The ectopic rhythm takes over by usurpation (the first fusion beat ends a measurably shorter cycle than the preceding sinus cycles); but it promptly slows again and, after the third fusion beat, surrenders control to the sinus pacemaker.

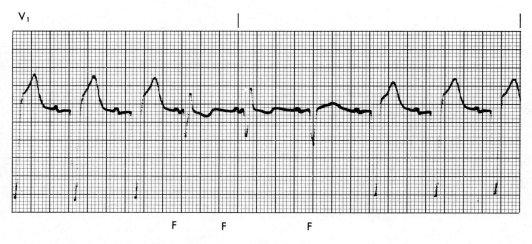

Fig. 13-13. An underlying LBBB with three fusion beats *(F)* due to an ectopic focus in the left ventricle.

Fusion beats in the diagnosis of ventricular tachycardia

The value of fusion beats in the diagnosis of ventricular tachycardia was emphasized by Dressler[3]; such beats are therefore often referred to as "Dressler beats." Their presence is considered excellent evidence in favor of ventricular tachycardia, since fusion almost always reflects ventricular ectopy. However, their value is limited because they are seldom seen if the rate is much over 150/min. All the examples published by Dressler had rates less than this. Another limiting factor is the fact that it is also possible for a junctional tachycardia with BBB (mimicking ventricular tachycardia) to produce fusion beats.[4]

In Fig. 13-14 there is a tachycardia of 150/min and fusion beats. The fusion beats occur when the sinus P wave is so placed that conduction occurs before the ventricular ectopic focus can completely activate the ventricles.

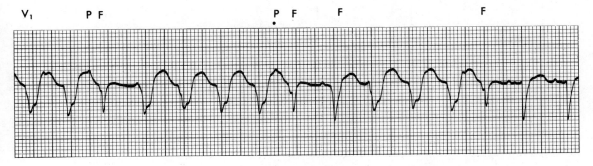

Fig. 13-14. Ventricular tachycardia (rate, 150/min) with fusion beats *(F)*.

Fig. 13-15, *A*, is a tracing that was erroneously diagnosed as ventricular tachycardia because of the fusion beat in the middle of the tracing; and it is indeed a tachycardia at 132/min with one fusion beat. The ventricular complexes are broad and resemble ventricular tachycardia; but, if you examine *B* from the same patient, you see two consecutive VPBs. The compensatory pause gives the P wave a chance to show up and identify the tachycardia as sinus with BBB and ventricular extrasystoles occasionally producing fusion.

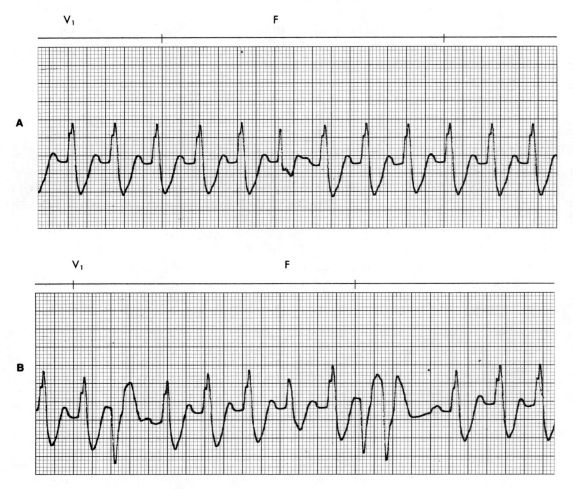

Fig. 13-15. A, A tachycardia (rate, 132/min) that was wrongly diagnosed as ventricular because of the fusion beat *(F)*. **B,** This tracing from the same patient establishes the tachycardia as sinus with BBB and frequent VPBs. A fusion beat *(F)* can also be seen.

Fusion with ventricular escape beats

Fig. 13-16, *A,* in both leads shows progressive slowing of the sinus rate until by the fourth complex a ventricular escape focus asserts itself at a rate of 48/min for three beats only. Then the SA node speeds up enough to recapture the ventricles. The first and third ectopic beats produce fusion complexes.

Fig. 13-16, *B,* begins with 2:1 AV block and ends with two idioventricular beats. The fourth beat in the strip is somewhat narrower than the idioventricular beats, is preceded by a P wave at a conductible interval, and is therefore a fusion beat.

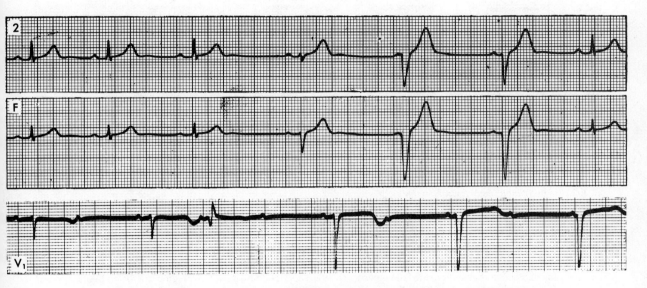

Fig. 13-16. Fusion with ventricular escape beats. **A,** In each strip the sinus rhythm slows and allows an idioventricular center to escape for three beats. The first and third of these escapes in each strip form fusion beats. **B,** The strip begins with 2:1 AV block (note the different PR intervals of the conducted beats—presumably type I block with RP-dependent PR intervals); then a ventricular extrasystole is followed by a longer cycle that enables an idioventricular pacemaker to escape. The first of the three escape beats is narrower than the last two, is preceded by a P wave at a conductible interval, and is clearly a fusion beat.

In Fig. 13-17 an idioventricular rhythm momentarily takes over because of a profound bradycardia secondary to 2:1 AV block. Note that the third and fourth beats in the top strip are fusion beats. Although the conducted pattern is LBBB, the fourth complex is actually normalized by the fusion—because the ectopic focus is on the same side as the BBB (see also Fig. 13-8).

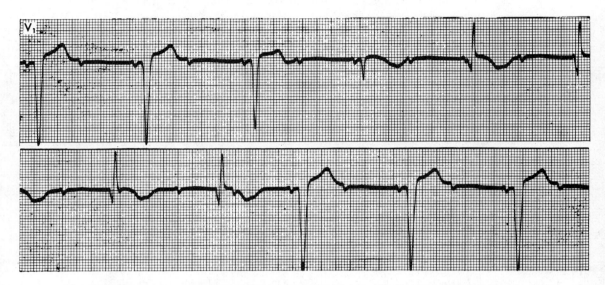

Fig. 13-17. The strips are continuous. The basic rhythm is sinus with AV block, probably type II, with 2:1 AV conduction and LBBB seen at the beginning of the top strip and in the second half of the bottom strip. The last two beats in the top strip and the first two in the bottom strip represent an idioventricular rhythm from the left ventricle. The third and fourth beats in the top strip are fusion beats (note the normalization of beat 4).

Fusion with paced beats

Artificial pacemakers are prolific factories of fusion beats, which may occur with both demand and fixed-rate pacemakers.

Fig. 13-18 shows a demand pacemaker producing fusion beats (*F*) as the sinus rhythm accelerates and takes control. When the sinus P wave emerges in front of the pacemaker spike, partial conduction occurs and fusion results.

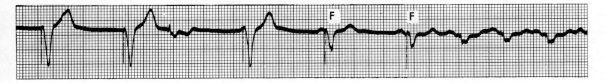

Fig. 13-18. Fusion between paced and sinus beats. In the second half of the strip a demand right ventricular pacemaker produces fusion with an accelerating sinus rhythm.

Fig. 13-19 shows a fixed-rate pacemaker ignoring and competing with the conducted sinus beats in the top strip; but toward the end of the bottom strip, fusion (*F*) finally occurs.

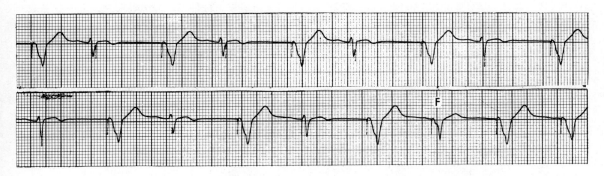

Fig. 13-19. The two strips are continuous. A fixed-rate right ventricular pacemaker beats relentlessly in competition with the sinus rhythm to produce a form of "escape-capture" bigeminy in the top strip. Toward the end of the bottom strip it at last achieves fusion (*F*).

Ventricular fusion in preexcitation

Although fusion is useful in the diagnosis of ventricular ectopy, it may also occur between two supraventricular impulses. In the presence of an accessory pathway (preexcitation), provided the orthodoxly conducted impulse reaches the ventricles before the accessory impulse has had time to activate the entire ventricular myocardium, the ventricular complexes will all be fusion beats.

In the bottom strip of Fig. 13-20 note the progressively widening QRS interval of the sinus beats, reflecting increasing degrees of preexcitation and resulting from changing contributions from each of the two wave fronts, both emanating from the SA node and reaching the ventricle via different pathways. Note that as the QRS broadens the PR shortens ("concertina" effect).

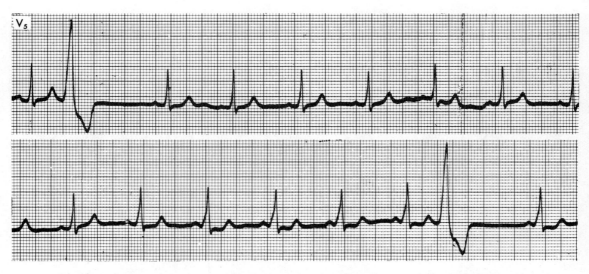

Fig. 13-20. The strips are continuous. Preexcitation syndrome interrupted by two ventricular extrasystoles. The "concertina" effect is seen at the beginning of the bottom strip, where the first three or four beats manifest progressive widening of the QRS with corresponding shortening of the PR.

Atrial fusion

When two impulses simultaneously invade the atria, atrial fusion results. This is most often seen when an accelerated junctional focus competes with the sinus rhythm. In such a case, if the junctional pacemaker sends its retrograde impulse into the atrium at the same time that the sinus impulse is also activating atrial muscle, an atrial fusion beat results (Figs. 13-21 and 13-22).

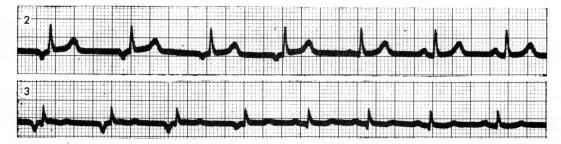

Fig. 13-21. In each lead a junctional rhythm with retrograde conduction shifts to sinus rhythm. In lead 2 the third, fourth, and fifth P waves are intermediate in form between retrograde and sinus Ps and presumably represent atrial fusion. In lead 3 only the fourth P wave is due to fusion.

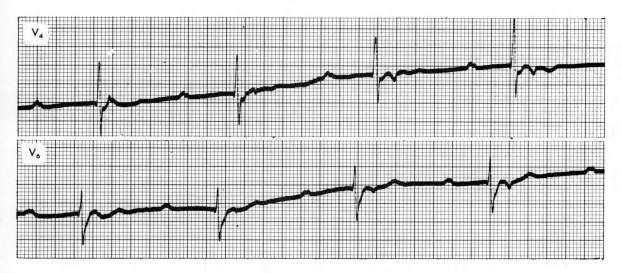

Fig. 13-22. Complete AV block, yet retrograde VA conduction occurs after the third and fourth beats in lead V_4 and after the fourth beat in V_6. Following the second QRS in V_4 and the second and third QRSs in V_6, sinus and retrograde P waves coincide to produce atrial fusion.

Atrial fusion may also be seen when an ectopic ventricular beat is followed by retrograde conduction to the atria at a time when the SA node has just discharged.

With an esophageal lead Kistin and Landowne[5] demonstrated that retrograde conduction to the atria was a common event following a ventricular extrasystole. They suggested that this is often missed in the clinical tracing because fusion produces a relatively isoelectric P wave.

References

1. Kistin, A.D.: Problems in the differentiation of ventricular arrhythmia from supraventricular arrhythmia with abnormal QRS, Prog. Cardiovasc. Dis. **9:**1, 1966.
2. Marriott, H.J.L., and others: Ventricular fusion beats, Circulation **26:**880, 1962.
3. Dressler, W., and Roesler, H.: The occurrence in paroxysmal ventricular tachycardia of ventricular complexes transitional in shape to sinoauricular beats. Am. Heart J. **44:**485, 1952.
4. Conover, M.B.: Understanding electrocardiography, ed. 3, St. Louis, 1980, The C.V. Mosby Co.
5. Kistin, A.D., and Landowne, M.: Retrograde conduction from premature ventricular contractions, a common occurrence in the human heart, Circulation **3:**738, 1951.

CHAPTER 14

Parasystole

Parasystole is an exquisitely simple arrhythmia, though usually classified as "complex." It has long been shrouded in an undeserved mystique that is immediately dispelled as soon as one realizes that its behavior is exactly like the behavior of the simplest of all pacemakers, the "fixed-rate."

The fixed-rate pacemaker fires regularly, regardless of the competitive sinus rhythm, because it cannot be shut off by a competing rhythm, with the result that the paced beats show a varying relationship to the sinus beats but are always a constant interval (or a multiple of that constant interval) from each other. The varying relationship to the dominant rhythm attests to one of its two cardinal characteristics, that it is *independent;* and the common denominator of the interectopic intervals declares that it is *undisturbable.* The only difference in the ECG between artificial (pacemaker) and natural parasystole is the "blip" that precedes and initiates all paced beats and, of course, also puts in lonely appearances whenever the pacemaker discharges during the refractory period of the ventricles.

Parasystole, then, is a rhythm in which the dominant pacemaker (usually sinus) coexists with, but never discharges, the ectopic pacemaker. Thus the ectopic focus maintains a fixed frequency independent of the normal pacemaker by virtue of some type of "protection," which may be loosely called *entrance block.*

In the context of parasystole, the term *exit block* describes the pathologic failure of an expected ectopic impulse to emerge from its focus of origin and propagate. Thus entrance block keeps extraneous impulses from invading and resetting the ectopic focus, and exit block limits the number of impulses propagated from the regularly firing ectopic pacemaker. Parasystole cannot exist unless the focus is protected by entrance block.

If the rate of the parasystolic focus is less than the sinus rate, it excites the heart only occasionally since only the impulses conducted to nonrefractory ventricles result in QRS complexes. If the rate of the focus were more than the sinus rate, the ventricular ectopic rhythm would dominate in the absence of exit block.

ECG criteria

Ventricular parasystole can be postulated in the presence of variable "coupling," interectopic intervals manifesting a common denominator, and (usually) fusion beats.

VARIABLE "COUPLING." Although the interval between the ectopic beat and the preceding beat of the dominant rhythm, often erroneously called the "coupling" interval, can vary, the term variable coupling is inappropriate. We shall continue to use it, however, since there is no acceptable pithy alternative. "Coupling" strictly refers to the interval between the dominant (usually sinus) beat and the coupled beat; and a coupled beat is one that is related to—dependent upon—the preceding beat to which it owes its existence. Since the quintessence of parasystole is *independence*, there is no coupling, constant or varying.

The ectopic impulse activates the ventricles if they are not refractory at the time of the parasystolic discharge. One should realize, however, as we shall later explain, that on rare occasions fixed "coupling" does not preclude a diagnosis of parasystole, any more than variable "coupling" proves parasystole. Exact coupling has been reported in arrhythmias assumed to be parasystolic[1-3]; and variable coupling is seen in those assumed to be supported by reentry.[4]

INTERECTOPIC INTERVALS. Interectopic intervals are simple multiples of a common denominator; that is, they reflect the cycle of the parasystolic focus although the QRS complexes themselves need not appear regularly. The times at which the parasystolic impulses activate the ventricles are not related to the sinus rhythm; however, they are related to each other, since the interval between any two parasystolic complexes depends upon the firing rate of the ectopic focus and therefore equals that interval or is some multiple of it. A play of ± 0.10 second is commonly allowed since the exit of the parasystolic impulse may occasionally be delayed because of refractoriness of the surrounding ventricular tissue due to the preceding sinus conducted impulse. In such a case the parasystolic impulse would be delayed in evoking a QRS complex because of local slow conduction.

Cranefield[13] also believes that entry block may be temporarily relieved because of summation (pp. 52-53). This would require that both ends of the depressed segment of tissue be activated simultaneously, evoking subthreshold action potentials. The two currents are then summated, reach threshold, and evoke an action potential that can propagate into the parasystolic focus and reset it.

FUSION BEATS. Fusion occurs between the dominant and the parasystolic impulses and is a mathematical certainty, eventually being seen if a long enough tracing is taken. Fusion beats are, however, not essential to the diagnosis. They occur when the fixed frequency of the parasystolic focus coincides with the activation of the ventricles by the sinus impulse.

We indicated earlier that a fixed-rate artificial pacemaker behaves just like a parasystolic focus. One is shown in Fig. 14-1 so that you can observe, as it were, the firing of the parasystolic focus and plot the interectopic intervals. It is easily appreciated in this tracing that the fusion beats *(F)* result from the simultaneous propagation within the ventricles of an ectopic impulse and a conducted sinus impulse.

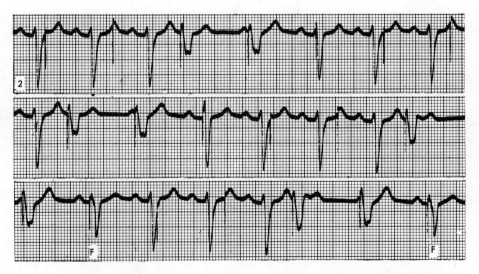

Fig. 14-1. The strips are continuous. Fixed-rate pacemaker for comparison with ventricular parasystole.

Note the parasystolic behavior of the fixed-rate pacemaker:

1. It is "protected," in the sense that nothing can shut it off.
2. Whenever its impulse falls at a time when the ventricles are responsive, a QRS accompanies the pacemaker blip.
3. Whenever it falls at a time when the ventricles are refractory, the blip appears but no ventricular complex results.
4. Therefore the longer interectopic intervals are multiples of the shortest interectopic interval; for example, in the second strip the long interectopic interval, 350, equals four times the shorter interval, 87 (hundredths of a second).
5. Whenever the artificial discharge coincides with sinus conduction into the ventricles, a fusion beat results (*F*).
6. Because parasystole represents an independent rhythm and is not beholden to the preceding beat, it will put in an appearance at varying intervals following the sinus beats (variable "coupling").

These six points are all characteristic of parasystole.

Parasystole is first suspected in the clinical tracing if ectopic beats show varying coupling intervals—as in Fig. 14-2, where the eye-catching feature is that the interval between the ectopic beat and the preceding sinus beat is never the same. It is a decided change from the exact coupling, thought to be due to reentry or afterpotentials, that characterizes unifocal extrasystoles.

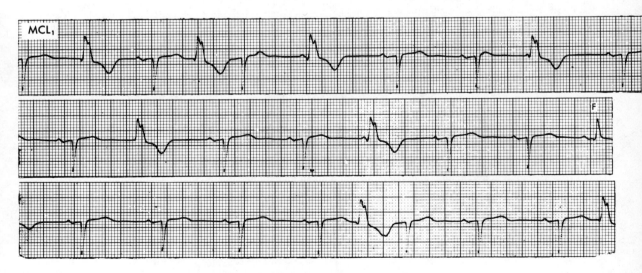

Fig. 14-2. Ventricular parasystole.

One then sets about demonstrating that the ectopic rhythm cannot be interrupted. This is accomplished by showing that the interectopic intervals have a common denominator. The first three ectopic beats in Fig. 14-2 indicate the shortest manifest interectopic intervals. They are 145 and 146 (hundredths of a second) respectively. All subsequent interectopic intervals are multiples of cycles between 143.5 and 156.5.

Fig. 14-3 illustrates the special pattern of fusion that occurs when, in the presence of BBB, the ectopic focus is on the same side as the BBB. Note that the third beat in the bottom strip looks remarkably normal. This is because the sinus impulse activated the unblocked ventricle while the ectopic impulse was simultaneously activating the side of the blocked branch, to produce a normally narrow QRS.

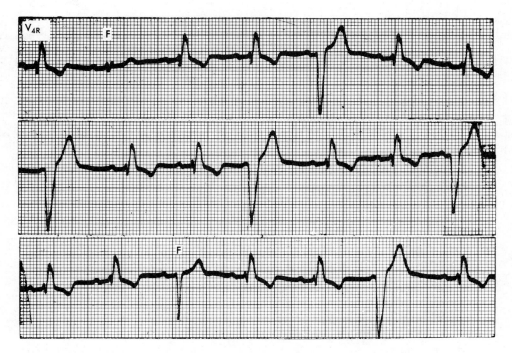

Fig. 14-3. The three strips are continuous and show a right ventricular parasystole competing with a sinus rhythm with RBBB.

Fig. 14-4 illustrates ventricular parasystole in the presence of atrial fibrillation. The diagnosis of fusion is made with less assurance in such a case since one never knows exactly when the next fibrillatory impulse is going to be conducted to the ventricles. However, in Fig. 14-4 it is reasonably certain that the third beat from the end of the second strip (*x*) is a fusion beat since, assuming parasystole, this is precisely where an ectopic beat was expected. It is therefore reasonable to conclude that the beat in question is mainly conducted from the fibrillating atria but contains a small distorting contribution from the ventricular ectopic focus.

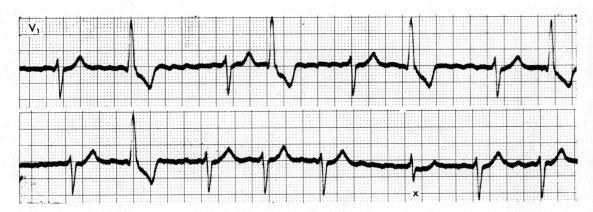

Fig. 14-4. Atrial fibrillation and parasystole.

Location of the ectopic focus

A parasystolic focus may be present in any part of the conductive system, and the morphology of the ectopic QRS will indicate whether the site of impulse formation is above or below the bifurcation of the His bundle.

Ventricular parasystole is more common and easier to diagnose than atrial or junctional parasystole because of the anomalous ventricular complex and because an atrial and possibly a junctional parasystolic discharge will interrupt and reset the sinus rhythm, producing what is called "reversed coupling."[5] This means that since the SA node is reset by the ectopic impulse the distance between the atrial or junctional parasystolic beat and the sinus P wave will be the same each time (exact coupling). However, instead of the usual situation in which the ectopic beat is coupled to the preceding sinus beat, the reverse is true; the sinus beat is "coupled" to the ectopic.

Fig. 14-5 shows an atrial parasystole. In *A* the parasystolic P waves are very similar to the sinus P waves. Note that the "coupling" interval between the atrial parasystolic beat and the preceding sinus P wave varies but that the interval between it and the following sinus P wave is identical in each case (reversed coupling). In this tracing the common denominator of the interectopic intervals is 56-57, making this a parasystolic tachycardia at a rate of 107/min with abundant exit block. In *B* you will note fusion beats. The "coupling" interval becomes longer and longer until the two impulses fuse within the atria.

In the presence of BBB, the parasystolic beats often arise on the side of the block and therefore have a shape characteristic of block of the opposite bundle branch[6] (Fig. 14-3). Some authorities[7-9] claim that the pathology responsible for the BBB also provides the conditions necessary for parasystole, that is, slightly to moderately injured Purkinje fibers with consequent enhancement of automaticity.[9]

This apparent relationship between BBB and parasystole might also explain the preponderance of ventricular parasystole over atrial and junctional and the common link between parasystole and organic heart disease.[7]

A

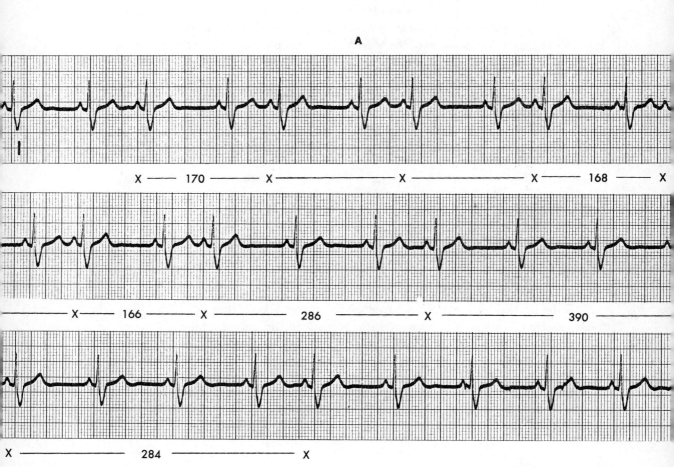

Fig. 14-5. A, Atrial parasystole with reversed coupling. Note that the atrial ectopic beats (very similar in shape to the sinus P waves) have an inconsistent relationship with the preceding sinus P wave but are precisely linked to the sinus P wave that follows. Since the common denominator for the interectopic intervals is 57, the rate of this atrial parasystolic focus is 107/min. (**A** and **B** courtesy Alan Lindsay, M.D., Salt Lake City.)

B

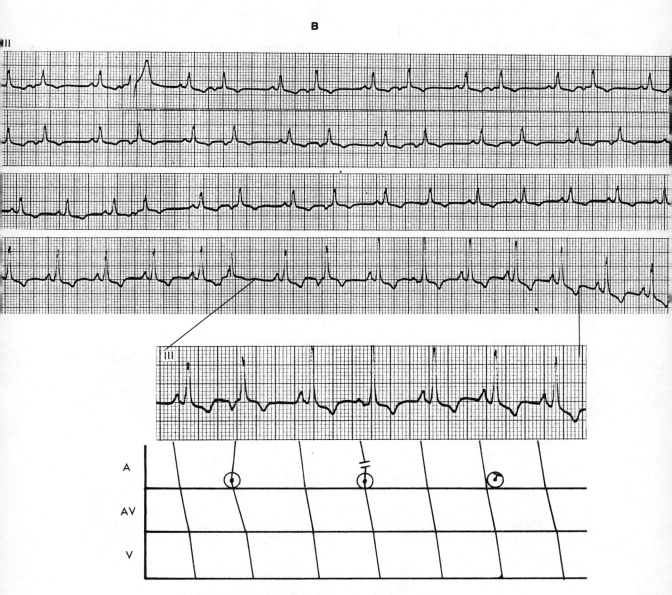

Fig. 14-5, cont'd. B, Atrial parasystole with fusion beats.

Mechanism of impulse formation

Phase 4 depolarization (automaticity) has been widely accepted as the mechanism responsible for the spontaneous impulse formation of parasystole.[10-12] This mechanism is operative without the need of a preceding impulse or extrinsic stimulation, and it thus fulfills the requirements for the independent impulse formation of the parasystolic rhythm.

Cranefield,[13] however, has another theory, which involves the creation of entrance block by some local depression resulting in one-way block: An automatic center thus is shielded from the sinus impulse so that the effect of overdrive suppression is withdrawn; that fiber may then become spontaneously active. If there is no exit block, a parasystolic rhythm would result. If the entrance block is resolved, the ectopic focus would be suppressed again by the sinus impulses and become latent.

Rate of discharge

The automatic discharge of ventricular parasystole is usually slow. Watanabe[6] reports the common range to be between 38 and 60/min. However, Scherf and Borneman[14] and Scherf and others[15] report that experimental ventricular parasystolic rates often reach 150 to 300/min. Clinically, supraventricular parasystole exhibits slower rates than those of ventricular parasystole, with the atrial variety even slower than the junctional.[15-17]

Mechanism of protection: entrance block

The concept of entrance block in parasystole was first introduced in 1912 by Fleming[18] and by Kaufmann and Rothberger,[19] who first defined parasystole and described its classical ECG criteria as we know them today. At this time a zone of unidirectional block surrounding the parasystolic focus was visualized and referred to as *Schutzblockierung*—"protective block." These same authors also postulated the possibility of a temporary loss of protection, thus implying what is known today as intermittent parasystole.[6,20-22]

In 1944 Vedoya[23] described the protection of parasystole in terms of two spherical zones, each having a different refractory period.

Scherf and Schott[24] in 1953 disagreed with the concept of a zone of unidirectional block completely surrounding the ectopic focus; they suggested that entrance block might be the result of disproportion between the excitability of the tissue surrounding the parasystolic focus and the strength of the sinus impulse, thus affording protection to the ectopic focus.

Since that time Singer[25] has suggested phase 4 block and Rosenbaum[9] a combination of phase 3 and phase 4 block as possible mechanisms.

Early studies by Scherf and Chick[26] suggested that the rapid rate of some parasystolic centers left the tissue surrounding it refractory. In these studies experimental parasystolic rates were as high as 300/min. Schamroth[27] also, independently, claimed that the "protection" enjoyed by a parasystolic focus was thanks to its own rapid discharge, its slow manifest rate being accounted for by a high-ratio (up to 9:1) exit block.

Finally, in 1973, Cranefield, Wit, and Hoffman[42] confirmed by microelectrode studies entrance block due to one-way block in depressed tissue. This concept is discussed in Chapter 3 (p. 52).

In the following paragraphs we describe in detail the other theories mentioned above: phase 4 depolarization, phase 3 and phase 4 depolarization, high-frequency discharge, and the electronic theory.

PHASE 4 DEPOLARIZATION.[25,28,29] This theory assumes that the mechanism responsible both for the activity of the ectopic focus and for its protection is phase 4 depolarization.

We know that the level of membrane potential at the time of excitation is among the variables that determine conduction velocity. Reduced membrane potentials exist during both phase 3 and phase 4 (see Chapter 11). If stimulation occurs during phase 4 in conjunction with a shift in the threshold potential toward zero and/or an impairment of membrane responsiveness, conduction disturbances can be expected. For example, if the threshold potential at the time of excitation is −60 instead of −70 mV, conduction is impaired or blocked altogether. Thus the ectopic focus would be surrounded with tissue in which there is an exit block that may become a two-way block. These facts could explain the intermittent nature of some parasystoles, in that any further enhancement of phase 4 depolarization (along with the shift in threshold potential and/or impairment of membrane responsiveness) could prevent propagation altogether; and by the same token, any reduction in phase 4 depolarization might permit the parasystolic beats to reappear because of a decrease in the degree of exit block.[25]

When phase 4 depolarization is not accompanied by such a shift in threshold potential and/or an impairment of membrane responsiveness, as would result from bradycardia, there is no significant conduction disturbance because the membrane potential at the time of excitation is normal.

If phase 4 depolarization exists in conjunction with impaired membrane responsiveness, irrespective of the threshold potential, the resulting action potential is reduced in V_{max} and dV/dt (the height and speed of the rise of phase 0). This results in decremental conduction, which may be enough to provide entrance or exit block.

PHASE 3 AND PHASE 4 DEPOLARIZATION. Rosenbaum and his group[9] have invoked both phase 3 and phase 4 as the mechanism of protection for the parasystolic focus—"perfect parasystole" having absolute protection and intermittent parasystole having a "window" of normal conduction through which the parasystolic focus can be invaded and reset.

These authors believe that the parasystolic focus is made up of a small group of moderately injured Purkinje fibers, or even a single fiber, in which phase 3 and phase 4 block each consecutively provides an entrance block through which no extraneous impulse may enter as long as there is no gap of normal conduction between the two phases. According to their tenet the critical factor determining the presence of parasystole is the duration of the period during which normal conduction can occur. If it is long, sinus impulses will repeatedly penetrate to discharge and reset the ectopic focus and the periods of protection will be limited (to the beginning and end of the parasystolic cycle). In such cases it would not be possible to document a parasystolic cycle.

With a greater degree of injury, protection of the focus may be absolute, producing two-way instead of one-way block (concealed parasystole).

To help visualize the parasystolic mechanism involving phase 3, phase 4, and a potential intermediate normal conduction range, Rosenbaum and others[30] have constructed an artificial parasystole that nicely illustrates two types of parasystole which deviate from the classical criteria.

Fig. 14-6 shows a parasystole in which the calculated ectopic cycles are not maintained with the expected regularity. In the top panel *P* represents the discharge rate of the parasystolic focus; at *X* the sinus impulse penetrates and resets this focus. Note that the sinus impulse penetrated before the refractory stage of phase 4 (dotted area) of the ectopic cycle was due to begin, squeezing in through a narrow range of normal conduction following phase 3 (squared area).

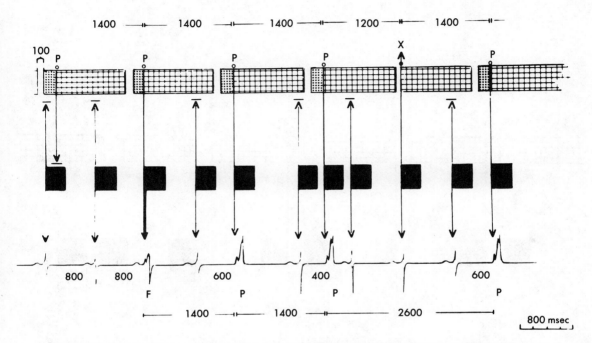

Fig. 14-6. "Artificial" ventricular parasystole. The squared bars represent the phase 3 block range of the parasystolic focus. The dotted bars represent the phase 4 block, which is always interrupted by a discharge of the parasystolic focus *(P)*. The interval between the phase 3 and phase 4 block ranges represents the opening of the parasystolic "accordion." The black bars represent the normal duration of refractoriness in the ventricular tissues around the parasystolic focus. *(F,* Fusion beat.) A sinus impulse may penetrate, discharge, and reset the parasystolic focus only when it falls during the intermediate normal conduction range, as in beat *X.* (From Rosenbaum, M.B., and others: In Wellens, H.J.J., Lie, K.I., and Janse, M.J., editors: The conduction system of the heart, Hingham, Mass., 1976, Martinus Nijhoff, Publishers.)

In Fig. 14-7, again in the top panel, note the discharge of the parasystolic focus (*P*). However, because of a broader gap of normal conduction and because of an ectopic rhythm that is harmonious with the sinus rhythm, every third sinus impulse penetrates and resets the parasystolic focus to produce a ventricular ectopic every third beat with the exact coupling intervals often thought to represent reentry or an afterpotential mechanism.

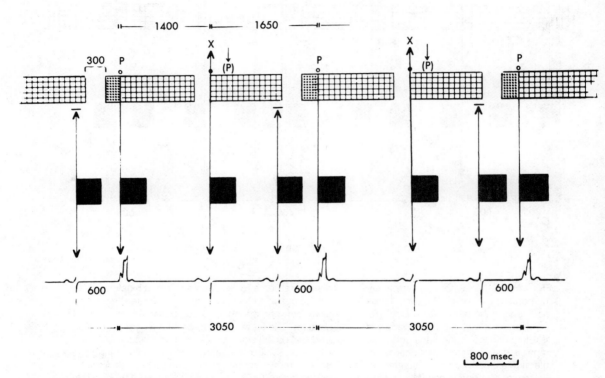

Fig. 14-7. Demonstration of how parasystole can give rise to a fixed coupling, if the variables of the model are properly adjusted. Symbols as in Fig. 14-6. (From Rosenbaum, M.B., and others: In Wellens, H.J.J., Lie, K.I., and Janse, M.J., editors: The conduction system of the heart, Hingham, Mass., 1976, Martinus Nijhoff, Publishers.)

In summary, according to Rosenbaum and colleagues,[30] the theory and clinical characteristics of parasystole can be reconciled as follows:

1. The parasystolic focus consists of a small group of slightly to moderately injured Purkinje fibers.
2. The rate of discharge of the parasystolic focus depends upon the degree of enhanced automaticity in the Purkinje fibers or injured fascicle.
3. Entrance block results from a combination of phase 3 and phase 4 block with a narrow, or absent normal conduction period between them. One-way block is common in phase 3 and also occurs during phase 4 if accompanied by slight hypopolarization and a shift of the threshold potential toward zero.

HIGH-FREQUENCY DISCHARGE FROM THE PARASYSTOLIC FOCUS.[14,15] Rapid impulse formation, keeping the focus almost continuously refractory, has been postulated as a mechanism of protection.[14,28,31-33] With rates of 150/min and above, exit block could be the explanation for the slow rates of most cases of parasystole.[14,33-35] Some investigators[36] do not support this theory because of the rare occurrence of manifest parasystolic tachycardia.

Scherf and Schott[24] suggest that entrance block may result from disproportion between the excitability of the surrounding tissue and the strength of the approaching sinus impulse.

THE ELECTRONIC THEORY.[37,38] Another possible explanation for the unusual finding of parasystole with fixed coupling is an electronic link across the zone of protection. Early studies demonstrating this electronic link were accomplished through computer model simulations[37,39,40] and were later confirmed in a biologic model.[38]

The electronic theory is based on the following premises:

1. The cycle length of a pacemaker can be altered by partial depolarization.
2. If this partial depolarization occurs early in phase 4 depolarization of the parasystolic focus, the next discharge will be delayed.[41]
3. If the partial depolarization occurs later in phase 4, the next expected discharge from the parasystolic focus will be early. This is because with the membrane potential closer to threshold potential an additional partial depolarization across the zone of protection would cause it to fire prematurely.[40]
4. In spite of the entrance block, the parasystolic focus is not entirely independent of the electrical influence surrounding it.
5. The parasystolic cycle may be modulated (prolonged or shortened) depending upon (a) the amplitude of the electronic events surrounding it and (b) the relationship of the two cycle lengths (parasystolic and sinus) to each other.

Thus the premise that the interectopic intervals are simple multiples of a common denominator clearly cannot be an obligatory feature of a parasystolic rhythm.[41]

EXIT BLOCK. In the presence of exit block no excitation of the heart from the parasystolic focus can arise. Exit block is therefore said to be present when an expected parasystolic impulse is not propagated even though the ventricles appear on the surface ECG to be nonrefractory. The concept of exit block has been experimentally confirmed time and again.[5,42-47]

Cranefield[13] proposes that the cause of exit block is concealed conduction in that the zone of protection around the parasystolic focus may be incompletely penetrated from both sides (the sinus conducted impulse and the parasystolic one). Every time a sinus impulse enters this zone but fails to traverse it, refractoriness is enhanced in the zone. Likewise every time a parasystolic impulse enters and is blocked, the same thing occurs. Therefore the period during which it is possible for an impulse to exit successfully from the zone surrounding the parasystolic focus may be shorter than appears on the surface ECG.

According to Cranefield[13] exit block may be relieved by a local increase in catecholamines, a local improvement in perfusion, sinus slowing, and summation.

The patterns of exit block that have been postulated are analogous to type I[5,38,48] and type II[5,8] second-degree AV block. First-degree and third-degree blocks would, of course, not be detected on the ECG.

Exceptions to the classical rules for parasystole

A diagnosis of parasystole is usually made when (1) there is no fixed coupling and (2) the interectopic intervals are simple multiples of a common denominator, implying an undisturbed cycle length. A diagnosis of parasystole may still be made even if all the classical criteria are not fulfilled.[5]

FIXED COUPLING IN PARASYSTOLE. If by chance rates of the parasystolic focus and the sinus node are mathematically related, fixed coupling may be seen.[1] For example, if the sinus rate is 70/min and the rate of the parasystolic focus is 35/min, there is a fixed relationship between the sinus beat and the parasystolic one, which is coincidental rather than real, and an ectopic beat will appear following every other normal beat at a fixed interval.

Supernormality is also recognized as a mechanism for fixed coupling in parasystole.[5,49-51] Fixed coupling may result when the impulse from the parasystolic focus is subthreshold and is effective only when it falls during the supernormal phase. An artificial example of fixed coupling due to supernormality can be seen in Fig. 14-8. A subthreshold fixed-rate pacemaker is firing at a regular rate throughout the tracing. It is effective only when it falls during the supernormal phase of excitability.

Reversed coupling and electronic influences have already been mentioned as possible causes of constant coupling in parasystole.

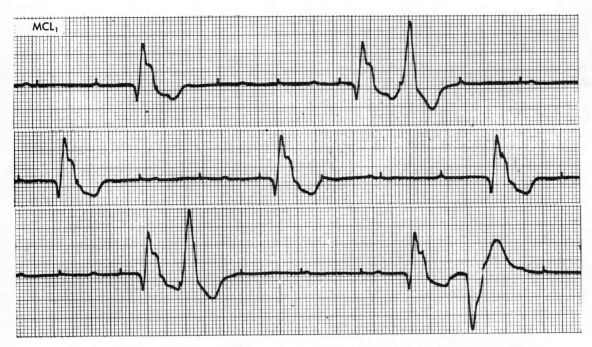

Fig. 14-8. Fixed coupling due to supernormality. In this tracing a subthreshold pacemaker is effective only when it fires during the supernormal period.

PAIRED ECTOPIC VENTRICULAR BEATS. Kuo and Surawicz[36] postulate that when paired ventricular ectopic beats are seen in parasystole the mechanism is that of reentry within the parasystolic focus or its vicinity. These authors noted that paired ventricular ectopic beats appeared more frequently in patients with no fixed coupling (presumably parasystole) than in those with fixed coupling.

Clinical significance of parasystole

Since parasystole is an independent, autonomous rhythm that cannot be interrupted, it follows that its impulses must (like the "blip" of a fixed-rate pacemaker) from time to time land on the T waves of the competitive sinus beats. Because of this inevitable R-on-T incidence, parasystole may be thought dangerous.

It is, however, an empiric observation that when a parasystolic impulse coincides with the T wave it seldom becomes a manifest beat. Moreover, there is no acceptable evidence that if parasystolic (automatic) beats arrive in the vulnerable period they will promote the same hazards as extrasystoles.

References

1. Langendorf, R., and Pick, A.: Parasystole with fixed coupling, Circulation **35**:304, 1967.
2. Levy, M.N., Lee, M.H., and Zieske, H.: Feedback mechanism responsible for fixed coupling in parasystole, Circ. Res. **31**:846, 1972.
3. Schamroth, L., and Marriott, H.J.L.: Intermittent ventricular parasystole with observations on its relationship to extrasystolic bigeminy, Am. J. Cardiol. **7**:799, 1961.
4. Mack, I., and Langendorf, R.: Factors influencing the time of appearance of premature systoles (including a demonstration of cases with ventricular premature systoles due to reentry but exhibiting variable coupling), Circulation **1**:910, 1950.
5. Pick, A.: The electrophysiologic basis of parasystole and its variants. In Wellens, H.J.J., Lie, K.I., and Janse, M.J., editors: The conduction system of the heart, Philadelphia, 1976, Lea & Febiger.
6. Watanabe, Y.: Reassessment of parasystole, Am. Heart J. **81**:451, 1971.
7. Pick, A.: Parasystole, Circulation **8**:243, 1953.
8. Rosenbaum, M.B., and others: Relationship between increased automaticity and depressed conduction in the main intraventricular conduction fascicles of the human and canine heart, Circulation **49**:818, 1974.
9. Rosenbaum, M.B., and others: The role of phase 3 and phase 4 block in clinical electrocardiography. In Wellens, H.J.J., Lie, K.I., and Janse, M.J., editors: The conduction system of the heart, Philadelphia, 1976, Lea & Febiger.
10. Hoffman, B.F., and Cranefield, P.F.: The physiological basis of cardiac arrhythmias, Am. J. Med. **37**:670, 1964.
11. Hoffman, B.F.: The electrophysiology of heart muscle and the genesis of arrhythmias. In Dreifus, L.S., and Likoff, W., editors: Mechanisms and therapy of cardiac arrhythmias, New York, 1966, Grune & Stratton, Inc.
12. Watanabe, Y., and Dreifus, L.S.: Newer concepts in the genesis of cardiac arrhythmias, Am. Heart J. **76**:114, 1968.
13. Cranefield, P.F.: The conduction of the cardiac impulse, Mount Kisco, 1975, Futura Publishing Co.
14. Scherf, D., and Bornemann, C.: Parasystole with a rapid ventricular center, Am. Heart J. **62**:320, 1961.
15. Scherf, D., and others: Parasystole, Am. J. Cardiol. **11**:527, 1963.
16. Scherf, D., Bornemann, C., and Yildiz, M.: AV nodal parasystole, Am. Heart J. **60**:179, 1960.
17. Eliakim, M.: Atrial parasystole, Am. J. Cardiol. **16**:457, 1965.
18. Fleming, G.G.: Triple rhythm of the heart due to ventricular extrasystoles, Q. J. Med. **5**:318, 1912.
19. Kaufmann, R., and Rothberger, C.J.: Beitrag zur Kenntnis der Entstellungsweise extrasystolischer Allorhythmien, Z. Ges. Exp. Med. **5**:3490, 1917; **7**:199, 1919; **9**:103, 1919; **11**:40, 1920; **13**:1, 1922.
20. Katz, L.N., and Pick, A.: Clinical electrocardiography. I. The arrhythmias, Philadelphia, 1956, Lea & Febiger.
21. Steffens, T.G.: Intermittent ventricular parasystole due to entrance block failure, Circulation **44**:442, 1971.
22. Cohen, H., Langendorf, R., and Pick, A.: Intermittent parasystole—mechanism of protection, Circulation **48**:761, 1973.
23. Vedoya, R.: Parasistolia, Buenos Aires, 1944, A. Lopez.
24. Scherf, D., and Schott, A.: Extrasystoles and allied arrhythmias, London, 1953, William Heinemann.
25. Singer, D.H., Lazzara, R., and Hoffman, B.F.: Interrelationships between automaticity and conduction in Purkinje fibers, Circ. Res. **21**:537, 1967.
26. Scherf, D., and Chick, F.B.: Experimental parasystole, Am. Heart J. **42**:212, 1951.
27. Schamroth, L.: Ventricular parasystole with slow manifest ectopic discharge, Br. Heart J. **24**:731, 1962.
28. Kao, C.Y., and Hoffman, B.F.: Graded and decremental responses in heart muscle fibers, Am. J. Physiol. **194**:187, 1958.
29. Van Dam, R.T., Moore, E.N., and Hoffman, B.R.: Initiation and conduction of impulses in partially depolarized cardiac fibers, Am. J. Physiol. **204**:1133, 1963.
30. Rosenbaum, M.B., and others: Paroxysmal atrioventricular block related to hypopolarization and spontaneous diastolic depolarization, Chest **63**:678, 1973.
31. Scherf, D., and others: Further studies on experimental parasystole and extrasystoles in groups, Proc. Soc. Exp. Biol. Med. **77**:28, 1951.

32. Chung, K.Y., Walsh, T.J., and Massie, E.: Ventricular parasystolic tachycardia, Br. Heart J. 27:392, 1965.
33. Delaye, J., Touboul, P., Delahaye, J.P., and Gonin, A.: Utilisation de la stimulation electrique endocavitaire dans le traitement des tachycardies ventriculaires, Arch. Mal. Coeur 63:205, 1970.
34. Watanabe, Y., and Dreifus, L.S.: Cardiac arrhythmias, New York, 1977, Grune & Stratton, Inc.
35. Rossi, P., Mololese, M., and Passaro, G.: Idioventricular parasystole with exit block in a subject with complete atrioventricular dissociation, Am. Heart J. 57:775, 1959.
36. Kuo, C.S., and Surawicz, B.: Coexistence of ventricular parasystole and ventricular couplets: Mechanism and clinical significance, Am. J. Cardiol. 44:435, 1979.
37. Moe, G.K., Jalife, J., Mueller, W.J., and Moe, B.: A mathematical model of parasystole and its application to clinical arrhythmias, Circulation 56:968, 1977.
38. Jalife, J., and Moe, G.K.: A biological model of parasystole, Am. J. Cardiol. 43:761, 1979.
39. Moe, G.K., Jalife, J., and Mueller, W.J.: Reciprocation between pacemaker sites. Reentrant parasystole. In Kulbertus, H.E., editor: Re-entrant arrhythmias: mechanisms and treatment, Baltimore, 1977, University Park Press.
40. Jalife, J., and Moe, G.K.: Effect of electronic potentials on pacemaker activity of canine Purkinje fibers in relation to parasystole, Circ. Res. 39:8101, 1976.
41. Weidmann, S.: Effect of current flow in the membrane potential of cardiac muscle, J. Physiol. (Lond.) 115:2277, 1951.
42. Cranefield, P.F., Wit, A.L., and Hoffman, B.F.: Genesis of cardiac arrhythmias, Circulation 47:190, 1973.
43. Cranefield, P.F., Klein, H.O., and Hoffman, B.F.: Conduction of the cardiac impulse. I. Delay, block, and one-way block in depressed Purkinje fibers, Circ. Res. 28:199, 1971.
44. Fisch, C., Greenspan, K., and Anderson, G.J.: Exit block, Am. J. Cardiol. 28:402, 1971.
45. Greenspan, K., Anderson, G.J., and Fisch, C.: Electrophysiologic correlate of exit block, Am. J. Cardiol. 28:197, 1971.
46. Hoffman, B.F.: The genesis of cardiac arrhythmias, Prog. Cardiovasc. Dis. 8:319, 1966.
47. Watanabe, Y.: Reassessment of parasystole, Am. Heart J. 81:451, 1971.
48. Langendorf, R., and Pick, A.: Mechanisms of intermittent ventricular bigeminy. II. Parasystole, and parasystole or re-entry with conduction disturbance, Circulation 11:431, 1955.
49. Soloff, I.A., and Fewell, J.W.: Supernormal phase of ventricular excitation in man: Its bearing on the genesis of ventricular premature systoles and a note on atrioventricular conduction, Am. Heart J. 59:869, 1960.
50. Spear, J.F., and Moore, E.N.: The effect of changes in rate and rhythm on supernormal excitability in the isolated Purkinje system of the dog. A possible role in re-entrant arrhythmias, Circulation 50:1144, 1974.
51. Pick, A., and Langendorf, R.: Parasystole and its variants, Med. Clin. North Am. 60:125, 1976.

CHAPTER 15

SA reentry, block, and sick sinus syndrome

SA node and perinodal fibers

The SA node is located superficially under the epicardium at the junction between the superior vena cava and the right atrium (Fig. 15-1). It is a crescent-shaped structure of specialized cells with a central body and tapering ends, and it may extend from epicardium to endocardium.

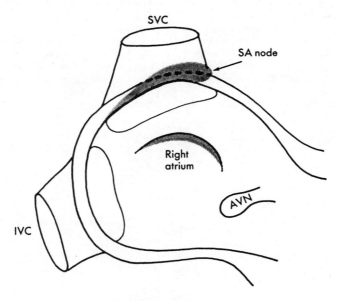

Fig. 15-1. The SA node.

The SA node is the dominant pacemaker of the heart because the maximal diastolic membrane potential is low (−60 mV) and phase 4 is steep. The means by which SA nodal cells depolarize and reach threshold (−30 to −40 mV) is discussed on p. 39.

Perinodal fibers with electrophysiologic characteristics distinct from those of atrial muscle and SA nodal cells have been found in the rabbit and are thought to be present in man.[1] Under pathologic conditions these fibers may act as a conduction barrier. It is known that conduction velocity in the sinus node and perinodal zone becomes slower and slower in response to more and more premature atrial extrasystoles, exhibiting behavior comparable to AV nodal tissue.[2] So it is that an atrial extrasystole may enter the perinodal zone and conduct slowly through it and the SA node, setting the scene for reentry. It may also rarely happen that the atrial extrasystole is early enough to arrive at the perinodal zone when the zone is in its absolute refractory period. In such a case the rhythm of the SA node remains undisturbed and the next sinus beat appears on time, resulting in an interpolated APB.

BLOOD SUPPLY. The blood supply to the SA node is from a large central artery with a rich supply of collateral vessels that are dense toward the center and thin out toward the periphery of the node. The large central SA node artery originates from the right coronary artery in 55% of cases and from the circumflex artery in 45% of cases. The disproportionately large size of the SA node artery is thought to be of physiologic importance[3,4] in that its perfusion pressure may affect the sinus rate.[5,6] Distention of the artery slows the sinus rate, whereas collapse causes an increase in rate.[2]

Role of the autonomic nervous system in SA node function

Parasympathetic and sympathetic influences modify the rate of spontaneous depolarization in the SA node as well as SA conduction time.

Vagal stimulation prolongs SA conduction time[6] and is thought to impede the normal falloff in K^+ conductance during phase 4[7-10] (the "pacemaker current"), causing sinus slowing, an increase in intranodal conduction time, and a lengthening of the effective and relative refractory periods of the SA node.[11]

Sympathetic stimulation shortens SA conduction time[2] and is thought to enhance the normal falloff in K^+ conductance during phase 4,[12] causing an increase in the sinus rate because of a steeper phase 4 depolarization.[10,13]

TEMPERATURE. Hypothermia inhibits the Na^+ pump, causing an accumulation of intracellular Na^+ and sinus slowing. Hyperthermia increases the sinus rate.

Paroxysmal sinus tachycardia due to SA nodal reentry

The possibility of reentry through the SA node as a cause of paroxysmal sinus tachycardia was first suggested in 1943[14] and conclusively documented by elaborate studies in the rabbit heart by Han, Malozzi, and Moe[15] in 1968. Experimental and clinical studies by others[16-25] have provided strong supportive evidence. Narula[20] in 1978 demonstrated SA nodal reentry to be the underlying mechanism in 8% of patients with PSVT. During programmed electrical stimulation of the heart the incidence ranged from 6% to 9.4% when a single atrial stimulus was introduced during the sinus rhythm.[22,23]

SA NODAL REENTRY MECHANISM. SA nodal reentry may develop without ectopic interference during a sinus rhythm or be initiated by an APB that arrives at the SA node before it has completely recovered excitability (during its relative refractory period). The premature impulse is then conducted slowly through the node and re-emerges to activate the atria in a normal manner. If the impulse then reactivates the incompletely recovered node, travels slowly through it, and again emerges, a reentry circuit is established (Fig. 15-2). Although reentry seems a likely mechanism, it is also possible that such a tachycardia could be caused by triggered activity from cells in the vicinity of the SA node.

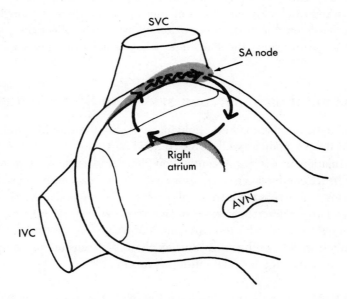

Fig. 15-2. SA nodal reentry.

The paroxysmal tachycardia resulting from SA reentry usually has a rate between 100 and 150/min, less than that of an AV reciprocating tachycardia.[21] It may go unnoticed by the patient, although in one study more than half the subjects complained of palpitations.

ECG FEATURES. This arrhythmia consists of what appears to be an inappropriate sinus tachycardia with sudden onset and ending. The P waves are usually similar to, but not always identical with, the sinus P waves and tend to precede rather than follow the QRS complexes.[26] Most attacks do not last longer than 10 to 20 beats[27]; but they are repetitive and sensitive to changes in autonomic tone, including those changes associated with normal breathing,[24] making distinction from sinus arrhythmia sometimes impossible.

Fig. 15-3 is an example of repetitive paroysmal sinus tachycardia. Most attacks go unnoticed or are only slightly bothersome. Others can cause angina, breathlessness, and syncope, especially when associated with heart disease and the sick sinus syndrome.[27]

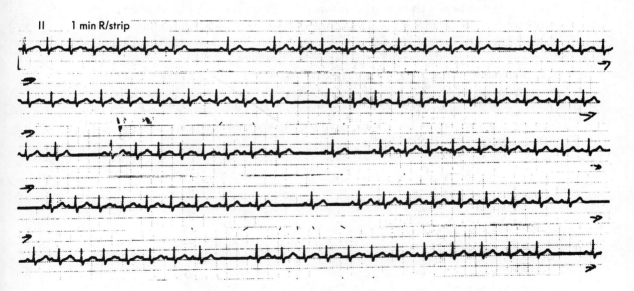

Fig. 15-3. Repetitive paroxysmal sinus tachycardia. (From Curry, P.V.L., and Shenasa, M.: In Mandel, W.J., editor: Cardiac arrhythmias; their mechanisms, diagnosis, and management, Philadelphia, 1980, J.B. Lippincott Co.)

.SA block

SA block is exit block and occurs between the actual discharge of the SA node and the arrival of the impulse in atrial tissue. The conduction barrier is assumed to be in the perinodal zone and the block may be first, second, or third degree.

FIRST-DEGREE SA BLOCK. First-degree SA block is, of course, concealed since the actual firing of the SA node is not seen on the surface ECG and since all impulses are conducted at a fixed interval. Uncomplicated first-degree SA block in the ECG is indistinguishable from normal sinus rhythm.

SECOND-DEGREE SA BLOCK. Second-degree SA block may be either type I or type II and is comparable to its second-degree AV block counterpart.

Type I. In type I second-degree SA block (sinus Wenckebach) there is progressive lengthening of SA conduction time until finally a sinus beat is not conducted to the atria. Since the sinus discharge is a silent event, this arrhythmia can be inferred only because of a dropped beat and the effect of the lengthening SA conduction times on the PP intervals. All the signs of AV Wenckebach except, of course, the lengthening PR intervals are present: (1) group beating, (2) shortening PP intervals, and (3) pauses that are less than twice the shortest cycle.

Fig. 15-4 is an example of SA Wenckebach with a 4:3 conduction ratio. Note the three above-mentioned clues to its diagnosis. The PR intervals are fixed, normal, and constant unless there is also a defect in AV conduction. The group beating is immediately apparent. The PP intervals shorten in classical Wenckebach fashion because the greatest increment in conduction time takes place between the first and the second beat. The pause of the dropped beat is less than two of the basic sinus cycles since conduction out of the SA node is better after the dropped beat than before it. Therefore the lengthened cycle is equal to two sinus cycles minus the conduction decrement out of the SA node. The cycle may be even further shortened if it ends with an escape beat (Fig. 15-5).

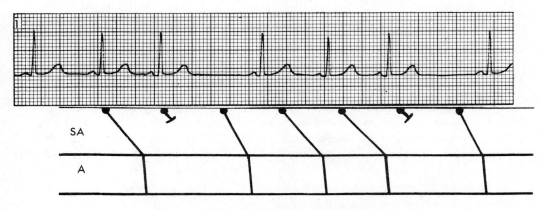

Fig. 15-4. Repeated 4:3 sinus Wenckebach periods.

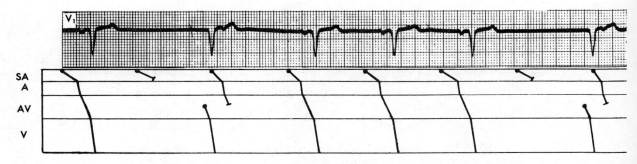

Fig. 15-5. Type I second-degree SA block producing a 5:4 Wenckebach. The two longer cycles of the dropped beats end with junctional escape beats (see laddergram).

Type II. In type II SA block there are dropped P waves without previous progressive prolongation of conduction times and therefore without progressive shortening of PP intervals. The cycle of the dropped P wave is exactly equal to two of the basic sinus cycles, as illustrated in Fig. 15-6.

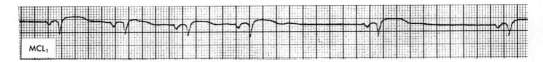

Fig. 15-6. Type II second-degree SA block. The longer cycles equal exactly two of the basic sinus cycles.

Sometimes two or more consecutive sinus impulses are blocked within the SA node, creating considerably longer pauses. In Fig. 15-7, *A*, the first pause equals four sinus cycles and the second equals three. In *B* the long pause is interrupted by a junctional escape beat, probably without retrograde penetration of the SA node, since the long PP interval equals exactly 4 sinus cycles. This implies an uninterrupted constant discharge rate with exit block.

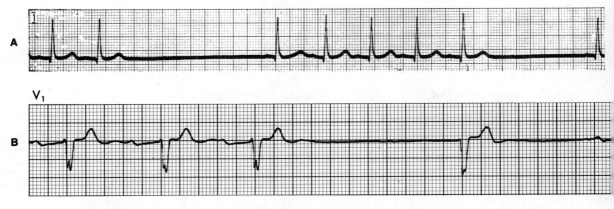

Fig. 15-7. A, Type II second-degree SA block. The first pause equals four sinus cycles (4:1 exit block), and the second pause equals three (3:1 exit block). **B,** Type II second-degree SA block with 4:1 exit block. The long pause is interrupted by a junctional escape beat without retrograde conduction to the atria.

THIRD-DEGREE SA BLOCK. Third-degree SA block is usually compensated by an atrial escape rhythm. With complete block in SA conduction there are no sinus P waves, although the SA node continues to discharge at regular intervals. This cannot be differentiated clinically from sinus arrest, which is a total cessation of impulse formation within the SA node.

Sick sinus syndrome

HISTORY. As early as 1827 Adams,[30] and then Stokes[31] two decades later, described syncopal attacks in patients with permanent bradycardia. In 1954[32] Short presented the diverse clinical picture of SA nodal dysfunction in his classical paper on the syndrome of alternating bradycardia and tachycardia. The catchy alliterative title of *sick sinus syndrome* was coined by Lown[33] in 1967, was later popularized by Ferrer[34,35] and by Rubenstein and others,[36] and was first used to characterize the situation following cardioversion for atrial fibrillation when there was unstable SA activity in the form of sinoatrial arrest or exit block.

Since that time many additional terms have been applied when SA nodal dysfunction is coupled with cerebral dysfunction, including "inadequate sinus mechanism," "sluggish sinus syndrome,"[37] "lazy sinus syndrome," and "sinoatrial syncope."[38]

ETIOLOGY. Sick sinus syndrome is usually encountered in the elderly although it may be seen at any age, even in children and adolescents.[39-42] It is the result of a combination of abnormalities of the SA node itself (automaticity and SA conduction) and interdependence between these intrinsic properties and extrinsic factors such as the integrity of the autonomic nervous system, endocrine system, atrial muscle, and blood supply to the SA node.

Although sick sinus syndrome is most commonly idiopathic, it has been described as being drug induced and in association with infiltrative disorders such as coronary atherosclerosis, atrial amyloidosis, diffuse fibrosis, collagen vascular disease, infectious processes, and pericardial disease.

During the acute stage of inferior and lateral wall myocardial infarction, sick sinus syndrome may be seen, especially in the form of profound sinus bradycardia or even sinus arrest.[43-45] It is not known whether this is secondary to ischemia or local edema or is the result of autonomic neural influences.

ECG MANIFESTATIONS. Some of the ECG manifestations of sick sinus syndrome
are

1. Sinus bradycardia that is persistent, severe, intermittent, or inappropriate
2. Sinus arrest with or without a new pacemaker arising
3. SA block
4. Failure of the sinus rhythm to follow termination of any supraventricular arrhythmia, whether the termination is spontaneous or electrically induced
5. Chronic atrial fibrillation with persistent slow ventricular rate, in the absence of bradycrotic drugs
6. Alternating bradycardia and tachycardia (bradycardia-tachycardia syndrome)

Many patients with sick sinus syndrome may also have BBB and AV conduction
abnormalities in the form of first-degree or second-degree AV block with prolonged
AH interval.[46,47]

Fig. 15-8 illustrates SA nodal dysfunction in the form of the bradycardia-tachycardia syndrome. The first part of the tracing shows atrial fibrillation. When the
paroxysm of atrial fibrillation ceases, a long pause ensues before the AV junction
escapes.

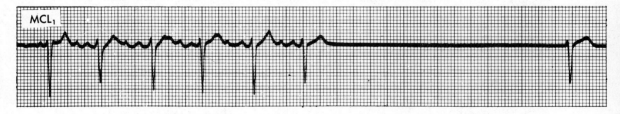

Fig. 15-8. Sick sinus syndrome in the form of a bradycardia-tachycardia syndrome.

Bradycardia-tachycardia is a freqent manifestation of the sick sinus syndrome; atrial tachycardia and atrial fibrillation are more frequently observed than atrial flutter. Other rhythms seen are accelerated junctional rhythm and AV nodal reentry tachycardia. These tachycardias terminate spontaneously. The response of the SA node and subsidiary pacemakers to this overdrive suppression is exaggerated, leaving the patient with a long period of asystole or bradycardia that may result in syncope.

Fig. 15-9 shows an unusual form of sick sinus. The top strip portrays a relatively excitable node beating at a rate of about 125/min. Yet, within a few seconds, the SA node becomes remarkably depressed and for several seconds perpetrates an irregular but marked bradycardia.

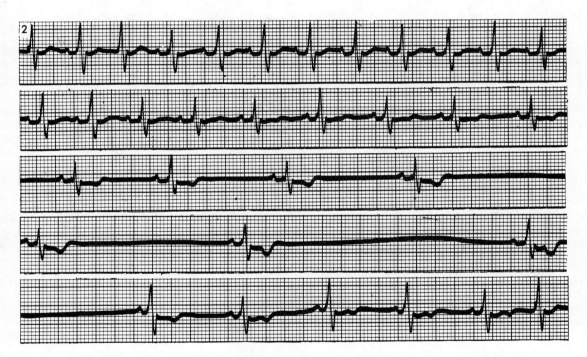

Fig. 15-9. The strips are continuous. Marked variation in rate manifested by a sick sinus node; soon after manifesting an excitable rate of about 125/min, it rapidly slows to reach a maximal cycle length of 3 seconds (= rate of 20/min).

Fig. 15-10 illustrates a sick sinus syndrome in the form of a marked and inappropriate sinus arrhythmia. The top tracing shows a rather consistent sinus rate of 98/min. Only a few seconds later there is a marked sinus arrhythmia with a cycle of almost 3 seconds in the bottom strip.

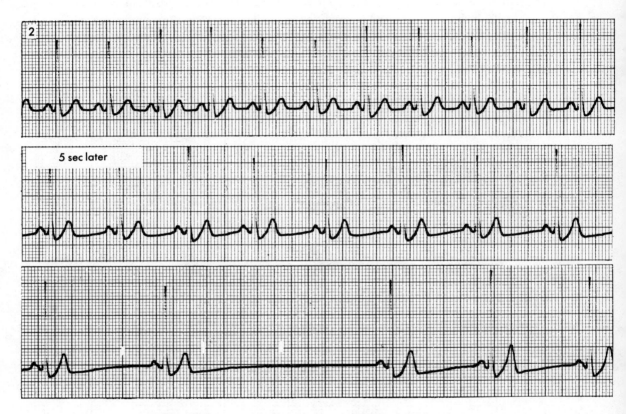

Fig. 15-10. Sick sinus syndrome in the form of a marked sinus arrhythmia.

In Fig. 15-11 there is an inappropriate overdrive suppression following an atrial premature beat.

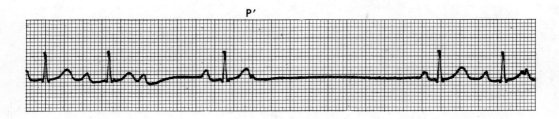

Fig. 15-11. Sick sinus syndrome with inappropriate overdrive suppression following an early APB (in the T before the pause). This patient also had AV and SA Wenckebach periods.

References

1. James, T.N., and Nadeau, R.A.: Sinus brady-cardia during injections directly into the sinus node artery, Am. J. Physiol. **204:**9, 1963.
2. Jordan, J.L., and Mandel, W.J.: Disorders of sinus function. In Mandel, W.J., editor: Cardiac arrhythmias; their mechanisms, diagnosis, and management, Philadelphia, 1980, J.B. Lippincott Co.
3. James, T.N.: Pulse and impulse formation in the sinus node, Henry Ford Hosp. Med. J. **15:**275, 1967.
4. Brooks, C.M., and others: Effects of localized stretch of the sinoatrial node region of the dog heart, Am. J. Physiol. **211:**1197, 1966.
5. Lang, G., and others: Effect of stretch on the isolated cat sinoatrial node, Am. J. Physiol. **211:**1192, 1966.
6. Brasil, A.: Autonomic sinoatrial block: a new disturbance of the heart mechanism, Arg. Bras. Cardiol. **8:**159, 1955.
7. West, T.C.: Ultramicroelectrode recording from the cardiac pacemaker, J. Pharmacol. Exp. Ther. **115:**283, 1955.
8. Harris, E.J., and Hutter, O.F.: The action of acetylcholine on the movements of potassium ions in the sinus venosus of the heart, J. Physiol. **133:**58, 1956.
9. Trautwein, W., Kuffler, S.W., and Edward, C.: Changes in membrane characteristics of heart muscle during inhibition, J. Gen. Physiol. **40:**135, 1956.
10. Musso, E., and Vassalle, M.: Inhibitory action of acetylcholine on potassium uptake of the sinus node, Cardiovasc. Res. **9:**490, 1975.
11. Hutter, O.F., and Trautwein, W.: Vagal and sympathetic effects on the pacemaker fibers in the sinus venosus of the heart, J. Gen. Physiol. **39:**715, 1956.
12. Tsien, R.W.: Effects of epinephrine on the pacemaker potassium current of cardiac Purkinje fibers, J. Gen. Physiol. **64:**293, 1974.
13. Kassebaum, D.G.: Membrane effects of epinephrine in the heart. In Krays, O., and Kovarikova, A., editors: Second International Pharmacologic meeting. Vol. 5. Pharmacology of cardiac function, Oxford, 1964, Pergamon Press.
14. Barker, P.S., Wilson, F.N., and Johnson, F.D.: The mechanism of auricular paroxysmal tachycardia, Am. Heart J. **26:**435, 1943.
15. Han, J., Malozzi, A.N., and Moe, G.K.: Sino-atrial reciprocation in the isolated rabbit heart, Circ. Res. **22:**355, 1968.
16. Hoffman, B.F., and Cranefield, P.F.: Electrophysiology of the heart, New York, 1960, McGraw-Hill Book Co.
17. Paulay, K.L., Varghese, P.I., and Damato, A.N.: Sinus node re-entry: an in vivo demonstration in the dog, Circ. Res. **32:**455, 1973.
18. Coumel, P., Attuel, P., and Flammang, D.: The role of the conduction system in supraventricular tachycardias. In Wellens, H.J.J., Lie, K.I., and Janse, M.J., editors: The conduction system of the heart, Philadelphia, 1976, Lea & Febiger.
19. Narula, O.S.: Sinus node reentry: mechanism of supraventricular tachycardia (SVT) in man [Abstract], Circ. Res. **32:**455, 1973.
20. Narula, O.S.: Sinus node reentry: a mechanism for supraventricular tachycardia, Circulation **50:**1114, 1974.
21. Paulay, K.L., Varghese, P.J., and Damato, A.N.: Atrial rhythms in response to an early atrial premature depolarization in man, Am. Heart J. **85:**323, 1973.
22. Wellens, H.J.J.: Role of sinus node re-entry in the genesis of sustained cardiac arrhythmias. In Bonke, F.I.M., editor: The sinus node: structure, function, and clinical relevance, The Hague, 1978, Martinus Nijoff.
23. Curry, P.V.L., Evans, T.R., and Krikler, D.M.: Paroxysmal reciprocating tachycardia, Eur. J. Cardiol. **6:**199, 1977.
24. Allessie, M.A., and Bonke, F.I.M.: Re-entry within the sino-atrial node as demonstrated by multiple micro-electrode recordings in the isolated rabbit heart. In Bonke, F.I.M., editor: The sinus node: structure, function, and clinical relevance, The Hague, 1978, Martinus Nijoff.
25. Narula, O.S.: Paroxysmal supraventricular tachycardia due to sinus node and intra-atrial reentry. In Narula, O.S., editor: Cardiac arrhythmias, Baltimore, 1979, The Williams & Wilkins Co.
26. Wu, D., and others: Clinical, electrocardiographic, and electrophysiologic observations in patients with paroxysmal supraventricular tachycardia, Am. J. Cardiol. **41:**1045, 1978.
27. Curry, P.V.L., and Shenasa, M.: Atrial arrhythmias: clinical concepts. In Mandel, W.J.,

editor: Cardiac arrhythmias, their mechanisms, diagnosis, and management, Philadelphia, 1980, J.B. Lippincott Co.

28. Reiffel, J., Gliklich, J., Gang, E., Weiss, M., Davis, J., and Bigger, J.T., Jr.: Human sinus node electrograms: transvenous catheter recorded technique and normal sinoatrial conduction times in adults [Abstract], Circulation **60** (suppl. II):63, 1979.

29. Hariman, R.J., Krongrad, E., Boxer, R.A., Bowman, F.O., Jr., Malm, J.R., and Hoffman, B.F.: Methods for recording electrograms of the sinoatrial node during cardiac surgery in man, Circulation **61**:1024, 1980.

30. Adams, R.: Cases of disease of the heart, Dublin Hosp. Rep. **4**:353, 1827.

31. Stokes, W.: Observations on some cases of permanent slow pulse, Dublin J. Med. Sci. **2**:73, 1846.

32. Short, D.S.: The syndrome of alternating bradycardia and tachycardia, Br. Heart J. **16**:208, 1954.

33. Lown, B.: Electrical reversion of cardiac arrhythmias, Br. Heart J. **29**:469, 1967.

34. Ferrer, M.I.: Electrocardiographic notebook, ed. 4, Mt. Kisco, N.Y., 1974, Futura Publishing Co.

35. Ferrer, M.I.: The sick sinus syndrome, Circulation **47**:635, 1973.

36. Rubenstein, J.J., Schulman, C.L., Yurchak, P.M., and DeSanctis, R.W.: Clinical spectrum of the sick sinus syndrome, Circulation **46**:5, 1972.

37. Tabatznik, B., Mower, M.M., Samson, E.B., and Prempree, A.: Syncope in the "sluggish sinus node syndrome" [Abstract], Circulation **40** (suppl. III):200, 1969.

38. Easley, R.M., and Goldstein, S.: Sino-atrial syncope, Am. J. Cardiol. **50**:166, 1971.

39. Bharati, S., Nordenberg, A., and others: The anatomic substrate for the sick sinus syndrome in adolescence, Am. J. Cardiol. **46**:163, 1980.

40. Radford, D.J., and Izukawa, T.: Sick sinus syndrome: symptomatic cases in children, Arch. Dis. Child. **50**:879, 1975.

41. Radford, D.J., and Izukawa, T.: Sick sinus syndrome in children, Arch. Dis. Child. **51**:100, 1976.

42. Yabeck, S.M., Swensson, R.E., and Jarmakani, J.M.: Electrocardiographic recognition of sinus node dysfunction in children and young adults, Circulation **56**:235, 1977.

43. Haden, R.F., and others: The significance of sinus bradycardia in acute myocardial infarction, Dis. Chest **44**:168, 1963.

44. Adgey, A.J.J., and others: Incidence, significance, and management of early bradyarrhythmia complicating acute myocardial infarction, Lancet **2**:1097, 1968.

45. Rokseth, R., and Hattle, L.: Sinus arrest in acute myocardial infarction, Br. Heart J. **33**:639, 1971.

46. Narula, O.S., Samet, P., and Javier, R.P.: Significance of the sinus node recovery time, Circulation **45**:140, 1972.

47. Gupta, P.K., and others: Appraisal of sinus nodal recovery time in patients with sick sinus syndrome, Am. J. Cardiol. **34**:265, 1974.

CHAPTER 16

Aberrant ventricular conduction

Aberrancy, the *temporary* abnormal intraventricular conduction of supraventricular impulses, was first described in 1910 by Sir Thomas Lewis.[1] He picturesquely stated: "I term the . . . beats aberrant because they are caused by impulses which have gone astray." Since that time "aberrancy," "aberrant ventricular conduction," and "ventricular aberration" have become interchangeable terms.

The clinical importance of aberration is that it widens the QRS complex and so simulates ectopic ventricular mechanisms; and this importance looms especially large in the differential diagnosis of the wide-QRS tachycardias.

Mechanism

We have already discussed the mechanism of aberration at length in Chapter 11 on phase 3 and phase 4 block. Phase 3 aberration is related to a shortening of the cardiac cycle; phase 4 aberration is associated with prolongation of the cardiac cycle. This chapter deals with phase 3 aberration, the most common form of which is RBBB.

Briefly the mechanism of phase 3 aberration consists of an impulse arriving in the bundle branches when one bundle branch can conduct and the other cannot. The BBB may be complete or incomplete depending upon the degree of repolarization. For example, if the impulse arrives when the membrane potential in the right bundle branch is only −50 mV, complete RBBB will result. However, if the membrane has repolarized to −60 or −65 mV, conduction may be only slowed rather than blocked, producing an incomplete RBBB.

Aberrant patterns

Wellens and co-workers[3] found that out of 70 episodes of aberration, 69% were RBBB. Others[4,5] have reported the incidence of RBBB aberration to be as high as 80% to 85%. In a relatively sick population, as in a coronary care facility, LBBB aberration assumes greater prominence and accounts for perhaps a third of the aberrant conduction encountered. Wellens and co-workers[3] found 31% to be LBBB aberration. In the study by Kulbertus and others[6] RBBB accounted for a smaller than expected proportion of the aberration produced experimentally whereas left posterior hemiblock occurred with surprising frequency. By inducing premature atrial beats in 44 patients, they were able to produce 116 aberrant configurations (Table 16-1).

Table 16-1. *Relative frequency of experimental aberration*

	Percent	
RBBB	24	i.e.:
RBBB + LAHB	18	RBBB = 52%
LAHB	15	LAHB = 33%
RBBB + LPHB	10	LPHB = 19%
LPHB	9	LBBB = 14%
LBBB	9	
ILBBB	5	
Trivial changes	6	
Marked anterior displacement	4	

From Kulbertus, H.E., and others: Br. Heart J. **38:**549, 1976.

ECG diagnosis

Sometimes the morphology of the aberrant complex is indistinguishable from an ectopic pattern; but at other times the aberrant shapes provide broad hints of their supraventricular origin. Morphology, especially when it includes signs such as the axis and the R:S ratio in V_6, may also point to ventricular ectopy. The heart rate during the tachycardia and the width of the QRS complex have also been found to contribute to the differential diagnosis.[3]

In 1965 and 1970 the classical RBBB pattern in V_1 (rSR′) was described[4,7] as being 10:1 in favor of aberration. This was later confirmed with His bundle electrocardiography by Vera and co-workers[8] and by Wellens and others,[3] who reported odds of 24:1 and 16:1 respectively.

In 1969 Rosenbaum[9] pointed out that right ventricular ectopy could be confidently diagnosed when there was a combination of a LBBB pattern in V_6 together with a wide r wave (>0.03 sec) in V_1 and right axis deviation in the limb leads. This was also later confirmed by Wellens.[10]

In 1972 Vera and others[8] used His bundle electrography to examine 1100 abnormal QRS complexes (750 ectopic, 350 aberrant) in patients with chronic atrial fibrillation. V_1 was found to be the most helpful lead in differentiating aberration from ectopy, the rSR′ pattern affording 24:1 odds in favor of aberration. These investigators also found that a monophasic R or a qR in V_1 favored ectopy 9:1 (later confirmed by Wellens and associates[3] with 12:1 odds). In the same study[8] previous findings[4] favoring ectopy were confirmed, that is, bizarre QRS axis (−90 to −180 degrees) and concordancy of the precordial leads. Of little diagnostic value in this study were coupling intervals, bigeminal rhythms, long-short cycle sequence, and a long pause following the anomalous beat.

In 1970 one of us[7] reported on the studies conducted by Gozensky and Thorne, which were later published by them,[11] describing the now widely accepted "rabbit ears" as an aid in distinguishing ventricular ectopy from aberration. Their findings were later confirmed by Wellens and co-workers,[3] who found their "rabbit ear" configuration (first peak taller than second in V_1) only in patients with ventricular tachycardia. However, in the Wellens study this configuration was seen in only 7 out of 65 cases of ventricular tachycardia with predominantly positive complexes in V_1.

The distinction between right ventricular ectopy and LBBB aberration has always been more difficult than between left ectopy and RBBB aberration. In their study of right ventricular ectopic beats, Swanick and co-workers[12] observed a number of helpful clues:

1. Two thirds of the observed examples of right ventricular ectopic beats had a negative QRS in lead I, a polarity that was not found in any of the LBBB patterns examined.
2. One third of the right ventricular ectopic beats had an initial r wave in V_1 that measured 0.04 second or more whereas only 3% of the LBBBs had this "fat" initial r wave.
3. More than half of the right ventricular ectopics had a more deeply negative QRS complex (QS or rS) in V_4 than in V_1 whereas only 6% to 7% of the examples of LBBB manifested a similar V_4/V_1 relationship.

Thus the presence of a negative QRS in lead I, a "fat" initial r in V_1, and a QRS in V_4 deeper than in V_1, singly or collectively, favor the diagnosis of ventricular ectopy rather than aberrancy.

SUMMARY: ABERRANCY VERSUS ECTOPY. The 1978 findings of Wellens and associates[3] are summarized below and in Tables 16-2 and 16-3.

Table 16-2. *Findings of Wellens and associates*[3,3a]

Complex	V₁	Aberrant	Ventricular tachycardia
1		—	15
2		11	17
3		19	3
4		38	3
5		—	7
6		1	16
7		—	4
		$\overline{69}$	$\overline{65}$

Table 16-3. *Findings of Wellens and associates*[3,3a]

Complex	V$_6$	Aberrant	Ventricular tachycardia
1		44	3
2		21	15
3		4	27
4		—	16
5		—	3
6		—	1
		$\overline{69}$	$\overline{65}$

1. A *heart rate* of >170/min in patients with predominantly positive QRS complexes in V_1 favored aberration. In ventricular tachycardia the heart rate was most frequently between 130 and 170/min. When the heart rate is greater than 220/min and irregular with wide uniform QRS complexes, one must immediately consider atrial fibrillation with aberrant conduction over an accessory pathway.
2. *AV dissociation* during the tachycardia favored ventricular ectopy. Dissociation is recognized by finding independent P waves, hearing varied intensity of the first heart sound, and observing irregular-occurring cannon waves in the jugular pulse.
3. *Ventricular rhythm* was usually regular in ventricular tachycardia (in 55 out of 70 cases [79%]). When it is irregular, one must differentiate between ventricular tachycardia and atrial fibrillation with aberrant conduction.
4. A *QRS width* of greater than 0.14 second was highly suggestive of ventricular ectopy (seen in 70% of the examples of ventricular tachycardia). A QRS width of only 0.12 second favored aberrant conduction (all patients with aberrant conduction had a QRS width of 0.14 sec or less). *Exception:* Patients with established BBB during sinus rhythm are likely to have QRS complexes of greater than 0.14 second during a supraventricular tachycardia.
5. A *left axis deviation and an R:S ratio of less than 1 in* V_6 strongly supported a diagnosis of ventricular ectopy.
6. A *monophasic R or qR in* V_1 suggested ventricular ectopy (Table 16-2).
7. A *classic rSR' RBBB pattern in* V_1 (complex 4 in Table 16-2) was highly suggestive of aberrant conduction, especially when combined with a narrow q wave in leads I and V_6 (complex 1 in Table 16-3). However, ventricular ectopy was favored when this pattern was combined with *left axis deviation and an R:S of less than 1 in lead* V_6.

8. *Triphasic and M-shaped patterns in* V_1 other than the classical RBBB configuration are found in both aberration and ectopy (complex 3 in Table 16-2). When combined with left axis deviation and an R:S of less than 1 in V_6, ventricular ectopy was favored.

9. The *taller left "rabbit ear"*[11] (predominantly positive QRS in V_1 with the first peak taller than the second) was seen only in ventricular tachycardia (complex 5 in Table 16-2).

10. A *concordant precordial pattern* (entirely upright or entirely negative QRS from V_1 to V_6) was seen in only 2 out of 62 patients with ventricular tachycardia, but never with aberration.

11. When the QRS complexes were LBBB shaped, no differences were observed in configuration between supraventricular and ventricular tachycardia in V_1. However, an initial fat r wave suggested a ventricular origin.[9,10]

12. In V_6 *a QS or QR* strongly suggested ventricular ectopy (complexes 4 and 5 in Table 16-3).

To illustrate the value of QRS morphology in the differential diagnosis of a wide-QRS tachycardia, Fig. 16-1 presents a junctional tachycardia—due to digitalis intoxication—with RBBB aberration. The rSR' pattern is virtually diagnostic of the supraventricular origin of the tachycardia (with odds of at least 16:1).

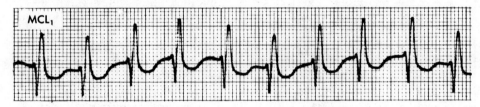

Fig. 16-1. Junctional tachycardia with RBBB aberration. Note the sagging ST segment due to digitalis.

On the other hand, Fig. 16-2 presents a pattern in V_1 that by itself is not diagnostic. It could be supraventricular with RBBB aberration or it could be a left ventricular tachycardia. However, even in a nonclassical RBBB pattern such as this the width of the QRS (0.12 sec) and the heart rate of greater than 170/min favor a diagnosis of supraventricular tachycardia with aberration. In this case V_6 is also available, demonstrating a qRs configuration giving 15:1 odds in favor of aberration. The narrow little q wave reflects normal septal activation, the tall thin R wave normal left ventricular activation, and the terminal s wave the late activation of the right ventricle expected in RBBB. This patient turned out to have a junctional tachycardia.

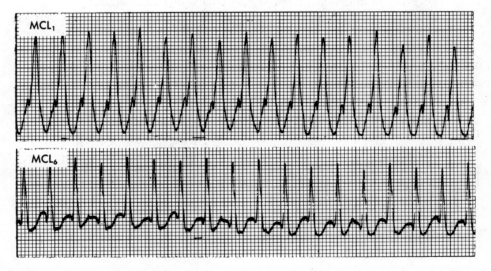

Fig. 16-2. A tachycardia not identifiable as supraventricular from the shape of the complex in MCL₁, but readily recognized in a left chest lead by its triphasic contour.

Other signs favoring aberrancy

In addition to morphology, other signs favoring aberration are as follows: preceding atrial activity and, to a much lesser extent an initial deflection identical with that of conducted beats (if RBBB), and an anomalous second-in-the-row beat.

PRECEDING ATRIAL ACTIVITY. Sometimes the diagnosis of aberration depends upon the recognition of P waves preceding the abnormal ventricular complex. Figs. 16-3 and 16-4 illustrate runs of tachycardia containing broad complexes whose shape is not the slightest use in distinguishing between ventricular tachycardia and supraventricular tachycardia with aberration, although the width of the QRS in both tracings points to aberration. The P′ waves are clearly visible before the aberration sets in.

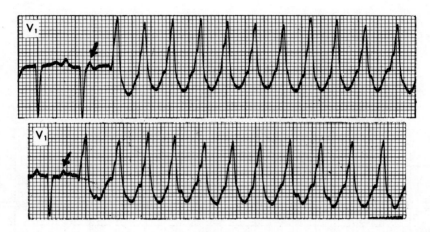

Fig. 16-3. Supraventricular tachycardia with RBBB aberration. P′ waves are clearly visible at the onset of the tachycardia and clinch the diagnosis.

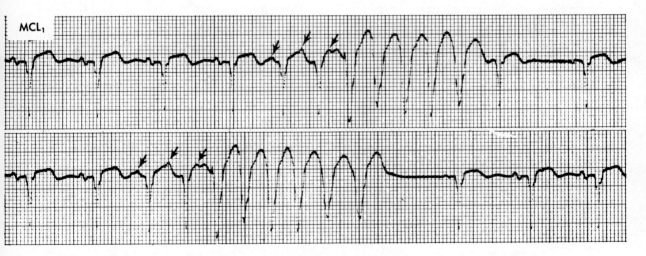

Fig. 16-4. Each strip contains a brief run of supraventricular tachycardia with LBBB aberration. The diagnosis is made because of antecedent P′ waves, the width of the QRS (0.12 sec) and the rate (200 beats/min). Note the momentary shift of pacemaker following each burst of tachycardia—the returning P wave differs from the sinus P waves.

Fig. 16-5 shows another tracing in which the diagnosis of aberration is mainly dependent upon preceding atrial activity. In each of the three strips the second in a row of rapid beats is anomalous. Is it an aberrant complex because it ends a suddenly shorter cycle or is it a ventricular extrasystole initiating a run of reciprocating tachycardia in the AV junction? The QRS morphology is of no assistance; but the T waves preceding the anomalous complexes, if carefully compared with the T waves of the other sinus beats, all contain a distortion—a superimposed P′ wave, which confirms aberration.

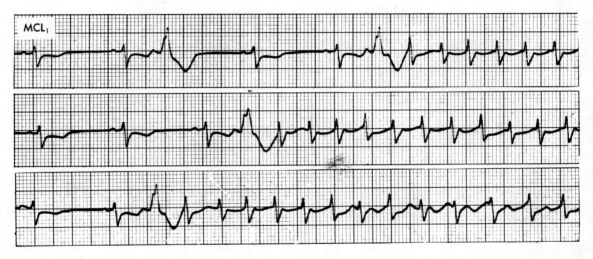

Fig. 16-5. Morphologically the anomalous beats in each strip could be either ectopic ventricular or aberrant. On three occasions they usher in a run of supraventricular tachycardia and so could be aberrant (second in the row) or ventricular extrasystoles initiating runs of reciprocating tachycardia. The differentiation is made by observing the slightly positive deformity (P′ waves) preceding each anomalous beat and not seen superimposed on the T waves of the isolated sinus beats.

INITIAL DEFLECTION IDENTICAL WITH THAT OF CONDUCTED BEATS. This rule applies only to RBBB aberration because the initial forces in uncomplicated RBBB are normal (septal) and are best seen in V_1 and in the lateral leads, I, aVL, and V_6. Fig. 16-6 contains both right and left BBB aberration. Note that the initial deflections of the RBBB aberration are almost the same as the sinus conducted beats whereas those of the LBBB aberration are not. The presence of P′ waves in front of the anomalous complexes secures the diagnosis of aberration.

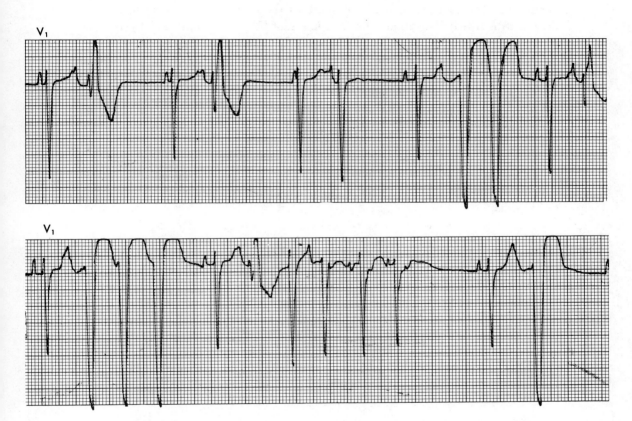

Fig. 16-6. The strips are not continuous. Right and left bundle-branch block aberration. When the aberration is RBBB, the initial deflection is often identical with that of the conducted sinus beats.

SECOND-IN-THE-ROW ANOMALY. The reason the second in a row of rapid beats is most likely to be aberrant is that it is the only beat that ends a relatively short cycle preceded by a relatively long one. The duration of the action potential and hence the refractory period are directly related to the cardiac cycle. As the cycle lengthens or shortens, so does the refractory period (this is reflected in the QT interval, which shortens as the heart rate increases).

Fig. 16-7 illustrates short bursts of supraventricular tachycardia in which only the first beat of the tachycardia (second in the row, counting the preceding sinus beat) is anomalous. The first premature beat shortens the cycle, causing itself to be conducted with RBBB aberration. Then the aberrant beat itself ends a relatively short cycle, giving the next beat a better chance of being conducted normally. Unfortunately, by the "rule of bigeminy,"[13] a lengthened cycle tends to precipitate a VPB and therefore the longer-shorter cycle sequence is inconclusive and the morphology and presence of a P′ wave preceding the onset of tachycardia are clearly of more help in making the diagnosis of aberration (as illustrated in Fig. 16-7). In Fig. 16-8 the alternative mechanism—a VPB initiating a run of reciprocating tachycardia in the AV junction—is diagrammed.

In this tracing the second in the row is also anomalous. However, the morphology of the anomalous beat (RS) and the absence of visible ectopic atrial activity strongly support a diagnosis of a ventricular extrasystole initiating a run of AV reciprocating tachycardia.

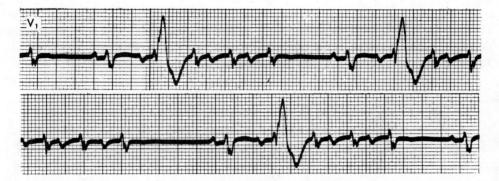

Fig. 16-7. The strips are continuous. Three short bursts of supraventricular tachycardia in which only the first beat (second in the row) develops ventricular aberration.

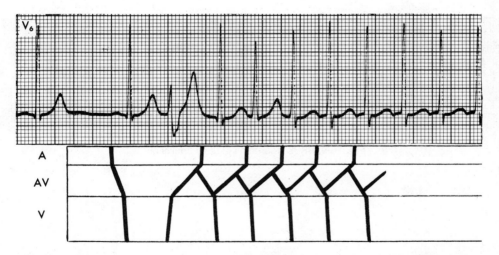

Fig. 16-8. Here the second in the row of rapid beats may be, and is diagrammed as, a ventricular extrasystole initiating a run of AV reciprocating tachycardia.

Aberrancy in atrial fibrillation

Since there is always preceding atrial activity in atrial fibrillation, one relies heavily on morphology, a reliance justified by the His bundle studies of Vera and co-workers[8] in 1972, who found the classical RBBB pattern in V_1 to be 24:1 in favor of aberration.

In Fig. 16-9, *A*, there is a single anomalous beat, a classical RBBB pattern with initial deflection the same as the normally conducted complexes, and a QRS width of only 0.12 second—all signs in favor of aberration. In Fig. 16-9, *B*, there is a run of RBBB aberration and two isolated RBBB complexes.

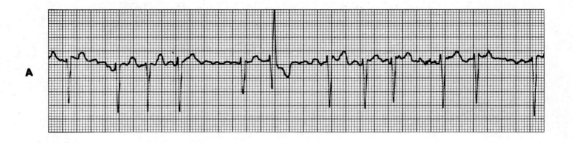

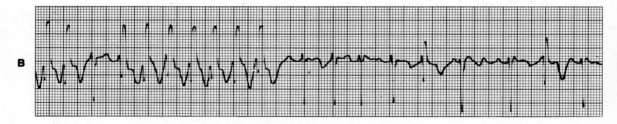

Fig. 16-9. RBBB aberration in atrial fibrillation.

ASHMAN'S PHENOMENON. In 1947 Gouaux and Ashman[5] said "aberration occurs when a short cycle follows a long one because the refractory period varies with cycle length." With a long cycle the refractory period lengthens; thus an impulse ending a short cycle preceded by a long one is more likely to encounter refractory tissue. This is most certainly an accurate statement; however, its application in atrial fibrillation is precarious since, because of concealed conduction, one never knows from the surface ECG exactly when a bundle branch is activated. It is known that the rampant electrical activity incompletely penetrates the bundle of His and bundle branches (concealed conduction) and that the irregular ventricular rhythm during atrial fibrillation is one result. This is why there are often pauses longer than the actual refractory period of the AV conduction system. Therefore, if an aberrant beat does end a long-short cycle sequence during atrial fibrillation, it may be due to refractoriness of a bundle branch secondary to concealed conduction into it rather than to changes in the length of the ventricular cycle. Note that in over 400 cases of atrial fibrillation and 1100 anomalous beats Vera and associates[8] did not find the long-short phenomenon to be helpful in the differential diagnosis between aberration and ectopy.

An equally important point establishing the invalidity of applying Ashman's phenomenon to atrial fibrillation is the "rule of bigeminy,"[13] which states that a long cycle tends to precipitate a VPB. Thus a long-short sequence ending with an anomalous beat is of no distinguishing value.

Fig. 16-10 shows an example of atrial fibrillation complicated by a rapid ventricular response (about 160/min). Toward the middle of the top strip four beats are conducted with RBBB aberration. Although the morphology of these anomalous beats may be either aberrant or ectopic (Table 16-1), a width of only 0.10 second in the QRS supports a diagnosis of aberration. The temptation is to misdiagnose and mistreat this short run of apparent ventricular tachycardia; but if this temptation is yielded to, the result can be similar to the effect on the patient in Fig. 16-11. The proper treatment aims at restoring a normal ventricular rate—the golden rule of antiarrhythmic therapy—and it applies whether the anomalous beats are aberrant or, in fact, ectopic ventricular. In either situation the four available options are digitalis, propranolol, verapamil, or cardioversion. In this case the bottom strip in Fig. 16-10 illustrates the prompt effect of 0.75 mg of digoxin intravenously.

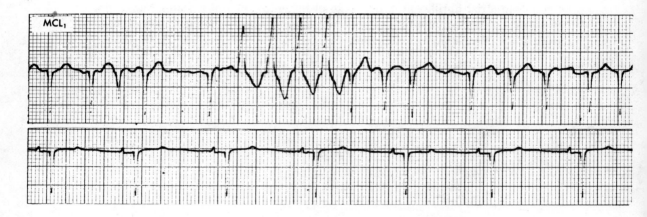

Fig. 16-10. The top strip shows atrial fibrillation with rapid ventricular response complicated by a four-beat run of aberrant conduction of RBBB type. The bottom strip was taken 30 minutes after 0.75 mg of digoxin was given intravenously.

Aberrancy in other arrhythmias

ATRIAL TACHYCARDIA. Fig. 16-11 illustrates aberration that was misdiagnosed and thus led to gross mismanagement. The top strip shows the patient's rhythm on admission: atrial tachycardia with 2:1 AV conduction (note the nonconducted P wave partially hidden in the QRS). This patient was started on digitalis and by the next morning (second strip) frequently manifested 4:1 conduction ratios. Because of this satisfactory "impairment" of conduction, digitalis was discontinued and quinidine started. The bottom strip was taken the following morning and shows the situation that developed at about midnight and led to night-long erroneous therapy for ventricular tachycardia; the bottom strip, in fact, represents atrial tachycardia with 1:1 AV conduction and RBBB aberration. The quinidine—perhaps partly by its antivagal effect but certainly through its slowing effect on the atrial rate (from 210 to 192/min)—enabled the AV junction to conduct all the ectopic atrial impulses. The resulting much-increased ventricular rate (from approximately 90 to 192/min) produced a dangerous hypotension from which the patient was finally rescued with the combination of pressor agent and countershock.

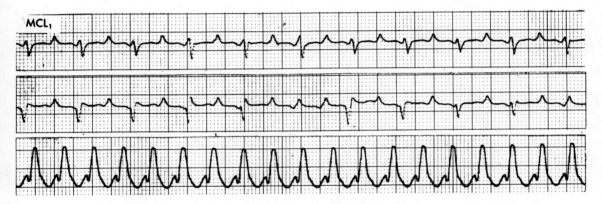

Fig. 16-11. The strips are not continuous. Top strip (on admission) shows atrial tachycardia with 2:1 AV conduction. Middle strip (next day) shows 2:1 and 4:1 conduction. Bottom strip (24 hours later) shows a slower atrial rate with 1:1 conduction and RBBB aberration—mistaken and treated for hours as ventricular tachycardia.

In 1958 Rosenblueth[14] documented the effect of atrial rate on normal AV conduction by pacing the atria of normal dogs. He found that at an average rate of 257 the animals developed Wenckebach periods and began to drop beats; and at an average rate of 285 they developed constant 2:1 conduction. Consider what this means in terms of ventricular rate. At an atrial rate of 286 the ventricular rate is 143. If the atrial rate slows by only 30 beats/min (to 256), conduction will be 1:1 with a ventricular rate of 256/min. Thus, with slowing of the atrial rate by only 30 beats/min, the ventricular rate increases by 113 beats/min. This is why it can be so dangerous to give atrial-slowing drugs such as lidocaine, quinidine, or even procainamide in the presence of atrial flutter or fibrillation when the ventricular response is already uncomfortably fast.[15] For example, if atrial flutter at a rate of 300 is associated with a 2:1 response, producing a ventricular rate of 150, and a drug such as lidocaine is administered, the atrial rate may slow to 250 and AV conduction may increase to 1:1, producing a dangerous ventricular rate of 250.

ATRIAL FLUTTER. From a therapeutic point of view an important form of aberration may complicate atrial flutter. Uncomplicated and untreated atrial flutter usually manifests a 2:1 AV conduction ratio. If digitalis or propranolol is then administered, the conduction pattern often changes to alternating 2:1 and 4:1, producing alternately longer and shorter cycles (Fig. 16-12). At this stage the beats that end the shorter cycles may develop aberrant conduction (Fig. 16-12); and if the patient is receiving digitalis, ventricular bigeminy secondary to digitalis toxicity is likely to be diagnosed. The drug is then wrongfully discontinued when, in fact, the situation calls for more digitalis to reduce conduction still further to a constant 4:1 and a *normal ventricular rate*—always the immediate goal of therapy.

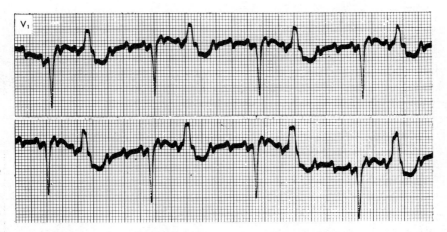

Fig. 16-12. Atrial flutter with alternating 2:1 and 4:1 conduction and RBBB aberration of the beats that end the shorter cycles—readily mistaken for ventricular bigeminy.

ALTERNATING ABERRANCY. It is not uncommon to see both right and left bundle branch aberration in the same patient. This is the case in Figs. 16-6 and 16-13. An interesting feature in each of these tracings is the abrupt switch from one BBB form of aberration to the other after a single intervening normally conducted beat. The mechanism of this phenomenon is unexplained but is sufficiently characteristic to assist in differentiating bilateral aberration from bifocal ectopy.

It is of interest that the first example of ventricular aberration to be published (Lewis, 1910[1]) was alternating aberration complicating atrial bigeminy (Fig. 16-14). Fig. 16-15 illustrates a contemporary example of similar alternating aberration.

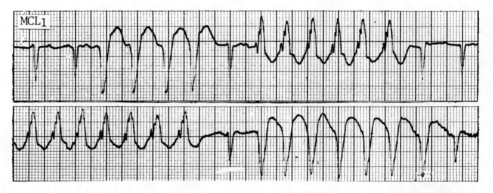

Fig. 16-13. Both strips illustrate the abrupt change from one BBB aberration to the other BBB, with a single intervening normally conducted beat.

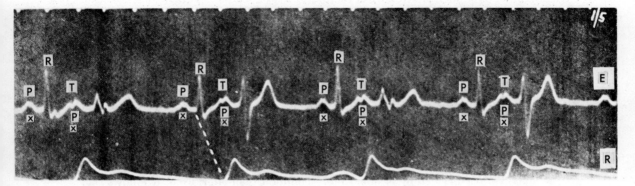

Fig. 16-14. The first example of ventricular aberration to be published (Lewis, 1910). Sinus rhythm with atrial bigeminy; each extrasystole is conducted aberrantly, but the form of aberration alternates.

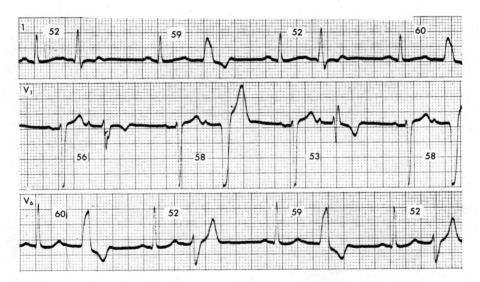

Fig. 16-15. Sinus rhythm with atrial bigeminy. The shorter extrasystolic cycles end in some form of RBBB aberration, whereas the longer ones end with LBBB aberration. The beats with RBBB, as evidenced by the slightly increased height of the R waves in lead I and the rS pattern in V_6, presumably manifest bifascicular aberration (RBBB + left anterior hemiblock). In V_1 the first atrial extrasystole shows only the earliest sign of RBBB, namely notching of the terminal upstroke.

Clinical implications

RBBB aberration is considered by many to be often physiologic (secondary to tachycardia or sudden shortening of the cycle). Phase 4 and/or LBBB aberration, on the other hand, are thought to indicate underlying cardiac disease. Whatever the cause, aberration is always secondary to another primary disturbance and of itself never requires treatment.

For the following reasons it is important to recognize ventricular aberration:

1. *It may be mistaken for ventricular ectopy*, causing unnecessary drugs to be given; or less commonly ectopy may be mistaken for aberration, with the result that therapeutic drugs are withdrawn.
2. *It may mask atrial ectopy* and thus, in the setting of acute myocardial infarction (MI), may deprive the clinician of a valuable clue to the onset of congestive heart failure, electrolyte imbalance, and/or oxygen deprivation.

Since ventricular ectopy is much more common than aberration, it follows that aberration should be diagnosed *only when there is positive evidence in favor of it*.

References

1. Lewis, T.: Paroxysmal tachycardia, the result of ectopic impulse formation, Heart 1:262, 1910.
2. Lewis, T.: Observations upon disorders of the heart's action, Heart 3:279, 1912.
3. Wellens, H.J.J., Bar, F.W.H.M., and Lie, K.I.: The value of the electrocardiogram in the differential diagnosis of a tachycardia with a widened QRS complex, Am. J. Med. 64:27, 1978.
3a. Wellens, H.J.J., and others: Medical treatment of ventricular tachycardia: considerations in the selection of patients for surgical treatment, Am. J. Cardiol. 49:187, 1982.
4. Sandler, I.A., and Marriott, H.J.L.: The differential morphology of anomalous ventricular complexes of RBBB type in lead V_1: ventricular ectopy versus aberration, Circulation 31:551, 1965.
5. Gouaux, J.L., and Ashman, R.: Auricular fibrillation with aberration simulating ventricular paroxysmal tachycardia, Am. Heart J. 34:366, 1947.
6. Kulbertus, H.E., and others: Vectorcardiographic study of aberrant conduction, Br. Heart J. 38:549, 1976.
7. Marriott, H.J.L.: Differential diagnosis of supraventricular and ventricular tachycardia, Geriatrics 25:91, 1970.
8. Vera, Z., Cheng, T.O., Ertem, G., Shoalehvar, M., Wickramasekaran, R., and Wadhwa, K.: His bundle electrography for evaluation of criteria in differentiating ventricular ectopy from aberrancy in atrial fibrillation, Circulation 46 (suppl. II):90, 1972.
9. Rosenbaum, M.B.: Classification of ventricular extrasystoles according to form, J. Electrocardiol. 2:269, 1969.
10. Wellens, H.J.J.: Personal communication, August, 1978.
11. Gozensky, C., and Thorne, D.: Rabbit ears: an aid in distinguishing ventricular ectopy from aberration, Heart Lung 3:634, 1975.
12. Swanick, E.J., LaCamera, F., and Marriott, H.J.L.: Morphologic features of right ventricular ectopic beats, Am. J. Cardiol. 30:888, 1972.
13. Langendorf, L.R., Pick, A., and Wintermitz, M.: Mechanisms of intermittent bigeminy. 1. Appearance of ectopic beats dependent upon the length of the ventricular cycle, the "rule of bigeminy," Circulation 11:422, 1955.
14. Rosenblueth, A.: Two processes for auriculoventricular and ventriculo-auricular propagation of impulses in the heart, Am. J. Physiol. 194:495, 1958.
15. Marriott, H.J.L., and Bieza, C.F.: Alarming ventricular acceleration after lidocaine administration, Chest 61:682, 1972.

CHAPTER 17

AV block

Everyone at all conversant with the language of cardiology is familiar with the conventional division of AV block into first, second, and third degrees. Few, however, appear to appreciate what confusion, misunderstanding, and mismanagement this oversimplified classification has created. The situation has been compounded by deficient definitions and multiple misconceptions. It is with these unfortunate aspects of the subject that much of this chapter is concerned.

The PR interval

The normal PR interval, measured from the beginning of the P wave to the beginning of the QRS complex, ranges between 0.12 and 0.20 second. This is not to say that somewhat longer and shorter intervals necessarily indicate abnormality; in a study of normal youths between the ages of 15 and 23 years,[1] 1.3% had PR intervals longer than 0.20 second and the same percentage had intervals shorter than 0.12 second. It may well be that these exceptions to the general rule represent merely the splayed extremities of a normal bell curve.

When all atrial impulses that should be conducted to the ventricles are so conducted, but with a PR interval of greater than 0.20 second, the term "first-degree" AV block is generally applied.

Nonconducted beats

The term "second-degree" block is applied when one or more (but not all) atrial impulses that should be conducted fail to reach the ventricles. It thus covers a great variety of conduction patterns of markedly variable significance.

When an atrial impulse fails to reach the ventricles, it is often referred to as a "dropped" beat. Usage of this term has been criticized, but it is difficult to find an adequate and appropriate substitute; it at least has the blessing of traditional use since Lewis.[2] Faute de mieux, we shall use it!

When an atrial impulse fails to reach the ventricles and a beat is "dropped," one must take the individual circumstances into account. If it arrives at the AV junction early in the cycle when the junction is still normally refractory, it is not conducted; but neither is it "blocked," for block implies a *pathologic* failure of conduction. Obviously one of the determinants of the prematurity with which an atrial impulse arrives at the junction is the atrial rate; and when the rate is exceedingly fast, as in atrial flutter, it is only proper that every other impulse should not be conducted. One of the normal functions of the AV node is to protect the ventricles from excessively rapid and therefore ineffective beating when the atria have gone berserk. Therefore 2:1 conduction resulting from normal refractoriness should not be called 2:1 *block*, which immediately places it in an abnormal category.

Before assessing the significance of a "dropped" beat, therefore, one must always take into consideration the atrial rate and its inseparable partner, the RP interval. The failure of an atrial impulse to reach the ventricles may have a quite different significance if its P wave lands after the end of the T wave from what it will have if it is perched upon the first part of the ST segment.

Type I and type II block

In 1899 Wenckebach,[3] without benefit of electrocardiograph and by simple observation of the pulses in the neck, described the form of AV block that bears his name in which the AV conduction time progressively lengthens until a beat is dropped (Fig. 17-1).

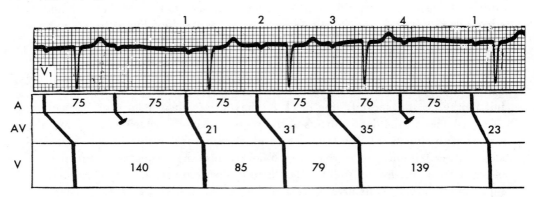

Fig. 17-1. A typical 4:3 Wenckebach period—of the four atrial impulses (*1, 2, 3, 4*), only three reach the ventricles. Characteristic features include the following: the first PR is slightly prolonged (0.21 sec); the larger PR increment is between the first and second PR (from 0.21 to 0.31 sec); as the increment decreases, the ventricular cycle shortens (from 0.85 to 0.79 sec); the longest cycle (of the dropped beat—1.39 sec) is less than twice the shortest ventricular cycle (0.79 sec); and there is no BBB.

Seven years later he in Vienna[4] and Hay in Scotland[5] both described a second form of AV block in which there was no progressive lengthening of the conduction time before conduction failed (Fig. 17-2).

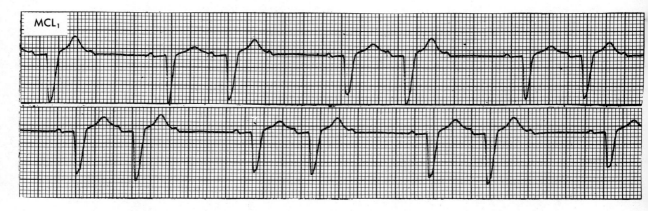

Fig. 17-2. A typical example of type II 3:2 AV block. Characteristic features include the following: consecutive atrial impulses are conducted with the same PR interval (0.18 sec) immediately before the dropped beat; the PR after the dropped beat is the same as the PR before it; the PR is of normal duration; and there is a BBB.

In 1924 Mobitz[6] correlated these earlier clinical findings with those in the electrocardiogram and suggested that the first type (1899) be called "type I" and the second type (1906) "type II." Hence they have since been frequently referred to as Mobitz type I and Mobitz type II block but are just as appropriately called Wenckebach type I and Wenckebach type II.[7,8] In later years His bundle recordings have repeatedly demonstrated that type I block is usually a manifestation of AV nodal block whereas type II is always infranodal block and is usually a manifestation of bilateral BBB.[9-12]

Useful as this classification has proved to be, and widely as the terms type I and type II are used, most authorities fail to fully explain how they are using them and the simple division into two types is beset with ambiguities.

If the terms are confined only to the basic patterns of block originally described, the terms are too restrictive and their usefulness is decreased. For example, if a patient has an atrial rate of 80/min with 3:2 Wenckebach periods, it is generally accepted as classical type I block. If the atrial rate increases to 100/min, however, with the result that the conduction ratio changes to 2:1, it is still the same type of block (that is, type I) although we no longer have the progressive increase in conduction times (PR intervals) before each dropped beat that is characteristic of the classical Wenckebach. Thus, if only examples with increasing PR intervals are included, important samples of type I block are excluded.

Anatomy versus behavior

Two ingredients blend indefinably to produce the recipe for both type I and type II block: pathophysiologic behavior and the anatomic level of the block. Unfortunately there is an irreconcilable dichotomy between anatomy and behavior. Most authorities, correctly following traditional usage, employ the terms type I and type II as behavioral descriptions.[13-16] Yet there is little doubt that the anatomic level of the lesion is clinically more important than its physiologic behavior; for example, Wenckebach periodicity in a bundle branch, in the presence of contralateral bundle-branch block, is behaviorally type I but clinically and prognostically is more appropriately considered type II.[8,17] Consequently a division into nodal and infranodal, or proximal and distal,[17] has much to commend it.

Table 17-1. *Established associations of type I and type II block*

	Type I	Type II
Clinical	Usually acute Inferior infarction Rheumatic fever Digitalis Propranolol	Usually chronic Anteroseptal infarction Lenegre's disease Lev's disease Cardiomyopathy

Anatomic	Usually AV nodal—
	  sometimes His bundle
		Always subnodal—usually
		  bundle branches

Electrophysiologic	Relative refractory period Decremental conduction	No relative refractory period All-or-none conduction
Electrocardiographic	RP/PR reciprocity Prolonged PR Normal QRS duration	Stable PR Normal PR Bundle-branch block

It would therefore be ideal if we could infallibly distinguish between AV nodal block (and call it type I) and infranodal block (and call it type II) from the clinical tracing. Unfortunately we cannot; and in many situations intracardiac recordings—the only sure way of accurately localizing the level of the block—are neither available nor desirable. Fortunately, with a knowledge of the attributes of both types of block (Table 17-1), aided at times by the result of carotid sinus massage and/or atropine administration,[17a] we can usually make an intelligent and correct guess; but we must always keep in mind that there are important exceptions to the usual findings such as the following:

1. Many Wenckebach periods are atypical[18] and fail to show all the classical features depicted in Fig. 17-1.
2. Rarely the classical Wenckebach period can develop in the bundle of His, and then the ECG is indistinguishable from the nodal Wenckebach.
3. The all-or-none conduction that characterizes the bundle branches may be found in the His bundle, and then type II block may be encountered with a narrow QRS complex.[8,19-22] This combination is said to occur almost exclusively in elderly women.[8]
4. In the presence of existing BBB, progressive lengthening of the PR interval before a dropped beat is due in perhaps 25% of cases[17] to progressive delay in the contralateral bundle branch.[23,24]

Despite such significant exceptions, "in most instances, the differentiation can be made easily and reliably from the surface ECG."[15] What it all seems to boil down to is that when we say type I we mean "probably nodal and usually benign" and when we say type II we mean "certainly infranodal and definitely malignant." Genuine type II block is an uneqivocal indication for an artificial pacemaker whereas type I block seldom is.

Wenckebach periodicity and RP/PR reciprocity

Although it may well prove to be an oversimplification, it is a convenient and practical concept to think of type I *behavior* as due to an abnormally long relative refractory period (RRP) and type II as the result of little or no RRP.[16] In the prolonged RRP the rate of conduction depends upon the moment of impulse arrival—the earlier it arrives at the AV node, the longer it takes to penetrate; the later it arrives, the shorter the penetration time (Fig. 17-3).

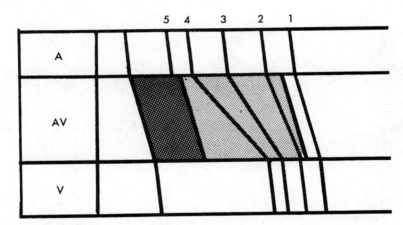

Fig. 17-3. Diagrammatic behavior of AV conduction during type I AV block. Dark stippling in the AV junction represents the absolute refractory period (ARP), light stippling the relative refractory period (RRP). If an atrial impulse *(1)* arrives at the AV node after the RRP is over, it is conducted normally. If it arrives a little earlier *(2)*, there will be some delay in AV conduction; and as it arrives earlier and earlier *(3 and 4)*, conduction time becomes longer and longer. Finally, the impulse arrives in the ARP *(5)* and is not conducted.

Thus it becomes obvious that the reason the Wenckebach type of conduction develops is that each successive impulse arrives earlier and earlier in the RRP of the AV node until, at last, one arrives during the absolute refractory period (ARP) and the impulse fails to get through.

A clinically practical concept results from translating this earlier and earlier arrival into terms of the surface tracing. Other things being equal, the earlier the impulse sets out from the sinus node the earlier it will reach the AV node and therefore the RP interval (measured from beginning of the QRS to beginning of the next P wave) gives us an approximate—and in practice highly satisfactory—indication of the relative earliness of arrival at the AV node. In terms of the clinical tracing the shorter the RP the longer the PR, and the longer the RP the shorter the PR; and so we can think and talk of "RP/PR reciprocity" and of "RP-dependent" PR intervals. If you can demonstrate such reciprocity in the clinical tracing, you can be sure that some part of the AV junction is exhibiting Wenckebach (type I) behavior.

In Fig. 17-4 the reciprocal relationship between RP and its associated PR is nicely demonstrated. After the first three beats, which are conducted normally with a PR of 0.17 complementing an RP of 0.48 second, the last four beats are all conducted with progressively shortening PR intervals (exactly the converse of what happens in a Wenckebach sequence) because they complement progressively lengthening RP intervals (again, exactly the converse of what happens in a Wenckebach).

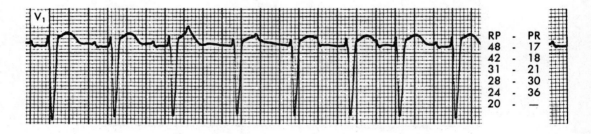

RP	-	PR
48	-	17
42	-	18
31	-	21
28	-	30
24	-	36
20	-	—

Fig. 17-4. This illustrates the reciprocal relationship between the RP interval and its complementing PR (see table at end of tracing). The last four conducted beats demonstrate the converse of what happens in a Wenckebach: as the RP gets longer with each successive beat, its complementary PR gets progressively shorter whereas in the Wenckebach the PR progressively lengthens in response to a progressively shortening RP.

In the classical Wenckebach (Fig. 17-1) the dropped beat fails to penetrate the diseased stratum of the AV node which therefore enjoys a relatively long rest (RP interval = 1.13 sec) with consequent optimal AV conduction (PR = 0.21 sec). Now, suddenly, the RP dramatically shortens—from 1.13 to 0.52 second—and the PR in consequence as dramatically lengthens—from 0.21 to 0.31 second. This explains why the second PR in the Wenckebach sequence almost always shows the largest increment over the preceding PR—because it follows the most dramatic shortening of the RP; that is, it arrives much earlier in the RRP of the sick AV node.

On the other hand, if there is virtually no RRP, it follows that beats that are conducted are conducted with the same facility, that is, with the same PR interval, whether early or late in diastole, provided they arrive after the ARP is over (Fig. 17-2); the PR is the same, regardless of the preceding RP, and RP/PR reciprocity is lacking.

It follows, in turn, from all this that when *consecutive* atrial impulses are conducted type I block is characterized by progressive lengthening of the PR before conduction fails altogether, whereas type II block has constant PR intervals when *consecutive* impulses are conducted before the dropped beat.

2 to 1 AV block

What of the situation, however, when only alternate beats are conducted with a resulting 2:1 ratio? With this ratio in both type 1 (Fig. 17-5) and type II (Fig. 17-6) the PR interval is, of course, constant in the beats that are conducted.

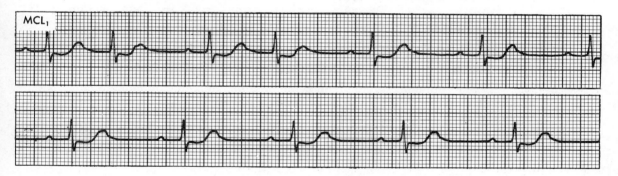

Fig. 17-5. From a patient with acute true posterior infarction. Note the prominent initial R wave with reciprocal ST depression. The strips are continuous and the atrial rate throughout is 103/min. At the beginning of the top strip there are two 3:2 Wenckebach periods; then through the bottom strip the conduction ratio changes to 2:1. Note that the PR interval is prolonged during the 2:1 conduction (0.25 sec).

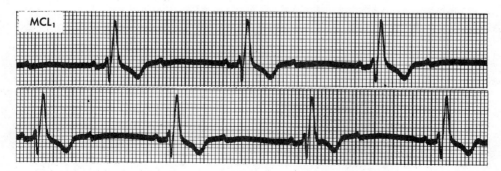

Fig. 17-6. The strips are continuous and show 2:1 AV block with RBBB. The atrial rate is 82/min, and the combination of a normal PR interval (0.15 sec) with BBB makes it likely that this is type II AV block.

This is true for type II since we have seen that all PRs are constant in this type of block; but it is also true of type I block since, provided the atrial rhythm is regular, the RP intervals will be constant and so therefore will the PRs (recall that in type I block the PR is RP dependent). This fact has been the source of much misunderstanding, with consequent misdiagnosis and mistreatment.

Although it no longer qualifies as the Wenckebach *phenomenon*, it must be obvious that when the classical form of Wenckebach conduction alternates with 2:1 conduction—as in Fig. 17-5—the type of block has not changed. Sometimes changes in the atrial rate produce changes in conduction ratios; sometimes the conduction ratios change spontaneously; but in such cases there can be no doubt that the type of block is unchanged. When the conduction ratio in Wenckebach periods changes from 5:4 to 4:3 or from 4:3 to 3:2, there is no doubt in anyone's mind that the type of block is unchanged; why, when it goes one stage further and becomes 2:1, should there be an immediate flurry to change the type and its prognostic significance?

If you look at Figs. 17-5 and 17-6, you will see two other features that are highly characteristic of the two types of second-degree AV block and that can be of assistance in differentiating types when only 2:1 conduction is present. The prolonged PR and the absence of BBB are typical of pure type I block, whereas the normal PR and the presence of BBB are characteristic of type II.

"Skipped" P waves

Another point that is not well appreciated and leads to faulty diagnosis is that the atrial impulse which is conducted to the ventricles is not always represented by the P wave that immediately precedes the QRS. In Fig. 17-7 the group beating and the other "footprints" clearly identify a Wenckebach.

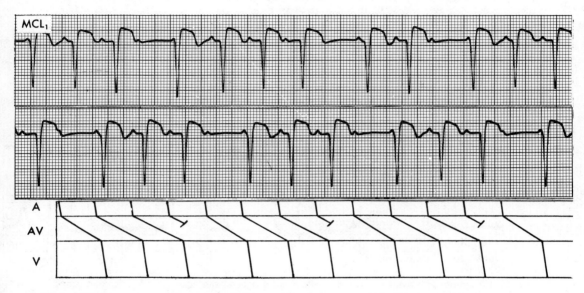

Fig. 17-7. The strips are continuous. Sinus tachycardia (rate, 125/min) with 3:2, 4:3, and 5:4 Wenckebach periods. Note that the PR intervals are longer than the PP intervals.

Moreover the increasing PR intervals in each group of beats are evident. However, in each group the first and second PR intervals are clearly too short for conduction and therefore conduction must come from the preceding P wave (see laddergram).

Furthermore, these rather long PR intervals—reaching 0.69 second—bring to mind the oft asked question: "How long can a PR be and still represent conduction?" There is no established answer to this; but at least it can be said that a PR of 0.60 second is not uncommon, one of 0.70 second is sometimes seen, and one of 0.80 to 0.90 second is rare. PR intervals of over 1 second have been published, but their validity is doubtful.

High-grade (or advanced) AV block

High-grade block represents a stage between the occasionally, or even alternately, dropped beats and complete block. High-grade block may be diagnosed when, *at a reasonable atrial rate* (say, 135/min or less) two or more than two consecutive atrial impulses fail to be conducted; and this failure of conduction must happen *because of the existing block itself*, not because an escaping junctional or ventricular pacemaker anticipates and prevents conduction. Fig. 17-8 presents two examples of high-grade AV block—the one probably type I, because of the inferior infarction and absence of BBB, and the other type II, because there is BBB as well as a normal PR interval in the conducted beats.

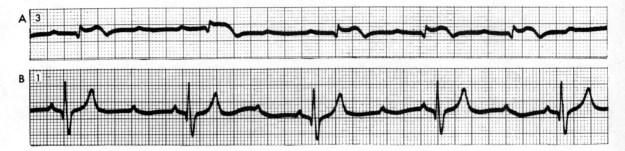

Fig. 17-8. High-grade (advanced) AV block. **A,** From a patient with acute inferior infarction, sinus tachycardia, and 3:1 and 2:1 AV block—presumably type I. **B,** From a 47-year-old patient with no history of heart disease presenting with Adams-Stokes attacks. There is sinus tachycardia (rate, 122/min) with 3:1 AV block. In this clinical context the normal PR (0.16 sec) with RBBB makes this likely to be type II block due to sclerodegenerative disease of the conduction system.

The two conditions italicized above are necessary ingredients in the definition because, for example, if the fluttering atria are beating at a frantic rate of 300/min it would be absurd to call 4:1 block (where three consecutive impulses are not conducted) high grade since a 4:1 ratio, producing a ventricular rate of 75, is exactly what the heart of both the therapist and the patient desires. Furthermore, the ventricular escape rate, quite apart from the block, can be a major determinant of nonconduction and cause of overdiagnosis, as we shall see later in this chapter.

Complete AV block

The block should be called complete when, and only when, the opportunity for conduction is optimal and yet none occurs. The key word here is opportunity since it is obvious that if there is no opportunity to do something one cannot be blamed for not doing it. If there is less than optimal opportunity for the AV conduction system to conduct, it cannot be regarded as a failure if it does not conduct; on the other hand, if it has every conceivable opportunity to conduct and invariably fails, it may well be blamed as a total failure. What then determines the presence or absence of opportunity for conduction? The several factors involved are listed on p. 287.

In order to make the diagnosis of complete block, there should be no conduction—recognized by the changing P-to-R relationship in the presence of a regular ventricular rhythm—but that absence of conduction must be in the presence of a slow enough ventricular rate, say, under 45/min, with P waves fully deployed across the RR intervals landing at every conceivable RP interval. Only then can one be satisfied that the opportunity for conduction is optimal and that the diagnosis of complete block is justified. These features require repeated emphasis because there is probably no entity in cardiology that is so often overdiagnosed and then overtreated.

Fig. 17-9 illustrates complete AV block: the ventricular rate is under 45/min, the ventricular rhythm is absolutely regular, and the P-to-R relationship is constantly changing as the P waves march resolutely through all phases of the ventricular cycle. Every possible chance for conduction is afforded, but none occurs; and so the diagnosis of the ultimate in block (complete) is warranted.

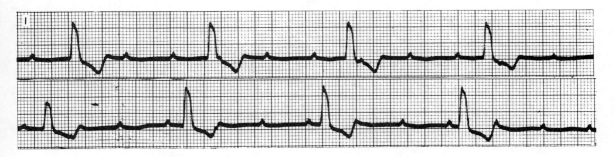

Fig. 17-9. Complete AV block. The strips are continuous. In the presence of sinus tachycardia (rate, 108/min) there is an independent idioventricular rhythm (rate, 36/min). Note that the ventricular rhythm is absolutely regular while the P to R relatonship is constantly changing.

Acute complete block is usually caused by a lesion in the AV node, as in acute inferior infarction and less often in severe digitalis intoxication. In acute anterior infarction complete block is more devastating and is almost always due to simultaneous block in both bundle branches. About 90% of chronic complete block is caused by bilateral BBB, the remaining 10% being caused by blockade at the level of the His bundle.

Ventricular asystole

As a rule, when AV conduction fails, an escaping pacemaker, junctional or ventricular, comes to the rescue. However, if the failure of conduction is associated with reluctant subsidiary pacemakers, ventricular asystole results. This sinister situation if unrelieved is obviously and rapidly fatal. The most common context for this occurrence is as an ominous and usually fatal climax of type II block; that is, it develops spontaneously against a background of existing BBB presumably because the other bundle branch is suddenly blocked (Fig. 17-10, *A*).

Ventricular asystole is not always so sinister. If it develops as a result of a vagal storm, as with vomiting (Fig. 17-10, *C*), the level of block is in the AV node and the disturbance may be relatively mild and transient. A third mechanism of asystole (Fig. 17-10, *B*) is tentatively assumed to be due to a phase 4 phenomenon since the block and the consequent asystole develop only after a lengthening of the atrial cycle, suggesting that the AV node may have spontaneously depolarized to an unresponsive level (p. 157).

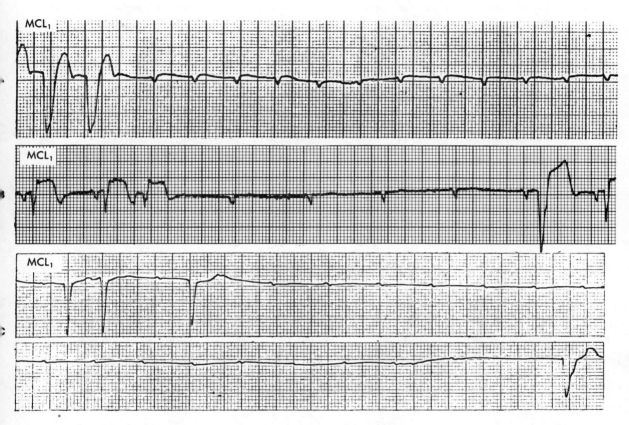

Fig. 17-10. Three examples of transient ventricular asystole due to sudden failure of AV conduction in the absence of an escaping pacemaker. **A,** *Spontaneous* asystole in the presence of LBBB, probably representing end-stage type II block. **B,** From a patient with acute anteroseptal infarction. The asystole is precipitated by an atrial premature beat (as were many repeated periods of asystole); the APB lengthens the ensuing sinus cycle, suggesting that the failure of conduction might be due to a *phase 4 phenomenon.* **C,** The strips are continuous. *Vagal* asystole, precipitated by vomiting, in a patient with acute inferior infarction.

NEED TO RECLASSIFY. There are several reasons why the diagnosis and management of the AV blocks are in a state of confusion.

Definitions wanting. The first is that most authors seem not to realize that there is any uncertainty in the current situation. In fact, in over 50 articles published in English since the advent of coronary care in 1962 dealing with the subject of complete AV block, not a single author considered it necessary to define it—presumably because it is tacitly, but erroneously, assumed that the term is uniformly used by and means the same to all. How far this is from the truth will become apparent.

Not only is complete block almost never defined; but on the rare occasions when it is, the definition is usually found wanting. And much the same is true of the usage and definition of other important categories of block such as "type II block" and "high-grade block."

Nondegrees of block. The second source of inconsistency resides in the usage of "degrees." The word, by definition, should indicate a measure of the severity of the AV conduction disturbance. However, this is not necessarily the case. Consider, for example, the rhythm strips in Fig. 17-11. By any criterion the top strip *(A)* is an example of 2:1 AV block, a ratio that some regard as "high-grade" block (see below),[8,25,26] while the second strip *(B)* shows no sign of any block. In fact, the owner of strip *B* has worse block than the patient in strip *A* because patient *B* develops 2:1 block when the atrial rate accelerates to only 84/min (strip *D*) whereas patient *A* is able to conduct 1:1 at a rate of 100/min (strip *C*). Obviously a patient who develops 2:1 conduction at a rate of 84 has worse block than one who can conduct every beat at a rate of 100/min. In evaluating the severity of AV block, RATE is far more important than RATIO; yet unfortunately our definitions of "degrees" have for decades been partially predicated upon ratios to the neglect of rate. Indeed, when the conduction ratio changes with an increase in rate, it may be described as a change for the worse in the degree of block[27] rather than recognizing it for what it is: a change in *rate* with a secondary and consequent change in the conduction *ratio,* not in the degree of block.

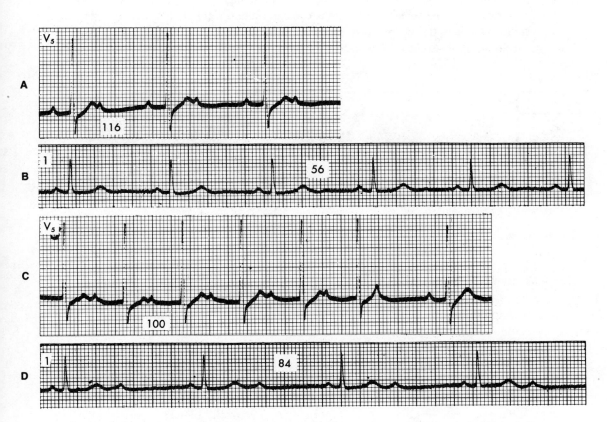

Fig. 17-11. Strips **A** and **C** are from one patient, **B** and **D** from a second. The first patient has 2:1 block at an atrial rate of 116/min (**A**) but can conduct 1:1 at an atrial rate of 100/min (**C**) whereas the second patient, though he conducts normally at 56/min (**B**), develops 2:1 block at a rate of only 84/min (**D**).

Let us hammer this point home with a diagram. In Fig. 17-12 each conducted beat is followed by an identical prolonged refractory period (shaded area); that is, the "degree" of severity of block is the same throughout the diagram. At the beginning of the strip the atrial cycle length is 100 (rate = 60/min), but after three beats the atrial cycle shortens to 76 (rate = 79/min) and 2:1 conduction develops; yet it is obvious that the severity, that is, "degree," of block has not changed. The primary change is the atrial rate and the secondary change is the conduction ratio. The message is that we should not assess the seriousness of any AV block from the conduction ratio alone without taking the associated rate into consideration.

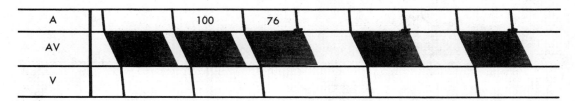

Fig. 17-12. Diagram illustrating the effect of atrial rate on the AV conduction ratio. Note that the abnormally long refractory period is identical throughout; that is, there is no worsening of the block, yet if the atrial cycle shortens from 100 (rate, 60/min) to 76 (rate, 79/min), the conduction ratio changes from 1:1 to 2:1.

Misconceptions rife. The third circumstance that fosters confusion is the prevalence of certain important misconceptions, some of which have been hinted at earlier in this chapter.

1. Some authorities[8,25,26] regard 2:1 AV block as high grade or advanced. The absurdity of using the conduction ratio as an index of severity is obvious when one stops to realize that 2:1 block can be anything from a disaster to a boon. At an atrial rate of 70, 2:1 block may be a disaster; at an atrial rate of 130, 2:1 block may prove a blessing. Clearly the ratio alone, in ignorance of the prevailing atrial and therefore ventricular rate, cannot give even an approximate idea of the block's severity.

2. A second misapprehension is the rather commonly encountered one that all 2:1 block is type II block. This is mainly owing to the fact that the PR intervals are constant and one does not have to look far to find defective definitions of type II block such as "AV block with constant PR intervals"[28] and "constant PR intervals for conducted sinus beats irrespective of the ratio of atrial to ventricular depolarizations."[29] It is because faulty definitions such as these so often omit the key word *consecutive*—which we carefully emphasized earlier in this chapter. It is only when *consecutive*—repeat, CONSECUTIVE!—atrial impulses are conducted with identical PR intervals immediately before the beat is dropped that the constant PR criterion can be applied. Another common, and appropriate, way of stating the constant PR rule is to say that the PR after the dropped beat is the same as the PR before it. In the classical example

of type II block in Fig. 17-2 the two consecutive PRs before the dropped beat are identical, and the PR immediately before the dropped beat is the same as the returning PR after it. What these variations of the rule are stating is simply that the PR is independent of the RP: it is the same after a short RP (before the dropped beat) as after a long RP (after the dropped beat); and, of course, the hallmark of type I block is RP/PR reciprocity.[30] Notice again the additional characteristic—but not invariable—features of type II block: the normal PR and the BBB.

In the acute setting of myocardial infarction, type I 2:1 block is, in fact, 20 or 30 times more common than type II 2:1 block—an important point to remember when temporary pacemakers are being brandished.

3. A third misconception is that, when AV block is evident and most of the atrial impulses are not conducted, the block is "high grade" or "advanced."

Fig. 17-13 shows an example of AV block in which there are 21 atrial impulses only one of which is completely conducted (there are possibly one or two fusion beats); yet, with so little conduction, the block is comparatively mild. The way to avoid the error of overdiagnosis in such cases is to focus on the conducted beat rather than on the numerous nonconducted ones, because the beat that is conducted tells you far more about the patient's conduction capability than do all the nonconducted beats together. It shows you quite specifically the patient's current requirements for conduction. Concentrate on the solitary capture beat (fifth beat in top strip). We recognize that when the RP interval reaches a length of 0.60 second the patient is able to conduct with a PR interval of 0.32 second. Thus we can deduce that at that time the patient had a 1:1 conduction capability if the atrial cycle equaled the cycle of the capture beat (that is, cycle length = 0.92 sec = 64/min). Furthermore, a person capable of conducting every beat at a rate of 64/min with but a prolonged PR interval certainly does not have an advanced degree of AV block. Add to this reasoning the fact that the patient has an inferior wall infarction and that the capture beat manifests no BBB and you know that the block is almost certainly in the AV node.

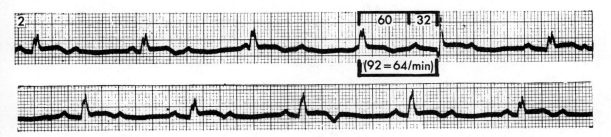

Fig. 17-13. The strips are continuous. From a patient with acute inferior myocardial infarction. Some (undetermined) degree of AV block (presumably type I), combined with an atrial rate of 88/min and a ventricular escape rate of 47/min, precludes conduction except for the one capture beat (fifth beat in the top strip) and two or three possible fusion beats in the bottom strip. The capture beat tells us that the patient is capable of conducting 1:1, with prolonged PR, at an atrial rate of 64/min (see text).

4. A fourth misconception is that, when AV block is clearly present and *none* of the atrial impulses is conducted, the block is necessarily complete.

In a tracing like that in Fig. 17-14, *A*, there is obvious block since P waves are seen in situations where conduction should occur and does not. In fact, there is no AV conduction since the junctional rhythm is absolutely regular. Thus we have AV block and complete AV dissociation, but this is by no means the same as complete AV block.[13] Such tracings should be diagnosed as "*some* (undetermined) degree of AV block which, combined with an accelerated junctional rhythm, produces complete AV dissociation." Yet more than half of 550 respondents to a questionnaire mailed to directors of cardiology departments and coronary care units asking how such a dysrhythmia should be described called it complete AV block[31]; and published examples of the same interpretative error are abundant.

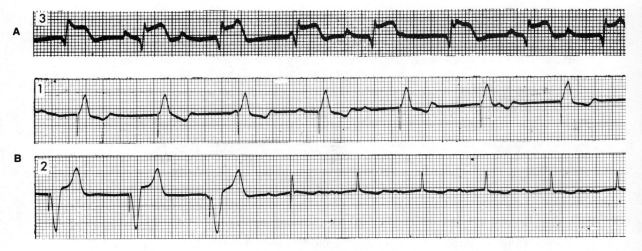

Fig. 17-14. A, Block/acceleration dissociation. Some (undetermined) degree of AV block (presumably type I), combined with an accelerated junctional rhythm at a rate of 68/min, produces complete AV dissociation. **B,** Illustration of how mild a degree of AV block, when combined with an accelerated ventricular rate, can produce complete dissociation. In lead 1 there is obvious AV block, the paced rhythm has a rate of 62/min, and there is complete AV dissociation. However, in lead 2, a few seconds later, an atrial impulse—represented by a P wave landing at a critical RP interval—captures the ventricles and reveals the mildness of the underlying conduction disturbance.

The argument here is that, although one cannot be sure that the block is not complete, there is a real possibility that it is relatively mild; and therefore it is a mistake to assume the worst, label it the ultimate in block, and run the attendant risks of overdiagnosis—especially since we know that patients with acute myocardial infarction who show this dysrhythmia as their worst manifestation of block usually have an excellent prognosis.

Fig. 17-14, *B*, shows how mild such a block may prove to be. In lead 1 there is a paced ventricular rhythm of 62/min. The P wave emerges from the QRS and marches backward across the RR interval without effecting capture—complete dissociation. However, in lead 2, after the third beat, the P wave happens to land at exactly the right RP interval and the atrial impulse captures the ventricles with a long PR interval. Once capture is effected, the atria remain in control for the rest of the strip with gradually lengthening PR intervals indicating that at the prevailing atrial rate the underlying block, far from being complete, is a mild form of type I block. The fundamental truth so poorly appreciated is that *the combination of quite mild block with a ventricular rate in the 50s or 60s can produce periods of complete AV dissociation*. Absence of conduction is not necessarily the same as block.

Therefore, when faced with a sample of AV block in which all or a significant majority of beats are not conducted, it is important to rehearse in one's mind the many influences that determine AV conduction and to assess the relative contribution of each:

1. State of AV junction and bundle branches
   a. Physiologic refractoriness
   b. Pathologic refractoriness
   c. Concealed conduction
2. Autonomic influences
3. Atrial rate
4. R/P relationships
5. Ventricular rate
6. Level of ventricular pacemaker

Dysrhythmias, such as that in Fig. 17-14, *A*, caused by the conspiracy of an undetermined degree of block with a subsidiary pacemaker beating at a rate faster than usual, clearly require a separate designation; and one of us[31] has therefore suggested the term "block/acceleration dissociation."

Remedial measures

To introduce some semblance of order from the current chaos, three modifications commend themselves: (1) disturbances of AV conduction must be classified into many more categories than the oversimplification into three misleading "degrees"; (2) "degrees" of AV block as presently defined (or not defined!) should be abandoned, or at least deemphasized, since they have caused more confusion than they have contributed precision; and (3) rates, both atrial and ventricular, in view of the major role they play in determining the frequency and ratio of AV conduction, must be included in all definitions and diagnostic categorizations of block.

With the above considerations in mind, we should divide the AV blocks into more meaningful categories—meaningful from the viewpoint of placing the site of the lesion, assessing the prognosis, and deciding upon the appropriate management. This can, as we have emphasized, usually be done from the surface tracing together with an informed appraisal of the clinical setting. As a short step in the right direction, we suggest that the disturbances of AV conduction be categorized and considered under at least the number of subdivisions listed below.

1. Prolonged PR interval
2. Block/acceleration dissociation
3. Occasional "dropped" beats
   a. Type I (Wenckebach periodicity)
   b. Type II
4. 2:1 AV block
   a. Type I
   b. Type II
5. High-grade block
   a. Type I
   b. Type II
6. Complete block
   a. Junctional escape
   b. Ventricular escape
7. Transient ventricular asystole
   a. Spontaneous
   b. Phase 4 (?)
   c. Vagal

References

1. Van Hemel, M.M., and Robles de Medina, E.O.: Electrocardiographic findings in 781 males between the ages of 15 and 23 years. I. Arrhythmias and conduction disorders, Excerpta Medica Cardiovasc. Dis. Cardiovasc. Surg., vol. 23 (abstract 981), 1975.
2. Lewis, T.: The mechanism and graphic registration of the heart beat, London, 1925, Shaw & Sons.
3. Wenckebach, K.F.: Zur Analyse des unregelmässigen Pulses. II. Ueber den regelmässig intermittirenden Puls, Z. Klin. Med. 37:475, 1899.
4. Wenckebach, K.F.: Beiträge zur Kenntnis der Menschlichen Herztätigkeit, Arch. Anat. Physiol., p. 297, 1906.
5. Hay, J.: Bradycardia and cardiac arrhythmia produced by depression of certain functions of the heart, Lancet 1:139, 1906.
6. Mobitz, W.: Ueber die unvollständige Störung der Erregungsüberleitung zwischen Vorhof und Kamme des menschlichen Herzens, Z. Ges. Exp. Med. 41:180, 1924.
7. Knoebel, S.B., Parsons, M.N., and Fisch, C.: The role of transvenous pacing in acute myocardial infarction, Heart Lung 1:56, 1972.
8. Narula, O.S.: His bundle electrocardiography and clinical electrophysiology, Philadelphia, 1975, F.A. Davis Co.
9. Damato, A.N., and Lau, S.H.: Clinical value of the electrogram of the conducting system, Prog. Cardiovasc. Dis. 12:119, 1970.
10. Rosen, K.M.: The contribution of His bundle recording to the understanding of cardiac conduction in man, Circulation 43:961, 1971.
11. Rosen, K.M., Gunnar, R.M., and Rahimtoola, S.H.: Site and type of second degree AV block, Chest 61:99, 1972.
12. Haft, J.I., Weinstock, M., and DeGuia, R.: Electrophysiologic studies in Mobitz type II second degree heart block, Am. J. Cardiol. 27:682, 1971.
13. Langendorf, R., and Pick, A.: Atrioventricular block, type II (Mobitz)—its nature and clinical significance, Circulation 38:819, 1968.
14. Barold, S.S., and Friedberg, H.D.: Second degree atrioventricular block: a matter of definition, Am. J. Cardiol. 33:311, 1974.
15. Zipe, D.P.: Second-degree atrioventricular block, Circulation 60:465, 1979.
16. Pick, A., and Langendorf, R.: Interpretation of complex arrhythmias, Philadelphia, 1979, Lea & Febiger.
17. Del Negro, A.A., and Fletcher, R.D.: Indications for and use of artificial cardiac pacemakers, Curr. Probl. Cardiol. 3(7):9, 1978.
17a. Mangardi, L.M., and others: Bedside evaluation of atrioventricular block with narrow QRS complexes; usefulness of carotid sinus massage and atropine administration, Am. J. Cardiol. 49:1136, 1982.
18. Denes, P., Levy, L., Pick, A., and Rosen, K.M.: The incidence of typical and atypical AV Wenckebach periodicity, Am. Heart J. 89:26, 1975.
19. Rosen, K.M., and others: Mobitz type II block without bundle branch block, Circulation 44:1111, 1971.
20. Gupta, P.K., Lichstein, E., and Chadda, K.D.: Electrophysiological features of Mobitz type II A-V block occurring within the His bundle, Br. Heart J. 34:1232, 1972.
21. Rosen, K.M., Loeb, H.S., and Rahimtoola, S.H.: Mobitz type II block with narrow QRS complex and Stokes-Adams attacks, Arch. Int. Med. 1342:595, 1973.
22. Puech, P., Grolleau, R., and Guimond, C.: Incidence of different types of AV block and their localization by His bundle recordings. In Wellens, H.J.J., Lie, K.I., and Janse, M.J., editors: The conduction system of the heart: structure, function, and clinical implications, Philadelphia, 1976, Lea & Febiger.
23. Rosenbaum, M.B., and others: Wenckebach periods in the bundle branches, Circulation 40:79, 1969.
24. Friedberg, H.D., and Schamroth, L.: The Wenckebach phenomenon in left bundle branch block, Am. J. Cardiol. 24:591, 1969.
25. WHO/ISC Task Force: Definition of terms related to cardiac rhythm, Am. Heart J. 95:796, 1978.
26. Josephson, M.E., and Seides, S.F.: Clinical cardiac electrophysiology. Techniques and interpretations, Philadelphia, 1979, Lea & Febiger.
27. Danzig, R., Alpern, H., and Swan, H.J.C.: The significance of atrial rate in patients with atrioventricular conduction abnormalities complicating acute myocardial infarction, Am. J. Cardiol. 24:707, 1969.
28. Stock, R.J., and Macken, D.L.: Observations

on heart block during continuous electrocardiographic monitoring in myocardial infarction, Circulation **38**:993, 1968.

29. Scheinman, M., and Brenman, B.: Clinical and anatomic implications of intraventricular conduction blocks in acute myocardial infarction, Circulation **46**:753, 1972.

30. Langendorf, R., Cohen, H., and Gozo, E.G.: Observations on second degree atrioventricular block, including new criteria for the differential diagnosis between type I and type II block, Am. J. Cardiol. **29**:111, 1972.

31. Marriott, H.J.L.: AV block: an overdue overhaul, Emerg. Med. **13**(6):85, 1981.

CHAPTER 18

An approach to arrhythmias

Many disturbances of rhythm and conduction are recognizable at first glance. For example, one can usually spot immediately atrial flutter with 4:1 conduction, atrial fibrillation with rapid ventricular response, or sinus rhythm with RBBB. There are, however, a significant number of dysrhythmias that defy immediate recognition and it is for these that we require a systematic attack. The following five-point approach evolved after analyzing the reasons for mistakes made in diagnosing arrhythmias and is therefore designed to avoid the common errors of omission and commission. Before outlining this systematic approach, it is worth making some observations about the principles of monitoring.

Principles of monitoring

USE A LEAD CONTAINING MAXIMAL INFORMATION. V_1, or an approximation thereof, clearly supplies the most information. Even though all the information gleaned from these leads is not immediately useful, why let available data go down the drain? An example of valuable information collected from monitoring in MCL_1 is the study of Thorne and Gozensky,[1] who monitored with this lead from the outset of the establishment of the coronary care unit in their hospital. They noted the taller left "rabbit ear" configuration in left ventricular ectopy, which was later confirmed by invasive studies[2] and today is widely used as an aid in the differential diagnosis between aberration and ectopy.

An example of lost information that might have been helpful is the fact that we do not yet really know whether there is any prognostic difference between left and right ventricular extrasystoles. If in the early years of the coronary care unit V_1 had been used as the monitoring lead, distinction between left and right ventricular premature beats would have been possible from the outset and this information might well be in hand today. However, a counterfeit lead II was used for many years—a lead in which LBBB, RBBB, and left and right ventricular ectopics *can* look identical (Fig. 18-1). For this reason if for no other, lead II is one of the least satisfactory leads for constant monitoring. What is the virtue of a monitoring lead that can look similar in these four conditions?

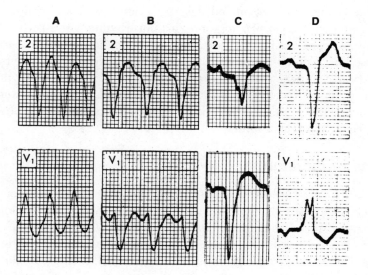

Fig. 18-1. Leads II and V_1. **A,** Left ventricular tachycardia; **B,** right ventricular tachycardia; **C,** LBBB; **D,** RBBB. Note that lead II has a QS configuration in all four conditions and that V_1 contains far greater morphologic contrast.

ENSURE A MECHANICALLY CONVENIENT MONITORING SYSTEM. For most systems a maximum of three wires and electrodes is appropriate, and these should be strategically placed so as not to interfere with physical examination of the heart or with the application of emergency countershock.

ONE LEAD IS NOT ENOUGH. In most situations it is obvious that a single monitoring lead is all that is convenient and practicable. However, it is important to appreciate the limitations of a single lead and to know when to obtain additional leads and which leads to obtain.

In Fig. 18-2 note that in V_1 and V_2 the pattern of the ventricular tachycardia is very similar to the conducted RBBB pattern—so much so that most observers would be content to call the tachycardia "supraventricular." However, another lead (aVF in this case) reveals the obvious and striking differences in the two patterns.

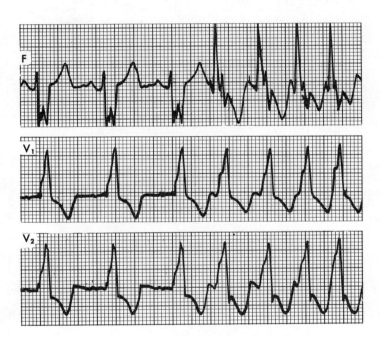

Fig. 18-2. The first three beats are sinus beats conducted with RBBB; the next four beats are ventricular tachycardia produced by artificially stimulating the left ventricle. Note the great similarity of the QRS complexes in V_1 and V_2 during both rhythms and the marked dissimilarity in aVF.

Another reason a single lead may be inadequate is that it may fail to reveal inconspicuous items in the tracing, such as P waves or pacemaker spikes. Fig. 18-3 illustrates the invisibility of a pacemaker spike.

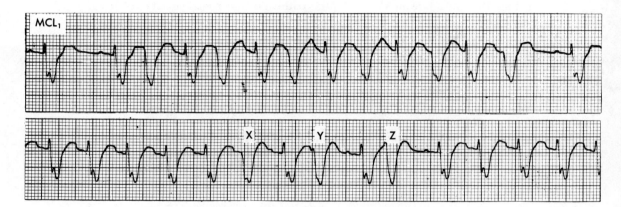

Fig. 18-3. The strips are not continuous. Beats *X, Y,* and *Z* are paced beats, as are the alternate ventricular complexes in the top strip beginning with the third beat; but the pacemaker blips are not visible in this monitoring lead, causing one to suspect spontaneous ventricular ectopy. An additional deception is that this is a demand pacemaker in which the demand mode is not functioning, so that it is behaving like a fixed-rate model imitating ventricular parasystole. The underlying rhythm is sinus tachycardia with sometimes 1:1 conduction (beginning and end of second strip), sometimes 2:1 (beginning and end of top strip).

More than one lead is helpful when the distinction between ectopy and aberration is uncertain in a right chest lead. In Fig. 18-4 the pattern of the tachycardia in MCL_1 could be either left ventricular or supraventricular with RBBB aberration. A look at MCL_6 indicates with reasonable certainty that the origin of the tachycardia is supraventricular (Chapter 16).

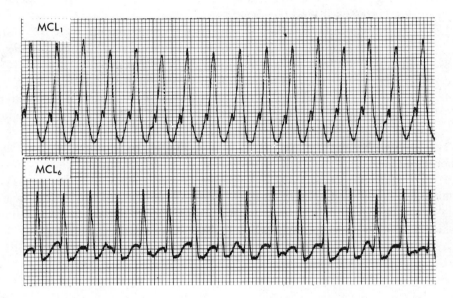

Fig. 18-4. Junctional tachycardia with RBBB aberration. From lead MCL_1 alone, one cannot make the distinction between left ventricular tachycardia and supraventricular tachycardia with RBBB aberration. However, the qRs pattern in MCL_6 immediately identifies it as supraventricular.

KNOW WHEN TO USE WHAT OTHER LEADS. A monitoring lead that satisfactorily fulfills most of the requirements is the modified CL_1 (MCL_1), introduced in 1968.[3] The positive electrode is placed at the C_1 (V_1) position, the negative electrode at the left shoulder, and the ground (which may be placed anywhere) usually at the right shoulder. This leaves a clear platform for emergency cardioversion and an unencumbered precordium for physical examination. In addition, since it closely imitates V_1, this lead affords several diagnostic advantages:

1. One can immediately distinguish between left ventricular ectopy (QRS mostly positive) and right ventricular ectopy (QRS mostly negative) in most instances.
2. RBBB and LBBB can be recognized with ease.
3. P waves are sometimes best or only seen in a right chest lead.
4. Most important of all, a right chest lead gives one the best shot at the differential diagnosis between left ventricular ectopy and RBBB aberration (Chapter 16).

The only disadvantages of lead MCL_1 are that it fails to recognize shifts of axis and is therefore useless for spotting the development of hemiblock and that the polarity of the P wave is not as informative as it is in lead II. However, these disadvantages are minor in comparison with the advantages, especially in view of the fact that many times in a right chest lead an ectopic P wave can easily be differentiated from a sinus P wave because of its shape. When it is diphasic, the sinus P wave is usually $+-$ (⋀⋁); the ectopic or retrograde P wave, when diphasic, is usually $-+$ (⋁⋀). This is illustrated in Fig. 18-5.

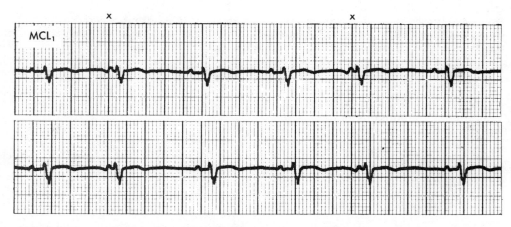

Fig. 18-5. The second and fifth beats in each strip are atrial premature beats. Note the $-+$ polarity of the ectopic P waves *(X)*.

When MCL_1 fails to provide the answer, try a left chest lead by placing the positive electrode at the C_6 (V_6) position to obtain an MCL_6, a reasonable imitation of V_6. If you want to simulate lead III (M_3) for the purpose of recording the polarity of the retrograde P', place the positive electrode low on the left flank below the diaphragm (leaving the negative electrode at the left shoulder). Fig. 18-6 illustrates a junctional rhythm in both MCL_1 and M_3.

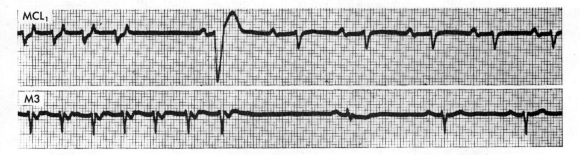

Fig. 18-6. Each lead shows the end of a run of junctional tachycardia with the retrograde P wave just following the QRS complex. In the second half of each strip, sinus rhythm resumes. Note that the retrograde and sinus P waves are both predominantly positive in MCL_1 whereas in M_3 the retrograde P waves show the more familiar inversion so characteristic of retroconduction in an inferior lead. On each occasion, after the tachycardia ceases, the returning beat is an escape beat.

A left chest lead (V_6 or MCL_6) is not reliable for distinguishing between left and right ventricular ectopy, since the QRS in both may be either positive or negative.

For examples of the sort of information that can be derived from a right chest lead that is not usually available in lead II, look at Fig. 18-7. In *A* the rSR′ pattern of the sinus beats is typical of RBBB; the qR pattern with early peak in the first extrasystole is typical of ectopy of left ventricular origin; and the rS pattern of the second extrasystole is typical of a right ventricular origin. In *B* the atrial fibrillation is interrupted by a burst of bizarre beats that are certain to evoke the "lidocaine reflex"; but the telltale shape (rSR′) of the first of these wide beats tell us that it is a run of aberrantly conducted beats rather than a run of ventricular tachycardia.

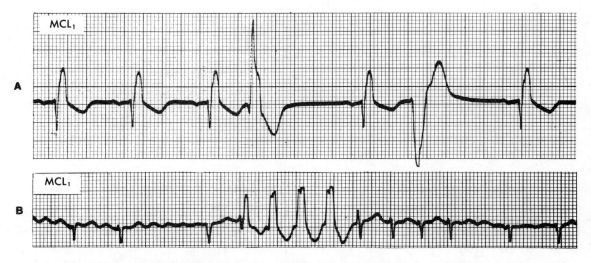

Fig. 18-7, A, The patterns of RBBB (sinus beats), left ventricular ectopy (fourth beat), and right ventricular ectopy (sixth beat) are readily recognized. **B,** A short run of aberrantly conducted beats during atrial fibrillation. The aberration is recognized by the characteristic triphasic (rSR′) contour of the first anomalous beat.

A systematic approach

Failing a diagnosis that falls in your lap a systematic 5-point approach is in order:
1. Know the causes
2. Milk the QRS
3. Cherchez le P
4. Who's married to whom
5. Pinpoint the primary

KNOW THE CAUSES. This is the first step in any medical diagnosis. It is part of the equipment that you carry around with you—prepared at a moment's notice to use when faced with an unidentified arrhythmia.

The eight basic dysrhythmias are early beats, unexpected pauses, tachycardias, bradycardias, bigeminal rhythms, group beating, total irregularity, and regular non-sinus rhythms at normal rates. Their most common causes, except for tachycardias, are outlined and illustrated below.

Causes of early beats

Extrasystoles (Fig. 18-8, *A* to *C*)

Parasystole *(D)*

Capture beats *(E)*

Reciprocal beats *(F)*

Better conduction interrupting poorer conduction *(G)*

Supernormal conduction during AV block *(H)*

Rhythm resumption after inapparent bigeminy *(I)*

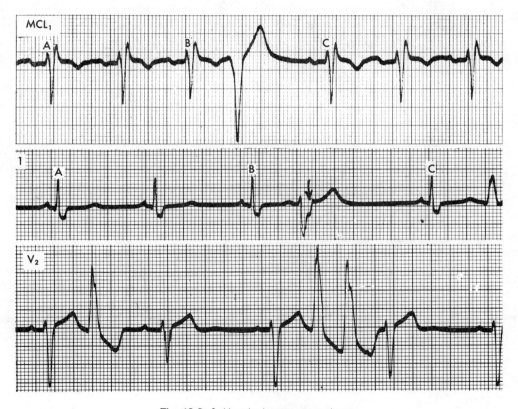

Fig. 18-8. A, Ventricular premature beats.

Continued.

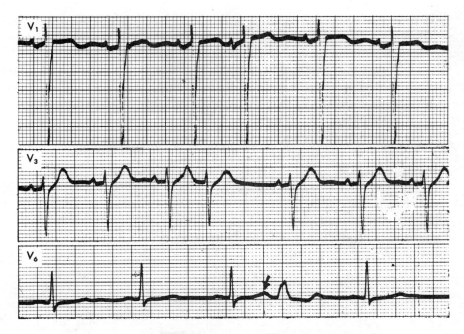

Fig. 18-8. B, Atrial premature beats.

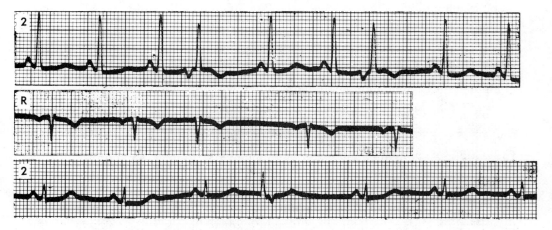

Fig. 18-8. C, Junctional premature beats.

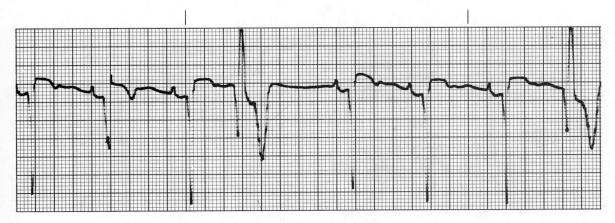

Fig. 18-8. D, Parasystole.

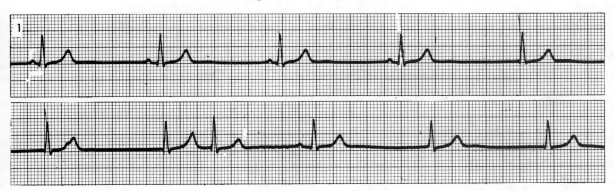

Fig. 18-8. E, A capture beat (bottom strip, third beat). The strips are continuous. Sinus bradycardia causing AV dissociation. The junction is escaping at a rate of about 43/min. One of the sinus beats in the bottom strip is conducted (capture).

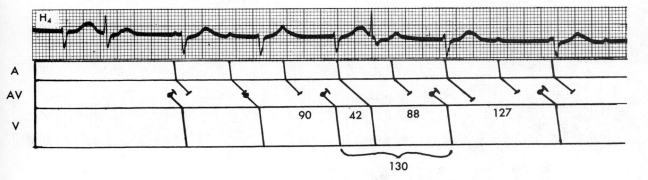

Fig. 18-8. F, Supernormal conduction during AV block. The junctional rhythm is interrupted twice by aberrantly conducted beats, both presumably due to supernormal conduction since later impulses fail to be conducted to the ventricles.

Continued.

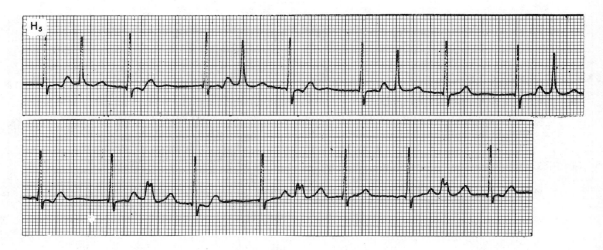

Fig. 18-8. G, Reciprocal beats. Continuous strips from a Holter monitoring lead. Throughout the tracing the beats are grouped in threes. The first of each trio is a junctional beat, which is followed by retrograde conduction to the atria and a reciprocal beat showing varying degrees of LBBB aberration. The third beat in each trio is probably a second reciprocal beat, with the preceding retrograde conduction failing to reach the atria.

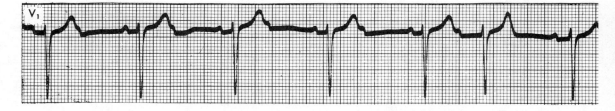

Fig. 18-8. H, Better conduction interrupting poorer conduction. The sixth beat is early because it is the second beat of a 3:2 Wenckebach interrupting 2:1 conduction. At a faster atrial rate the early beat might develop aberration and be difficult to distinguish from a VPB.

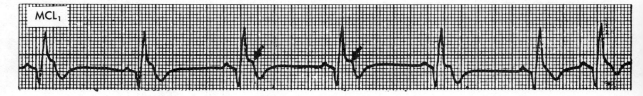

Fig. 18-8. I, Sinus rhythm with nonconducted atrial bigeminy. The atrial extrasystoles deform the shoulder of the ST segment (arrows). In the penultimate beat the deformity disappears and two consecutive sinus beats result in a shorter cycle.

Causes of pauses

Nonconducted atrial extrasystoles (Fig. 18-9, *A*)
Second-degree AV block (*B* and *C*)
Second-degree SA block (*D* and *E*)
"Sick sinus" variants (*F*)
Concealed conduction (*G*)
Concealed junctional extrasystoles (*H*)
Pacemaker pauses (*I*)

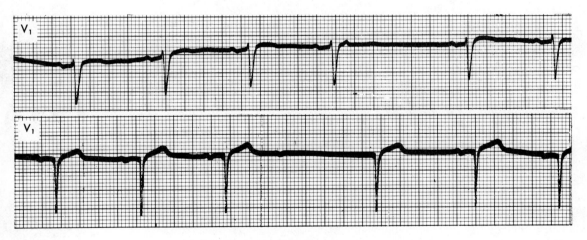

Fig. 18-9. A, Nonconducted atrial extrasystoles.

Continued.

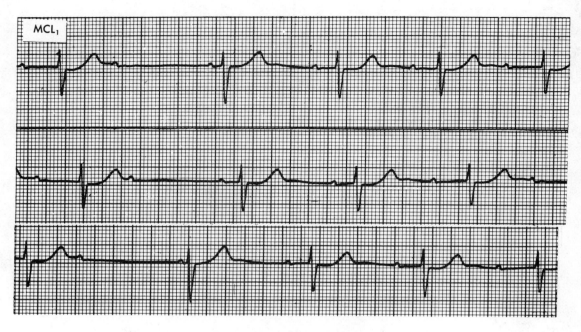

Fig. 18-9. B, Type I second-degree AV block.

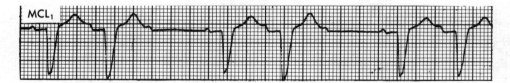

Fig. 18-9. C, Type II second-degree AV block.

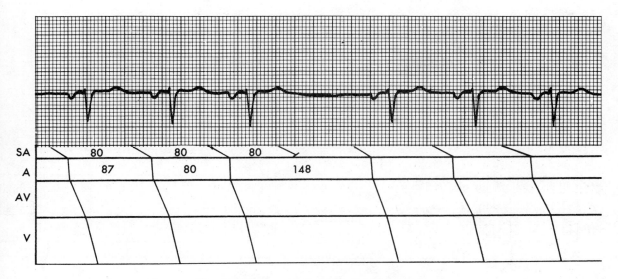

Fig. 18-9. D, Type I second-degree SA block.

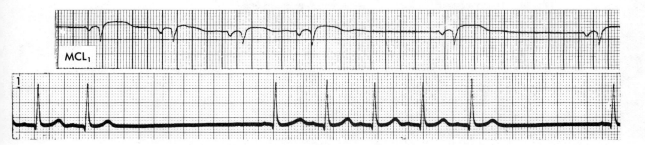

Fig. 18-9. E, Type II second-degree SA block.

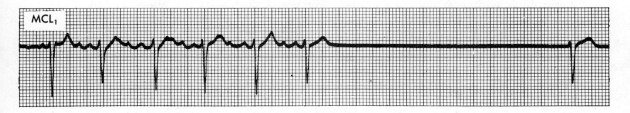

Fig. 18-9. F, Sick sinus (tachycardia-bradycardia) syndrome.

Continued.

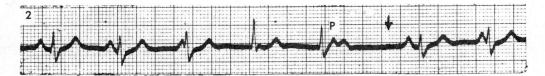

Fig. 18-9. G, Concealed conduction. The missing beat (arrow) results from incomplete penetration into the AV junction by a sinus impulse postponing the next beat of an accelerated idiojunctional rhythm (rate, 86/min).

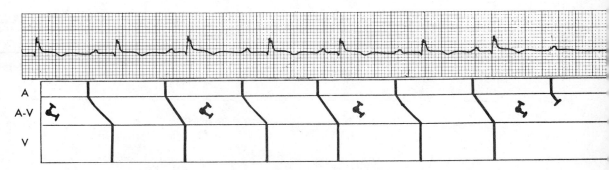

Fig. 18-9. H, Concealed junctional extrasystoles every third beat, causing lengthening of the subsequent PR and preventing AV conduction altogether toward the end of the strip (laddergram).

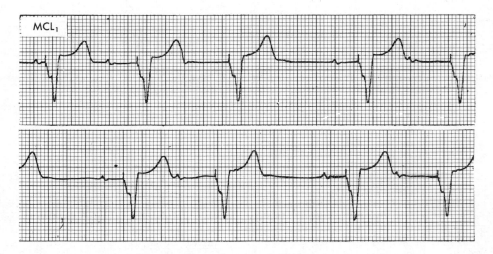

Fig. 18-9. I, Pacemaker pauses. The pauses in this tracing result from the pacemaker's sensing the T wave.

Causes of bradycardia

Sinus bradycardia (Fig. 18-10, *A*)
SA block *(B)*
Nonconducted atrial bigeminy *(C)*
AV block *(D)*

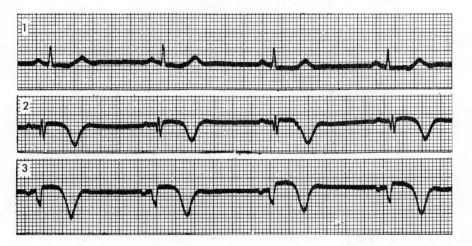

Fig. 18-10. A, Sinus bradycardia.

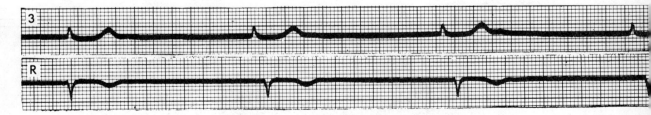

Fig. 18-10. B, Sick sinus. No atrial activity is visible, and the idiojunctional escape rate is 29/min. Absence of the P waves could be due to generator failure, exit block, atrial paralysis, or an inadequate sinus impulse.

Continued.

Lead II   Basic pattern

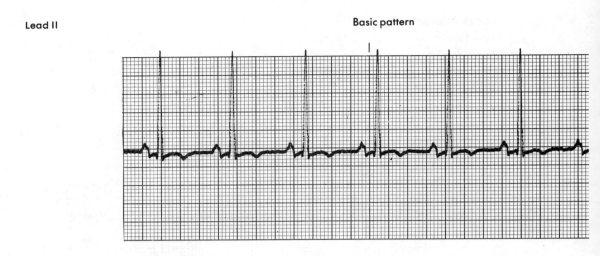

Lead II   Moment later

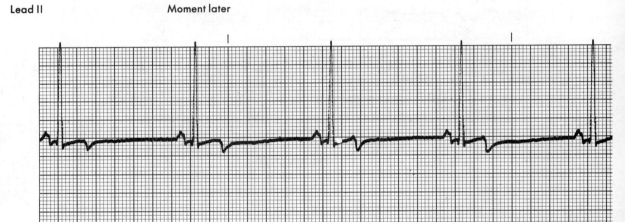

Fig. 18-10. C, Nonconducted atrial bigeminy. (Courtesy Janet Bacon, R.N., Portland, Oregon.)

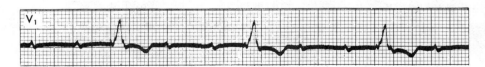

Fig. 18-10. D, AV block. Sinus rhythm (rate, 126/min) with 3:1 block producing a ventricular rate of 42/min.

Skeleton classification of bigeminy

Extrasystoles (Fig. 18-11, *A*)
Parasystole *(B)*
3:2 conduction *(C* to *F)*
Reciprocal beating *(G)*
Fortuitous pairing in atrial fibrillation *(H)*

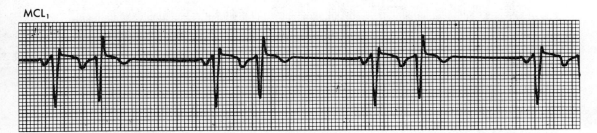

Fig. 18-11. A, Extrasystoles (bigeminal APBs with RBBB aberration).

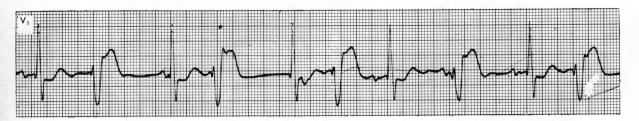

Fig. 18-11. B, Parasystole producing bigeminy with varying "coupling." Note that although the relationship of the ventricular ectopic beats to the preceding supraventricular beats varies markedly the interval between consecutive ectopic beats is constant.

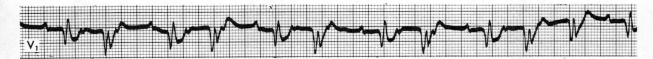

Fig. 18-11. C, 3:2 conduction of Wenckebach type during sinus tachycardia (rate, 132/min), leaving the ventricular complexes in pairs except for one threesome. The beats ending the shorter cycles are conducted aberrantly compared with the first beat of each pair.

Continued.

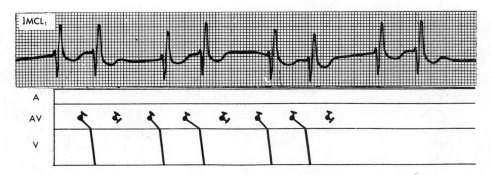

Fig. 18-11. D, 3:2 conduction. Junctional tachycardia with no sign of atrial activity; 3:2 Wenckebach conduction below the junctional pacemaker, leaving the ventricular complexes paired.

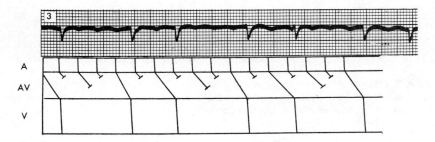

Fig. 18-11. E, 3:2 conduction. Atrial flutter with alternating 2:1 and 4:1 conduction, resulting in paired ventricular complexes; there is 2:1 "filtering" at a higher level in the AV junction combined at a lower level with 3:2 Wenckebachs of the alternate beats that pass the filter.

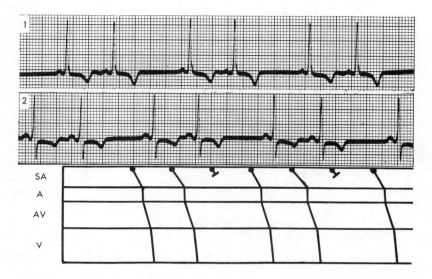

Fig. 18-11. F, 3:2 sinus Wenckebachs result in pairing of sinus beats.

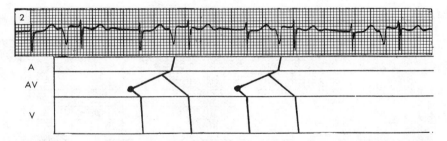

Fig. 18-11. G, Reciprocal beating during a junctional rhythm with delayed retrograde conduction produces bigeminy.

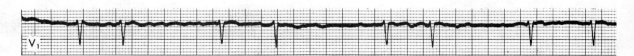

Fig. 18-11. H, Fortuitous pairing in atrial fibrillation. Occasionally, presumably by chance or by some nuance of concealed conduction, the beats in atrial fibrillation are conducted after alternately longer and shorter cycles.

Common causes of group beating

Supraventricular tachycardia with Wenckebach periods (Fig. 18-12, *A*)

Atrial flutter with 2:1 "filtering" at upper level in junction and Wenckebach periodicity below *(B)*

Sinus rhythm with two or more consecutive extrasystoles *(C)*

Recurrent bursts of tachycardia, ventricular or supraventricular *(D)*

Every third beat an interpolated ventricular extrasystole

Common causes of chaotic irregularity

Atrial fibrillation

Atrial flutter with varying AV conduction

Chaotic (multifocal) atrial tachycardia

Shifting (wandering) pacemaker with atrial extrasystoles

Sinus rhythm with multifocal extrasystoles

Mixed ventricular rhythms

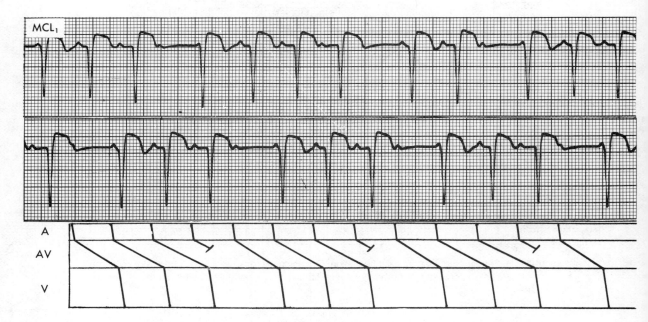

Fig. 18-12. A, Supraventricular (sinus) tachycardia with Wenckebach periods.

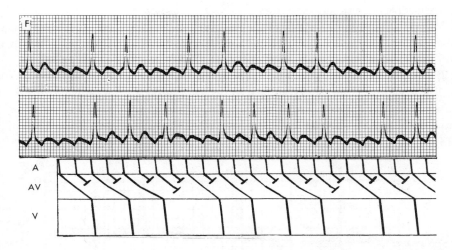

Fig. 18-12. B, Atrial flutter with 2:1 "filtering" at upper level in the junction and Wenckebach periodicity below (see laddergram).

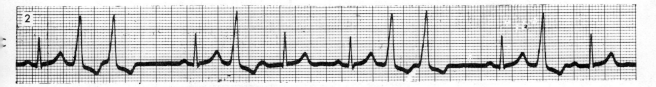

Fig. 18-12. C, Sinus rhythm with two consecutive extrasystoles. The first and third trios consist of a sinus beat followed by a pair of ventricular extrasystoles; the second and fourth consist of a ventricular extrasystole interpolated between two sinus beats.

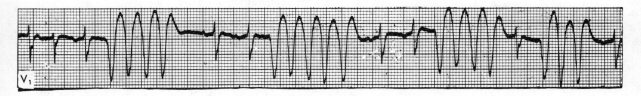

Fig. 18-12. D, Recurrent bursts of ventricular tachycardia.

MILK THE QRS. In arrhythmia detection give priority to ventricular behavior. In general, it matters little what the atria are doing so long as the ventricles are behaving themselves.

When measuring the QRS duration, be sure to check in at least two leads because it may be that initial or terminal forces are isoelectric in a particular lead, causing the QRS to appear narrow in that lead only (Fig. 18-13).

If the QRS is of normal duration, you know that the rhythm is supraventricular; but if it is wide and bizarre, you have to decide whether it is supraventricular with ventricular aberration or ectopic ventricular. Your knowledge of the ECG in the distinction between aberrancy and ectopy will enable you to get the most out of the QRS milking process (Chapter 16).

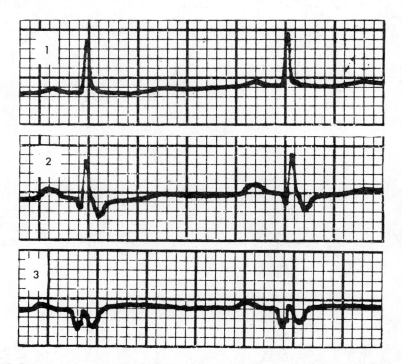

Fig. 18-13. From lead 1, no one would think that this patient has intraventricular block with a QRS interval of 0.11 second, as seen in leads 2 and 3. By Einthoven's equation, since the terminal 0.06 second of the QRS in lead 2 and that in lead 3 are almost identical negative deflections, this part of the QRS in lead 1 is isoelectric.

CHERCHEZ LE P. If the shape of the QRS does not help you make a diagnosis, turn to the P wave for help. In the past the P wave, as the key to arrhythmias, has certainly been overemphasized. However, there are times when it holds the diagnostic clue and must be accorded the starring role.

In one's search for P waves, there are several clues and caveats to bear in mind.

The S₅ lead. This lead was introduced by French cardiologists in 1952. It is obtained by placing the positive electrode at the fifth right interspace close to the sternum (just below the C_1 position) and the negative electrode on the manubrium of the sternum. This will sometimes greatly magnify the P wave, rendering it readily visible when it may have been virtually indiscernible in other leads. Fig. 18-14 illustrates this amplifying effect and makes the diagnosis of atrial tachycardia with 2:1 block immediately apparent. If it succeeds, this technique is certainly preferable to invasive ones (atrial wire or esophageal electrode).

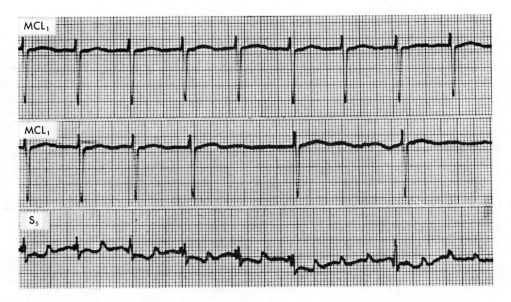

Fig. 18-14. The S₅ lead. The top strip of MCL₁ shows barely perceptible P′ waves of an atrial tachycardia. The second stirp shows the effect of carotid sinus stimulation: the ventricular rate halves because of increased AV block, and additional P′ waves become barely visible through the artifact. In contrast, the strip of lead S₅ has prominent P waves.

The Bix rule. Whenever P waves of a supraventricular tachycardia are exactly halfway between the ventricular complexes, you should always suspect that additional P waves are hiding within the QRS complex—a point emphasized by the late Harold Bix of Vienna and Baltimore. In the top strip of Fig. 18-15 the P′ wave is midway between the QRS complexes. Moments later the conduction pattern alters (middle strip) and exposes the lurking P′ waves. It is clearly important to know if there are twice as many atrial impulses as are apparent because, if there are, there is the ever present danger, especially if the atrial rate should slow somewhat, that the ventricular rate may double or almost double. It is better to be forewarned and take steps to prevent such potentially disastrous acceleration.

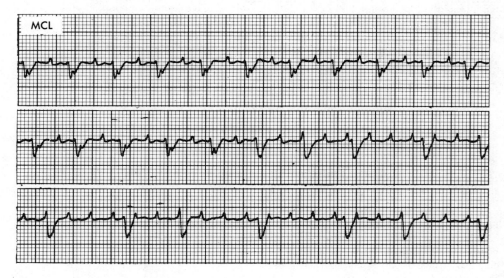

Fig. 18-15. The Bix rule (top strip). The P waves are midway between the ventricular complexes, making one suspicious of a hidden P′ wave.

The haystack principle. If you were searching for a needle in a haystack, you would obviously prefer a small to a large haystack. Therefore, whenever you can't find an elusive P wave or pacemaker spike, give the lead with the least disturbance of the baseline (the smallest ventricular complexes) a chance to help you. There are some leads that no one would think of looking at to solve an arrhythmia (aVR, for example). The patient whose tracing you see in Fig. 18-16 died because no one thought to apply the haystack principle and look in aVR. He had a runaway pacemaker at a discharge rate of 440/min with a halved ventricular response of 220/min. Lead aVR was the lead with the smallest ventricular complex, and it was the only lead in which the pacemaker "blips" were plainly visible (arrows). The patient went into shock and died because none of the attempted therapeutic measures affected the tachycardia, when all that was necessary was to disconnect the wayward pulse generator.

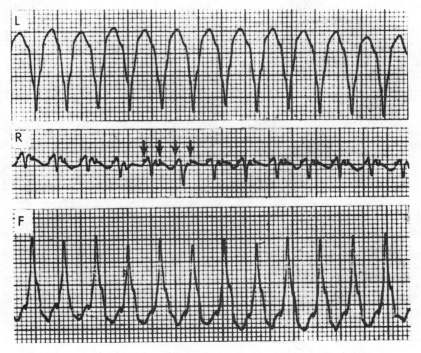

Fig. 18-16. The haystack principle. The patient's runaway pacemaker is recognizable only in the lead with the least disturbance of the baseline, in this case aVR.

Mind your "Ps." This means to be wary of things that look like P waves and particularly applies to P-like waves that are adjacent to the QRS complex—they may turn out to be part of the QRS complex. This is a trap for the unwary sufferer from the P-preoccupation syndrome, to whom anything that looks like a P wave is a P wave. For example, the strips of V_1 and V_2 in Fig. 18-17 would be diagnosed by many as a supraventricular tachycardia for the wrong reasons. In V_1 the QRS seems not to be very wide and appears to be preceded by a small P wave. In V_2 an apparently narrow QRS is followed by what appears to be a retrograde P wave. In fact, the P-like waves in both these leads are part of the QRS complex. If the QRS duration is measured in V_3 it is found to be 0.14 second. To attain a QRS of that duration in V_1 and V_2, one needs to include the P-like waves in the measurement.

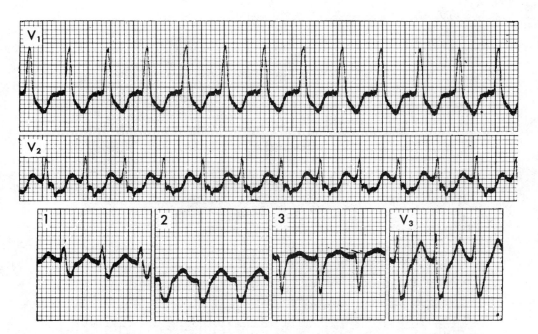

Fig. 18-17. Mind your "Ps." The QRS duration in leads 1 and V_3 measures 0.14 second. Therefore the P-like waves in the other leads must be part of the QRS.

Find a break. It is at a break in rhythm that you are most likely to spot the solution. For example, look at Fig. 18-18. At the beginning of the strip, where the rhythm is regular at a rate of 200/min, it is impossible to know whether the tachycardia is ectopic atrial, ectopic junctional, or reciprocating in the AV junction. A fourth possibility is that the little peak is part of the QRS and not a P wave at all. Further along the strip there is a pause in the rhythm. The commonest cause of a pause is a nonconducted atrial extrasystole; and, sure enough, there at the arrow is the culprit—in this situation a diagnostic ally. As a result of the pause the P wave can be seen in front of the next QRS; therefore the mechanism is atrial tachycardia.

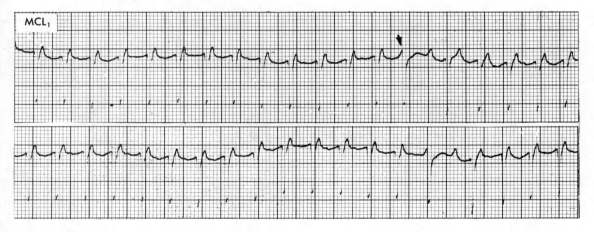

Fig. 18-18. Focus on the break in rhythm, and it gives you the answer: the P' wave precedes the QRS rather than follows it.

WHO'S MARRIED TO WHOM? Establishing relationships is often the crucial step in arriving at a firm diagnosis. This principle is illustrated in Fig. 18-19, where a junctional rhythm is dissociated from sinus bradycardia. On three occasions there are bizarre early beats of a qR configuration that is nondiagnostic. The fact that they are seen *only* when a P wave is emerging beyond the preceding QRS tells us that they are "married to" the preceding P waves and establishes them as conducted (capture) beats with RBBB aberration rather than ventricular extrasystoles.

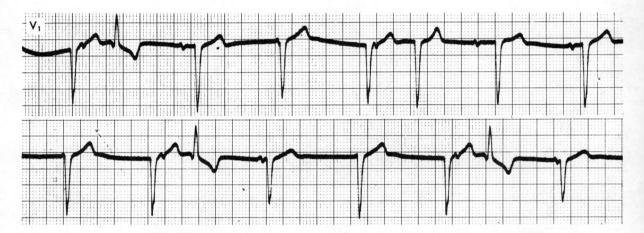

Fig. 18-19. Who's married to whom? The strips are continuous. The early beats are consistently preceded by a sinus P wave just emerging beyond the QRS and are therefore conducted (capture) beats. The underlying rhythm is sinus bradycardia producing AV dissociation.

PINPOINT THE PRIMARY. One must never be content to let the diagnosis rest with a phenomenon such as AV dissociation, escape, or aberration, which are always secondary to some primary disturbance.

In Fig. 18-20 there is a junctional rhythm with retrograde conduction at a rate of 31/min. Show this to most observers and ask for a *diagnosis*. Almost certainly the answer will be "junctional rhythm." But this is not a diagnosis. No junctional rhythm could possibly hold sway in the presence of a normal sinus node. The diagnosis—the primary disturbance—is a sick SA node; and junctional rhythm is a secondary escape mechanism.

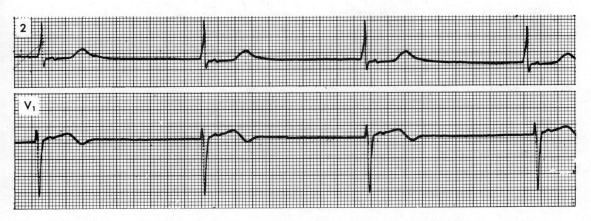

Fig. 18-20. Pinpoint the primary condition, which is sick sinus syndrome with resulting AV junctional escape (rate, 31/min) with retrograde conduction.

Fig. 18-21 gives us a chance to review several of the points under "A systematic approach," p. 298. This tracing was sent thousands of miles with the note: "This patient needed a pacemaker for this funny sort of block—what is it?"

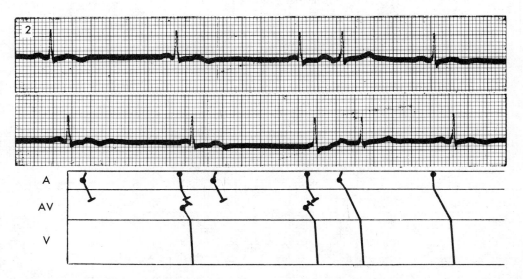

Fig. 18-21. The strips are continuous. Sinus rhythm with atrial bigeminy; most of the APBs are not conducted, with resulting junctional escape.

After observing the presence of bradycardia and of two premature supraventricular beats, probably the first thing that you notice is AV dissociation and the different shapes of the Ts. The P′ wave is a common reason for such distortion, and the diagnosis "falls into your lap": conducted and nonconducted bigeminal APBs with junctional escape beats.

Failing this approach the diagnosis could have been arrived at by any of the following methods:

1. Review the causes of bradycardia. Nonconducted atrial bigeminy is third on the list and elicits from you a careful examination of the T waves, in which you find the nonconducted APBs.

2. If you were motivated by the injunction to "find the break," you would concentrate on the early beats, since they represent the "break" in the otherwise regular rhythm. Attention would then be directed to the T waves and the hidden Ps.

3. If you had recited the causes of early supraventricular beats, you would have thought first of atrial extrasystoles.

References

1. Thorne, D., and Gozensky, C.: Rabbit ears: an aid in distinguishing ventricular ectopy from aberration, Heart Lung 3:634, 1974.
2. Wellens, H.J.J., and others: The value of the electrocardiogram in the differential diagnosis of a tachycardia with a widened QRS complex, Am. J. Med. **64**:27, 1978.
3. Marriott, H.J.L., and Fogg, E.: Constant monitoring for cardiac dysrhythmias and blocks, Mod. Concepts Cardiovasc. Dis. **39**:103, 1970.

CHAPTER 19

Digitalis dysrhythmias

Digitalis intoxication can produce virtually every disturbance of rhythm or conduction. However, whether a particular dysrhythmia is, in fact, due to the drug is always a *clinical* diagnosis, never a purely electrocardiographic one. There are, of course, circumstances in which the clinician may suspect the diagnosis on the basis of the ECG, especially when one of the disturbances so typical of digitalis overdosage (such as ventricular bigeminy, accelerated idiojunctional rhythm or AV Wenckebach) is seen along with the typical sagging ST-T changes. Even in the face of such arrhythmias, however, the diagnosis of toxicity is made only after weighing all the evidence.

When digitalis is given in excess or when its toxic effects are felt because of a lowered potassium, the dysrhythmic manifestations can be divided into two categories: the excitant and the suppressant effects. Often, there is a combination of the two.

Excitant effects

The main excitant disturbances caused by digitalis intoxication are listed below.

1. Ventricular extrasystoles, especially bigeminal and multiform
2. Atrial tachycardia
3. AV junctional tachycardia
4. Accelerated junctional rhythm
5. Ventricular tachycardia
6. Bidirectional tachycardia
7. Ventricular fibrillation

VENTRICULAR EXTRASYSTOLES. Ventricular extrasystoles are the most frequently seen cardiac manifestation of digitalis overdosage, except in children in whom supraventricular disturbances are more common. One should note, however, that ventricular arrhythmias are in no sense diagnostic of digitalis intoxication, being common in both health and disease of any kind. Furthermore, digitalis is often an effective drug for reducing or eliminating ventricular extrasystoles that are not caused by the drug.[1,2] When they are caused by digitalis, they tend to be bigeminal. Of interest is the fact that digitalis has been found to cause afterdepolarizations,[3] which, if they attain threshold, would produce precisely coupled ventricular extrasystoles (p. 140). Scherf and Schott[4] claim that the ventricular ectopic beats of a digitalis-induced bigeminy will always show variation in morphology if long enough strips are taken, a concept that agrees with the afterdepolarization theory as a digitalis-induced arrhythmogenic mechanism, since a precise focus (and therefore uniform VPBs) need not be involved. Sometimes the bigeminy due to digitalis is "concealed"; that is, bigeminal runs are not seen, but all interectopic intervals contain only odd numbers of sinus beats[5] (see p. 66).

ATRIAL TACHYCARDIA. Atrial tachycardia caused by digitalis tends to possess P' waves of normal sinus polarity but of smaller than average amplitude, and they may be somewhat irreglar in time and variable in shape ("multifocal atrial tachycardia" or "chaotic atrial tachycardia"). The arrhythmia is often associated with varying ratios of AV conduction ("PAT with block").

Atrial flutter and atrial fibrillation have only occasionally been described as manifestations of digitoxicity.[1,11]

AV JUNCTIONAL TACHYCARDIA. AV junctional tachycardia is another fairly common manifestation of digitalis intoxication. Although the drug usually slows sinus pacemakers, it tends to enhance the automaticity of junctional pacemakers. Sometimes it produces a genuine tachycardia, as in Fig. 19-1. At other times it induces a more modest enhancement to a rate between 60 and 100/min; and the disturbance is then appropriately termed accelerated AV or junctional (or idionodal) rhythm, illustrated in Fig. 19-2.

The patient whose tracing is seen in Fig. 19-1 had atrial fibrillation. An excess of digitalis produced an AV junctional tachycardia, recognized because of its almost precise regularity at a rate of 140/min.

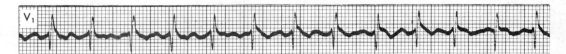

Fig. 19-1. AV junctional tachycardia (rate, 140/min) with incomplete RBBB in the presence of atrial fibrillation.

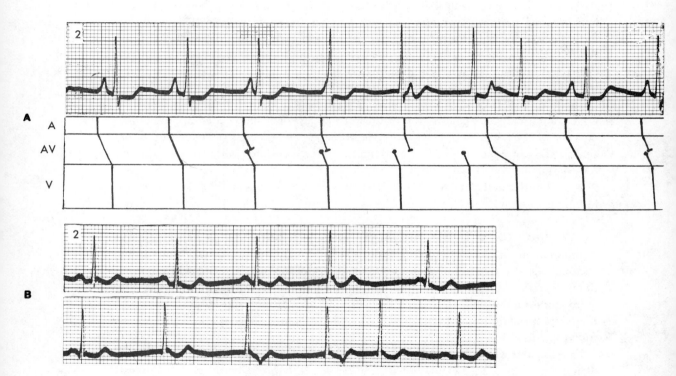

Fig. 19-2. A, An accelerated idiojunctional rhythm (rate, 78/min) usurps control from a sinus rhythm (rate, 70 to 75/min). The seventh beat is a capture beat conducted with prolonged PR interval. **B,** The strips are continuous. An irregular accelerated junctional rhythm usurps control from the sinus rhythm. Beats 3 and 4 in the bottom strip are followed by retrograde conduction to the atria. Beat 5 is a ventricular "echo" (reciprocal beat).

ACCELERATED JUNCTIONAL RHYTHM (AJR). The accelerated junctional rhythm (rate, 60 to 100/min) is an early manifestation of digitalis intoxication and is secondary to enhanced automaticity in the AV junction.

Fig. 19-2, *A*, is the tracing of a 12-year-old girl who required a mitral commissurotomy. After successful surgery her digitalis dosage was not reduced, and signs of intoxication soon developed in the form of the AJR seen in this tracing. This arrhythmia commonly leads to AV dissociation, seen in the same tracing.

Fig. 19-2, *B*, illustrates another case of AJR resulting from digitalis overdosage. The patient was a young woman with a rheumatic heart who was 1 day postpartum. By mistake, she received an extra dose of 0.5 mg of digoxin intravenously and began to show the somewhat irregular junctional rhythm illustrated.

VENTRICULAR TACHYCARDIA. Fig. 19-3 is the tracing of a patient who was being relentlessly nudged toward his death by repeated intravenous doses of digoxin. His RBBB was present on admission, and the first evidence of intoxication was the junctional tachycardia. In the second strip ventricular tachycardia of the "swinging" variety (the polarity of the QRS swings between positive and negative) develops, another excitant manifestation of digitalis toxicity.

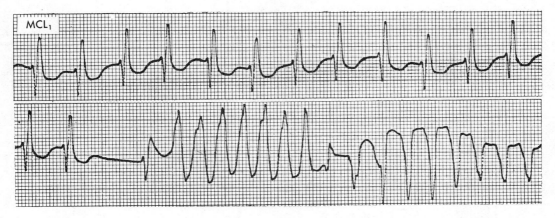

Fig. 19-3. The strips are continuous. Two excitant manifestations of digitalis intoxication: AV junctional tachycardia (rate, 125/min) (upper strip) and ventricular tachycardia of the "swinging" variety (lower strip). There is also an underlying RBBB. In the lower strip the junctional tachycardia suddenly pauses (?exit block), and the lengthened cycle precipitates the ventricular tachycardia.

DOUBLE TACHYCARDIA. Digitalis toxicity is the most common cause of "double tachycardia"[6]: the simultaneous existence of two rapidly firing but independent foci, such as the simultaneous atrial and junctional tachycardia seen in Fig. 19-4.

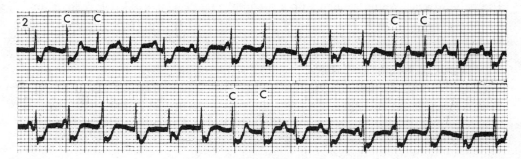

Fig. 19-4. The strips are continuous. Simultaneous but independent atrial tachycardia (rate, 172/min) and junctional tachycardia (rate, 154/min). Pairs of captured beats (*C*) are recognized by the slight shortening of the ventricular cycles.

BIDIRECTIONAL TACHYCARDIA. This term is purely descriptive and does not imply a mechanism; His bundle studies have shown the mechanism to be sometimes bifocal ectopic ventricular[7,8] and sometimes AV junctional with RBBB and alternating hemiblocks.[9] A bidirectional or alternating tachycardia is seen in Fig. 19-5.

Another possibility in some cases is an interpolated ventricular bigeminy with fortuitously equal coupling and postectopic intervals.

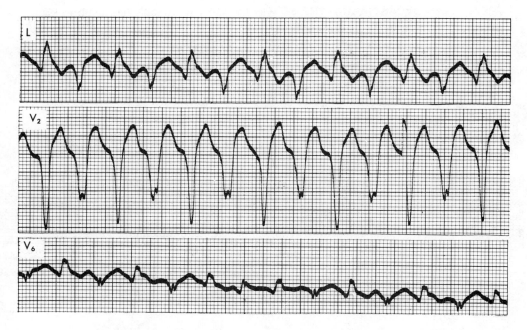

Fig. 19-5. Bidirectional tachycardia. In aVL and V₆, there is a tendency for the ventricular complexes to be alternately positive and negative. In V₂ the QRS amplitude alternates (alternating tachycardia).

Suppressant effects

The main suppressant disturbances caused by digitalis intoxication are listed below.

1. Sinus bradycardia
2. SA block
3. Type I second-degree AV block
4. Complete AV block

SINUS BRADYCARDIA AND THE SA WENCKEBACH. Digitalis has a suppressant effect both on impulse formation in the SA node and on conduction out of the node. Fig. 19-6, *A*, shows both sinus bradycardia and a simultaneous 5:4 SA Wenckebach (see laddergram).

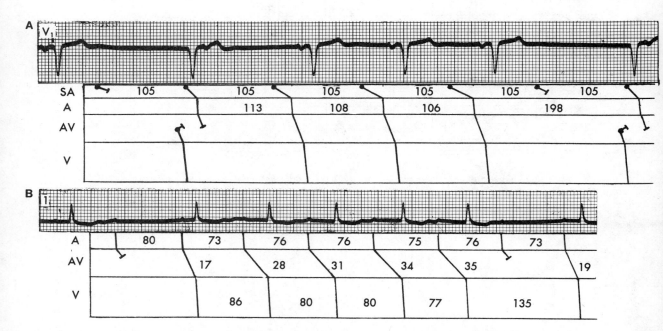

Fig. 19-6. A, Sinus bradycardia complicated by a sinus exit block of the Wenckebach type. The second and last beats are junctional escape beats (see laddergram). Wenckebach-type conduction is inferred from the progressive shortening of the atrial (PP) interval (*113, 108, 106*)—"footprints" of the Wenckebach. **B,** Second-degree AV block, type I. This typical Wenckebach period shows progressive lengthening of the PR interval until the sixth beat is dropped (6:5 AV block)—see laddergram.

AV BLOCK. When digitalis impairs conduction in the AV junction, its effect is on the AV node itself; and therefore, if there is significant AV block, it is of the type I variety and complete block results in an escaping junctional pacemaker. Fig. 19-6, *B*, presents a 6:5 Wenckebach period in a patient with mild digitalis toxicity.

It is doubtful whether digitalis ever produces type II AV block or BBB. However, in advanced stages of intoxication in severely diseased hearts it is possible that digitalis may impair conduction in the Purkinje fibers.

Combined effects

The common combined disturbances caused by digitalis intoxication are as listed.

1. Atrial tachycardia with AV block ("PAT with block")
2. Sinus bradycardia with AV junctional tachycardia
3. Regular accelerated junctional rhythm in the presence of atrial fibrillation
4. Double tachycardias, atrial and AV junctional

ATRIAL TACHYCARDIA WITH AV BLOCK. Atrial tachycardia with AV block is one of the most common combinations of excitant and suppressant effects of digitalis toxicity. It carries a high mortality rate if the drug is not immediately discontinued. It is said to be more likely to develop in patients with cor pulmonale and hypoxia.[12]

Fig. 19-7 is a classical example of this combined arrhythmia. The P′ waves are variable in shape, irregular in rhythm, and of normal polarity most of the time; and the conduction ratio is variable. The sagging ST segments are characteristic of digitalis effect.

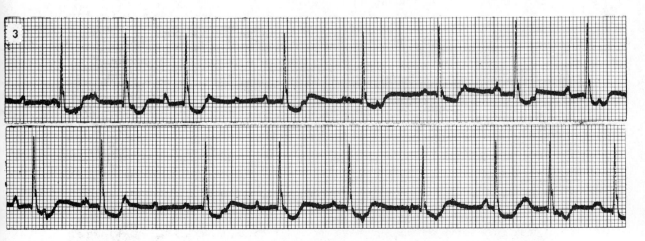

Fig. 19-7. The strips are continuous. Multifocal atrial tachycardia with varying AV block. Note the variable P wave morphology, irregular atrial rhythm, changing AV conduction ratio, and sagging ST segments characteristic of the digitalis effect.

Fig. 19-8 also shows this combination but, in addition, contains ventricular extrasystoles. This patient was mistakenly given 2 mg of digoxin intravenously, with the disturbing results you see.

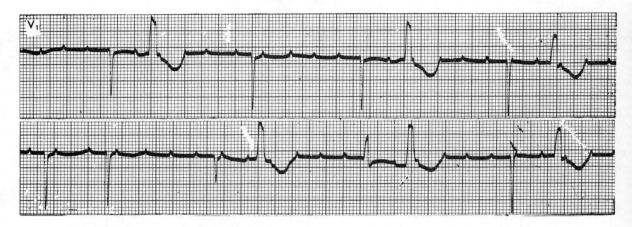

Fig. 19-8. The strips are continuous. Atrial tachycardia with varying AV block and numerous ventricular extrasystoles tending to bigeminy. Note the irregularity of the atrial rhythm. From a 30-year-old woman with postpartum cardiomyopathy who was mistakenly given an overdose of intravenous digoxin.

SINUS BRADYCARDIA WITH AV JUNCTIONAL TACHYCARDIA. Fig. 19-9, *A*, illustrates another threefold effect of digitalis overdosage: sinus bradycardia, a minor degree of AV block, and junctional tachycardia.[13]

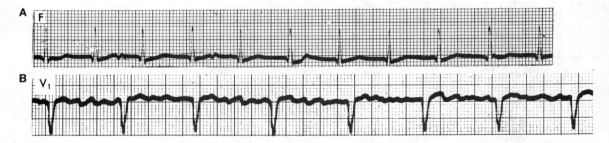

Fig. 19-9. A, Sinus bradycardia (rate, 55/min) with some degree of AV block and junctional tachycardia—all due to digitalis. The third and the fifth beats end slightly shorter cycles and are presumably conducted with prolonged PR intervals; elsewhere the two rhythms are dissociated. **B,** Atrial fibrillation with some degree of AV block and independent accelerated idiojunctional rhythm (rate, 70/min). The degree of block and the enhancement of AV automaticity necessary to produce the dissociation are both due to digitalis.

REGULAR ACCELERATED JUNCTIONAL RHYTHM WITH ATRIAL FIBRILLATION.

Fig. 19-9, *B*, illustrates a patient with atrial fibrillation in whom the digitalis has produced some degree of AV block and an accelerated idiojunctional rhythm, the combination of which has caused complete AV dissociation.

Fig. 19-10 is from a patient with atrial fibrillation, true posterior infarction, and digitalis intoxication. Lead V_3 shows the accelerated junctional rhythm resulting from the toxicity. Leads V_2 and V_4 have the same accelerated rhythm but with Wenckebach periods out of or below the AV pacemaker causing group beating. In V_2 there are 5:4 and 4:3 Wenckebach periods whereas in V_4 there is the more common 3:2 ratio producing bigeminal grouping (see laddergram).

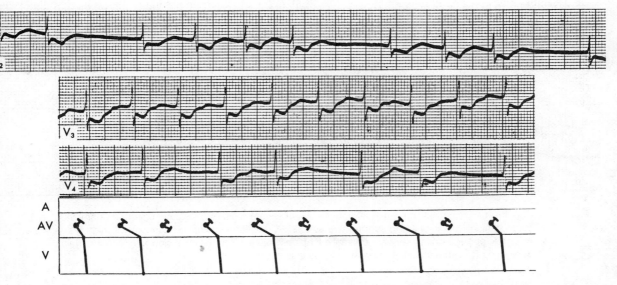

Fig. 19-10. Lead V_3 shows the accelerated AV junctional rhythm (rate, 98/min) resulting from digitalis toxicity. Leads V_2 and V_4 show the same accelerated junctional rhythm complicated by Wenckebach periods out of (exit block) or below the AV pacemaker. V_2 shows the even more common 3:2 ratio producing bigeminal groupings.

Fig. 19-11 is from a patient with atrial fibrillation and severe digitalis intoxication. There is at least high-grade and probably complete AV block with resultant escaping idionodal rhythm at the slow rate of about 40/min. There is ventricular bigeminy and, as is always the case,[4] the extrasystolic complexes vary in shape ("multiform" or "variform"). A nondysrhythmic sign said to be diagnostic of digitalis intoxication is also seen in this tracing: sagging ST segments in leads in which the QRS is predominantly negative.[14]

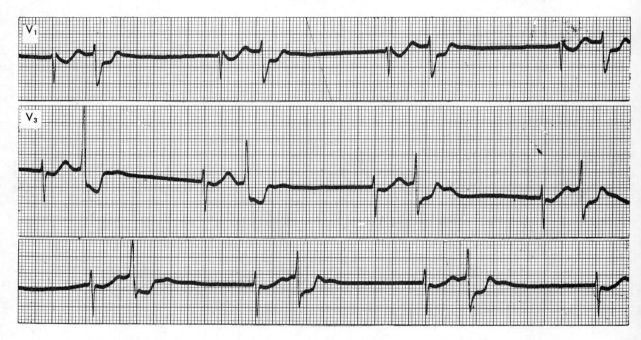

Fig. 19-11. From a patient with atrial fibrillation and severe digitalis intoxication, showing combined manifestations of excitant and suppressive actions: **1,** multiform ventricular bigeminy; **2,** high-grade AV block, perhaps complete, with resultant escaping idiojunctional rhythm at slow rate (about 40/min); **3,** sagging ST segments in leads with a dominantly negative QRS.

Fig. 19-12 is from a 10-year-old boy who, after mitral valve surgery, was mistakenly maintained on a double dose of digitalis. On 8/8/68 he manifested an accelerated idioventricular rhythm, dissociated from his sinus rhythm, with ventricular bigeminy. There is also some degree of block since the atrial impulses in lead 1 land beyond the T wave and yet are not conducted. Four days later, after discontinuance of the digitalis, the rhythm has reverted to sinus uncomplicated except for residual first-degree AV block.

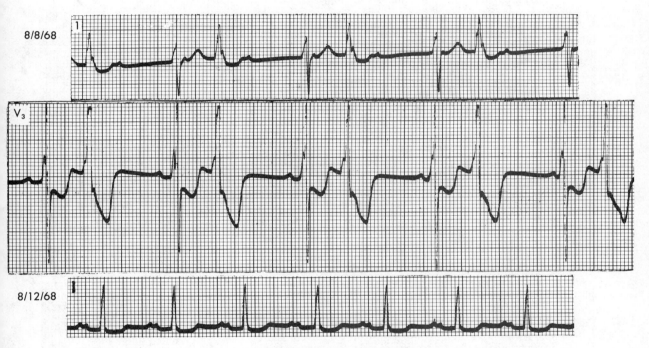

Fig. 19-12. From a 10-year-old who was mistakenly maintained on a double dose of digitalis preparations after mitral valve surgery. The combined effects of digitalis toxicity are seen in the first tracing (8/8/68): accelerated idioventricular rhythm (rate, 64/min) with ventricular bigeminy dissociated from the sinus rhythm (rate, 90/min). There is some degree of AV block—note the P waves in lead 1 landing beyond the T waves, which should be conducted but are not. Digitalis was discontinued, and 4 days later the rhythm reverted to sinus (rate, 80/min) with first-degree AV block. Note the P-mitrale in lead 1 on both days.

Fig. 19-13 is from a 50-year-old woman with acute inferior infarction in whom sinus tachycardia developed at a rate of 130/min. She was given 0.75 mg of digoxin intravenously, and the dose was repeated 1 hour later. During the subsequent several hours many manifestations of digitalis intoxication appeared, including severe vomiting and the cardiotoxic effects illustrated in Fig. 19-13.

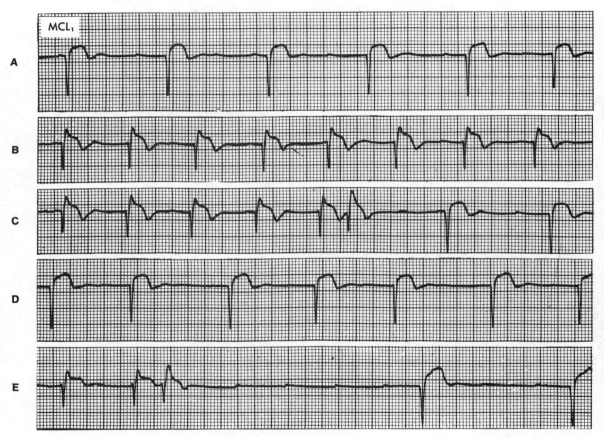

Fig. 19-13. The strips are not continuous but were selected during several hours of severe digitalis intoxication. From a patient with acute inferior infarction who received 1.5 mg of digoxin intravenously in 1 hour; 6 hours later the digoxin level was 7.4 ng. **A,** Sinus tachycardia (rate, 135/min) with significant AV block and a junctional escape rhythm (rate, 50/min). The final beat, since it ends a shorter cycle, is probably conducted with a polonged PR interval. **B,** Accelerated idiojunctional rhythm (rate, 72/min) with incomplete RBBB, dissociated from the persisting sinus tachycardia. The incomplete RBBB may be rate dependent, or it may be due to the form of aberration that results from an eccentric location of the junctional pacemaker. **C,** More of the same, terminated by a junctional premature beat with a greater degree of RBBB aberration. The fact that a premature stimulus interrupts the accelerated rhythm suggests that the mechanism of the rhythm is reciprocating. **D,** The third and sixth beats are escape beats, but the rest end shorter cycles and are probably conducted. **E,** The ending of another run of faster idiojunctional rhythm (as in the third strip). This time the escaping pacemaker is less alive, reveals an advanced degree of AV block, and "wakes up" only after 3 seconds.

DOUBLE TACHYCARDIAS. Fig. 19-14 is from the same patient as in Fig. 19-1, *B*, at a later stage of intoxication. It shows a combination of the same AV junctional tachycardia with RBBB but now with intermittent AV block below the level of the AV pacemaker and, in the middle strip, the development of a right ventricular tachycardia at a modest rate. The fusion beats *(F)* in the middle of the bottom strip are a nice example of the "normalization" that results when BBB is present and a ventricular impulse, arising on the same side as the BBB, fuses with a simultaneous supraventricular impulse (p. 215).

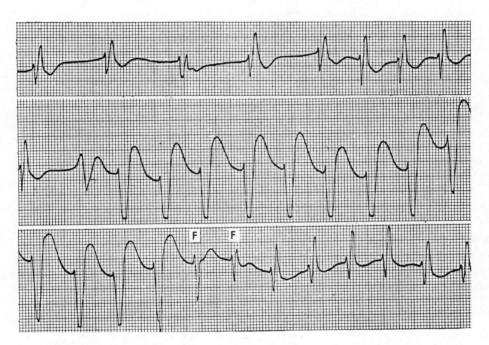

Fig. 19-14. The strips are continuous. The top strip begins with the same irregular junctional tachycardia seen in Fig. 19-1, at first with probable 2:1 exit block or block below the AV pacemaker. The strip ends with 1:1 conduction. After another blocked beat at the beginning of the second strip, a right ventricular tachycardia takes over (rate, 112/min). In the bottom strip there are two "normalized" fusion beats (*F*) between the impulses of the two tachycardias

References

1. Scherf, D., and Schott, A.: Extrasystoles and allied arrhythmias, ed. 2, pp. 592, 990, 993, London, 1973, William Heinemann Medical Books, Ltd.
2. Lown, B., and others: Effect of a digitalis drug on ventricular premature beats, N. Engl. J. Med. **296:**301, 1977.
3. Cranefield, P.F.: Action potentials, afterpotentials, and arrhythmias, Circ. Res. **41:**415, 1977.
4. Scherf, D., and Schott, A.: Extrasystoles and allied arrhythmias, ed. 2, London, 1973, Heinemann Medical Books.
5. Schamroth, L., and Marriott, H.J.L.: Concealed ventricular extrasystoles, Circulation **27:**1043, 1963.
6. Castellanos, A., and others: Digitalis-induced arrhythmias: recognition and therapy, Cardiovasc. Clin. **1**(3):108, 1969.
7. Cohen, S.I., and others: Infra-His origin of bidirectional tachycardia, Cirulation **47:**1260, 1973.
8. Morris, S.N., and Zipes, D.P.: His bundle electrocardiography during bidirectional tachycardia, Circulation **48:**32, 1973.
9. Rosenbaum, M.B., and others: The mechanism of bidirectional tachycardia, Am. Heart J. **78:**4, 1969.
10. Gavrilescu, S., and Luca, C.: His bundle electrogram during bidirectional tachycardia, Br. Heart J. **37:**1198, 1975.
11. Agarwal, B.L., and others: Atrial flutter: a rare manifestation of digitalis intoxication, Br. Heart J. **34:**392, 1972.
12. Agarwal, B.L., and Agrawal, B.V.: Digitalis induced paroxysmal atrial tachycardia with AV block, Br. Heart J. **36:**330, 1972.
13. Kastor, J.A.: Digitalis intoxication in patients with atrial fibrillation, Circulation **47:**888, 1973.
14. Lepeschkin, E.: Modern electrocardiography, Baltimore, 1951, The Williams & Wilkins Co.

Glossary

A wave (HBE) Represents atrial activation.

aberrant ventricular conduction The *temporary* abnormal intraventricular conduction of supraventricular impulses; also called "ventricular aberration" or "aberrancy."

absolute refractory period The period during which the cell will not respond to a second stimulus of even greater strength or duration than was necessary to discharge it in its nonrefractory state.

accelerated idiojunctional rhythm An ectopic junctional rhythm at a rate exceeding the normal firing rate of the junction without retrograde conduction to the atria.

accelerated idioventricular rhythm A rhythm of ectopic ventricular origin, faster than the normal rate of the His-Purkinje system but slower than 100/min without retrograde conduction to the atria.

accelerated junctional rhythm An ectopic junctional rhythm at a rate exceeding the normal firing rate of junctional tissue and with or without retrograde atrial conduction.

accessory pathway An extra muscular tract between atrium and ventricle.

afterdepolarization (delayed) A slow channel depolarization following in the wake of an action potential.

AH interval (HBE) Represents AV nodal conduction time, measured from the A wave on the HBE to the earliest onset of the His-bundle potential.

allorhythmia A repetitive arrhythmic sequence.

alternating aberration Ventricular aberration assuming alternate forms of intraventricular block.

Ashman's phenomenon Aberrant ventricular conduction in atrial fibrillation that results when a short cycle follows a long one.

automaticity The capability of a cell to depolarize spontaneously, reach threshold potential, and initiate an action potential.

AV junctional tachycardia An ectopic junctional rhythm at a rate exceeding 100 beats/min.

AV reciprocating tachycardia A supraventricular tachycardia supported by AV nodal reentry or reentry using the AV junction and an accessory pathway.

AV tract A muscular pathway between atrium and ventricle with one end inserted into conductive tissue.

bidirectional tachycardia Tachycardia in which the wide QRS complexes alternate in polarity in the observed lead.

bradycardia-tachycardia syndrome Any dysrhythmia characterized by alternating slow and fast heart rates.

cardiac action potential The very precise rapid sequence of changes in the electrical potential across the cell membrane.

chaotic atrial tachycardia Atrial tachycardia with P′ waves that are irregular in time and variable in shape; multifocal atrial tachycardia.

concealed accessory pathway An accessory pathway that conducts only in a retrograde direction, often producing a "concealed WPW syndrome."

concealed bigeminy Although the mechanism producing the bigeminal rhythm continues in effect, it is not always manifested on the ECG; recognized by finding only odd numbers of P waves between manifest extrasystoles.

concealed conduction The propagation and block of an impulse, usually within the specialized conduction system, that can be recognized only from its effect on the subsequent beat or cycle.

concealed junctional extrasystole A junctional impulse arising in and discharging the AV junction but failing to reach either atria or ventricles.

concealed reentry The reentrance and block of an impulse in a depressed pathway leaving the pathway refractory to the passage of a subsequent impulse.

concealed supernormal conduction Supernormal conduction that is recognized only by its effect on subsequent conduction or impulse formation.

concentration gradient The gradient that exists across a membrane that separates a high concentration of a particular ion from a low concentration of the same ion.

connection A muscular pathway between atrium and ventricle apart from the conductive system.

coupling interval The interval between the dominant (usually sinus) beat and the coupled extrasystole.

decremental conduction Conduction that slows progressively because the effectiveness of the propagating impulse progressively decreases.

delta wave Slurring of the initial part of the QRS due to preexcitation.

depolarization The reduction of a membrane potential to a less negative value.

depressed fast response action potential The action potential produced when only some of the fast sodium channels are used to depolarize the fiber, resulting in decreased velocity and amplitude of phase 0 and consequent reduction in conduction velocity.

double tachycardia The simultaneous operation of two rapidly firing but independent foci, one controlling the atria and one the ventricles.

dV/dt The rate of change of voltage with respect to time; its units are in volts/sec.

echo beat A reciprocal beat, that is, one that results from the return of an impulse to a chamber to reactivate it; may be either atrial or ventricular.

effective refractory period The period during which a fiber may respond at the cellular level to a stimulus but this response will not be propagated.

electrical potential gradient The gradient that exists when an electrical voltage difference exists across a membrane.

entrance block A zone of block surrounding a pacemaker focus, protecting it from discharge by an extraneous impulse.

excitability The property by which a cardiac cell can give rise to an action potential when driven by an adequate stimulus.

exit block The pathologic failure of an expected impulse to emerge from its focus of origin and propagate.

fast response action potential The action potential produced when all of the fast sodium channels are available for depolarization, resulting in rapid upstroke velocity and maximal amplitude for phase 0, and consequent optimal conduction velocity.

functional refractory period The shortest interval at which a tissue is capable of conducting consecutive impulses; measured by the time intervening between the arrival of an initial impulse and the earliest subsequent conductible (premature) impulse at the distal end of the conducting tissue in question.

fusion The complex (ventricular or atrial) that results when two impulses collide within the same pair of chambers (ventricles or atria).

gap phenomenon A zone in which a premature stimulus encounters block, whereas an earlier or later stimulus is conducted.

gating mechanism The increasing duration of the action potential from the AV node to a point in the distal Purkinje system, beyond which point it again decreases.

H deflection (HBE) Represents His bundle activation.

His bundle electrogram (HBE) A direct recording of the electrical activity in the bundle of His.

His-Purkinje system The conduction system from the bundle of His to the distal Purkinje fibers inclusive.

HV interval (HBE) The conduction time through the His-Purkinje system, measured from the earliest onset of the His potential to the onset of ventricular activation recorded on either the intracardiac bipolar His bundle lead or any of the multiple surface ECG leads.

inhibition The effect of weaker impulse, unable to conduct through a depressed segment, leaving that segment refractory so that a subsequent stronger impulse is also blocked.

interpolated VPB A ventricular extrasystole sandwiched between two consecutive beats of the dominant—usually sinus—rhythm.

Kent bundles Accessory AV pathways.

longitudinal dissociation The insulation of parallel pathways from each other, usually in the AV junction.

Lown-Ganong-Levine syndrome A form of preexcitation characterized by a short PR interval and a normal QRS; associated with a tendency to supraventricular tachycardia.

macroreentry Reentry involving a large circuit, for example both bundle branches.

Mahaim fibers Paraspecific conductive tracts running between AV node or His bundle and the muscle of the ventricular septum.

maximal diastolic membrane potential The greatest degree of negative transmembrane potential achieved by the cell during diastole.

maximum diastolic potential The most negative level of transmembrane potential achieved by the cell.

membrane conductance The degree of permeability of the membrane to particular ions.

membrane responsiveness The relationship between the membrane potential at the time of stimulation and the maximal rate of depolarization of the action potential.

microreentry Reentry involving a small circuit, for example within Purkinje fibers.

multifocal Arising from more than two foci.

multiform Of varied shape; variform.

Nernst equation Relates the electrical potential across a membrane to the concentration ratio of permeable ions across that membrane.

overdrive suppression The inhibitory effect of a faster pacemaker on a slower pacemaker.

P′ Conventional label for any P wave that is not a sinus P wave.

PA interval (HBE) A measurement of intraatrial conduction time, measured from the onset of the P wave on the standard ECG or from the atrial deflection of the high right atrial electrogram to the A wave on the HBE.

pacemaker current The time dependent decrease in outward potassium current that is peculiar to the pacemaking cell and causes it to reach threshold potential.

parasystole An independent and undisturbable ectopic rhythm whose pacemaker cannot be discharged by impulses of the dominant (usually sinus) rhythm.

perinodal fibers Atrial fibers surrounding the SA node.

phase 0 The upstroke of the action potential.

phase 1 The initial rapid repolarization phase of the action potential.

phase 2 The plateau of the action potential.

phase 3 The terminal rapid repolarization phase of the action potential.

phase 3 aberration Ventricular aberration resulting from the arrival of the impulse in the ventricular fascicle during phase 3 of its action potential.

phase 4 aberration Ventricular aberration resulting from the arrival of the impulse in a spontaneously depolarizing ventricular fascicle late in diastole.

preexcitation Activation of part of the ventricular myocardium earlier than would be expected if the activating impulses traveled only down the normal routes.

reentry Reactivation of a tissue for the second or subsequent time by the same impulse.

reflection A form of reentry in which, after encountering delay in one fiber, the impulse enters a parallel fiber and returns retrogradely toward its source.

refractoriness The inability of a fiber to respond to a second stimulus after it has responded to a prior stimulus.

resting membrane potential The transmembrane voltage that exists when the heart muscle is at rest.

relative refractory period The period during phase 3 when a fiber can produce a propagated action potential provided the stimulus is of greater strength and duration than is necessary at full repolarization.

retrograde Wenckebach Progressively lengthening conduction from the ventricles or AV junction to the atria until an impulse fails to reach the atria.

"rule of bigeminy" The tendency of a lengthened ventricular cycle to precipitate a ventricular premature beat.

SA conduction time Conduction time from the sinus node to the atrial musculature, measured from the SA deflection in the SA nodal electrogram to the beginning of the P wave in the bipolar records or to the beginning of the high right atrial electrogram in the unipolar record.

SA electrogram A direct recording of the electrical activity of the SA node.

short-PR-normal-QRS syndrome Describes itself; when associated with supraventricular tachycardia, sometimes called "Lown-Ganong-Levine syndrome."

sick sinus Sinus node dysfunction characterized by marked sinus bradycardia, SA block, sinus arrest, prolonged SA pauses, or the bradycardia/tachycardia syndrome.

sick sinus syndrome Sinus node dysfunction complicated by cerebral dysfunction secondary either to failure of escape mechanisms or to a tachycardia.

slow response action potential The action potential produced when none of the fast sodium channels are available for depolarization and the fiber is depolarized only via slower Na^+/Ca^+ channels to produce an action potential with a slow upstroke velocity, low amplitude, and consequent slow conduction.

summation The merging of weaker impulses to form a stronger wave front.

supernormal conduction: Conduction that occurs when block is expected.

supernormal excitability The ability of the myocardium to respond to a stimulus that is ineffective when applied earlier or later in the cycle.

supernormal period A period at the end of phase 3 during which activation can be initiated with a lesser stimulus than is required at maximal repolarization.

"swinging" ventricular tachycardia Tachycardia in which the polarity of the wide QRS complexes swings between positive and negative; les torsades de pointes.

threshold potential The transmembrane potential that must be achieved before an action potential can be initiated.

triggered activity Rhythmic activity that results when a series of afterdepolarizations reach threshold potential.

triggered impulse An impulse that results when an afterdepolarization reaches threshold potential.

type A preexcitation Preexcitation in which the R wave is dominant in V_1, V_2, and/or V_E.

type B preexcitation Preexcitation in which the S or Q wave is dominant in V_1, V_2, and/or V_E.

unidirectional block Pathologic failure of conduction in one direction while conduction is possible in the other direction.

V deflection (HBE) Represents ventricular activation.

Index

DON JUAN VALERA, CRÍTICO LITERARIO

BIBLIOTECA ROMÁNICA HISPÁNICA

DIRIGIDA POR DÁMASO ALONSO

II. ESTUDIOS Y ENSAYOS

MANUEL BERMEJO MARCOS

DON JUAN VALERA, CRÍTICO LITERARIO

BIBLIOTECA ROMÁNICA HISPÁNICA
EDITORIAL GREDOS, S. A.
MADRID

© MANUEL BERMEJO MARCOS, 1968.

EDITORIAL GREDOS, S. A.
Sánchez Pacheco, 83, Madrid. España.

Depósito Legal: M. 17890 - 1968.

Gráficas Cóndor, S. A., Sánchez Pacheco, 83. Madrid, 1968. — 3155.

A la memoria de mi padre.

A mi madre y hermanos, con emocionada
gratitud.

EL CRÍTICO

*"Yo he criticado siempre más
como aficionado que como profesor, aspirando no a enseñar nada
a mis lectores, cuando los tenía,
sino a entretenerlos un rato con
mi charla".*

J. VALERA.

("Homenaje a Echegaray", 1905.
O. C., II, p. 1179).

NOTA: Para la realización del presente trabajo hemos manejado la
segunda edición de las Obras Completas de don Juan Valera, Editorial
Aguilar, 1949. En las notas a pie de página nos referimos a ellas consig-
nando solamente las siglas O. C. y el volumen correspondiente. Los trabajos no incluidos en dicha edición van citados en detalle.

INTRODUCCIÓN

Conocíamos y admirábamos a don Juan Valera como prosista. Como dueño de uno de los estilos más tersos, más hermosos y cuidados de nuestras letras.

Al enfrentarnos por primera vez con su tarea crítica, al dejarnos llevar de la mano de su ingenio, a través de temas que en sí mismos eran en ocasiones insignificantes y que, tratados por Valera, resultaban auténticas joyas como ensayos críticos, empezamos a sospechar que el crítico literario tenía una importancia mayor de la que ordinariamente se le había concedido.

En los artículos y trabajos consagrados a Valera que habíamos estudiado (¡sin descontar, claro está, los manuales más al uso de nuestra Historia de la Literatura!) se le tachaba siempre de "crítico benévolo en exceso" [1].

Después de las consabidas alabanzas para el novelista, o por mejor decir, para el prosista magnífico, se dedicaban unos párrafos, por lo general muy breves, en los que se acababa por decir, más o menos veladamente, que don Juan no fue nunca verdadero crítico porque no tuvo valor para castigar como hubiera debido.

---

[1] En el apéndice bibliográfico se hallará una lista de los trabajos que hemos revisado, dedicados a estudiar la obra valerina. Salvo el de la Sra. Fishtine —de cierta extensión— y el de Araujo Costa, todos los demás son estudios de conjunto y no conocemos ninguno dedicado exclusivamente al análisis detallado de la crítica literaria de Valera.

Sospechamos que quienes opinan así no se han tomado nunca la molestia de estudiar, con un poco más de espacio, la treintena larga de volúmenes que ocupa la obra crítica de Valera en la Edición de la Imprenta Alemana.

Seguramente dichos autores se han limitado a repetir lo que afirmaron, tal vez sin mala intención, quienes conocían en persona la bondadosa condición y la elegancia de carácter que adornaban a don Juan.

Antes de pasar a discutir lo que haya de verdad en la "cuestión de la bondad valerina" conviene que nos detengamos unos instantes a analizar cómo y cuándo surgió esta tan extendida idea hoy en día de que don Juan Valera no es un gran crítico (para muchos que le niegan el pan y la sal, ¡no es ni siquiera crítico!) a causa de su falta de coraje para censurar.

¿Cómo nació esta idea entre sus contemporáneos? Sencillamente porque el mismo don Juan Valera, desde sus primeros estudios publicados en la prensa periódica, declara abiertamente que no cree en la crítica severa. Que no pretende "deshacer" sino ayudar a hacer. Que no son los remedios a sangre y fuego los que él tratará de emplear, sino antes al contrario, la frase de aliento y el consejo amable [2]. Análisis amoroso, no tremebunda disección, sin anestésico de ningún género, o, lo que era muy corriente en la crítica del último tercio del siglo XIX, autopsias crueles. En otras palabras: que Valera quería hacer crítica positiva [3].

---

[2] Vid. "Poesías de F. de Zea", O. C., II, p. 125 (artículo de 1858) y O. C., II, p. 787, III, p. 1185, III, p. 64, idem, 224, idem, 438.

[3] Veremos más adelante que, justamente por esta "peculiar postura" y por la manera tan personal de ejercer el oficio de crítico, haciendo siempre una labor con vistas al futuro (y no hacia el pasado, como lo estaba haciendo la crítica punitiva), Valera se adelanta en muchos años a la tarea de sus contemporáneos. Don Juan Valera no sólo no es el crítico benévolo que muchos han querido ver en él, sino que, visto a la luz real de una crítica auténticamente constructiva, es el primer crítico español realmente

El hecho de que Valera se ocupe de una obra literaria indica que él la considera como de mérito suficiente pues, de lo contrario, "las obras necias o pedestres" no son para tenidas en cuenta ni siquiera para hablar mal de ellas.

Y, en efecto, desde sus primeros artículos hasta los que escribiera en sus últimos días fue siempre fiel a estas consignas. El lector actual, como el de su tiempo, no encontrará jamás críticas feroces ni crueles torniscones, como en la obra de muchos que pasan hoy por críticos reputados.

En la crítica de Valera no se encuentra ese ingrediente corrosivo que por desgracia suele abundar en las de sus coetáneos: la amarga bilis del castigo. Juez severísimo que se preocupa más de señalar los defectos que de mejorar y estimular las calidades positivas de una obra.

Con todo, no fueron solamente las declaraciones de Valera —ni la misma comprensiva bondad que se reflejaba en sus artículos— las únicas que contribuyeron a crear esta fama (o leyenda, que casi nos atrevemos a calificarla de tal). Colaboró también a ello un elemento que pudiéramos llamar externo: el contraste violento que ofrecían los moderados ensayos de don Juan con las encendidas diatribas que salían de la pluma de Revilla, primero, y de Clarín, más tarde.

Si bien es cierto que Valera comenzó a escribir sus artículos periodísticos cuando los otros dos grandes críticos del siglo XIX, Leopoldo Alas y don Marcelino Menéndez Pelayo, contaban muy pocos años de edad, no lo es menos que hasta 1870 la labor crítica de don Juan no fue ni muy regular ni muy abundante. A partir de esta fecha, pasada ya la cuarentena, la labor creadora del novelista, primero, y del crítico, más tarde, se regulariza. Sus artículos y sus

---

moderno con que contamos. Volveremos a este punto con más calma. Vid. artículos citados en la nota precedente, O. C., II, p. 1073 y O. C., III, páginas 610 y siguientes.

libros van apareciendo con cierta periodicidad. El triunfo como novelista (año 1874, recordémoslo, con *Pepita Jiménez*) le consagró
definitivamente como gran escritor ante el público y... ante sí
mismo.

Precisamente en la década que va del año 1870 al 1880 es
cuando otro gran escritor, profesor en la Universidad de Oviedo,
comenzó sus campañas de crítica en periódicos y revistas de la capital de España. Muy pronto adquirió gran fama y el propio Valera
reconocía en él, públicamente, gran talento, buen gusto y cualidades excelentes de crítico.

Los artículos de Clarín —por su severidad y su especial sentido
del humor— se hicieron popularísimos. Los juicios críticos, cada vez
más violentos, alcanzaban caracteres de auténticos ataques lanzados
contra los escritores que él consideraba dignos de castigo. En muy
pocos años puede decirse que Clarín se levantó con el cetro de la
crítica española.

Don Juan siguió publicando —al par que Clarín— sus ensayos
críticos. El lector, que se encontraba con dos maneras tan diferentes, tan radicalmente opuestas, pese a tener ambas el mismo fin, no
podía por menos de establecer comparaciones, de enfrentarlas. Y de
este confrontar a la ligera nacieron las conclusiones fáciles, que se
convertirían muy pronto en generalizaciones vaguísimas: la ferocidad de Clarín y la bondad de don Juan[4].

De lo que no se percataban quienes llegaban a tan sencillas conclusiones es de que muchas veces se engañaban: que ni Valera era
tan bondadoso como a primera vista pudiera parecer, ni los toni-

---

4   Hemos de señalar, antes de seguir adelante, que la crítica de don
Marcelino no fue nunca crítica tan popular como las de Clarín y Valera.
Menéndez y Pelayo fue, antes que nada, investigador, y si hoy es considerado, con razón, como nuestro primer crítico, su labor no fue prácticamente conocida por el mero lector de periódicos. Su tarea, más profunda,
más de erudito verdadero, iba dirigida a un público más formado y por
tanto más reducido.

tronantes varapalos de Clarín, que rasgaban las carnes de sus víctimas propiciatorias, eran siempre tan eficaces.

Los caminos de las dos tareas críticas eran más complicados y laberínticos de lo que aparentaban. Recorriéndolos podía uno fácilmente extraviarse. Por el bosque frondoso de los ataques de Clarín, como por el deleitoso campo de las infinitas digresiones valerinas, coloreadas con el mejor ingenio andaluz, podía el lector poco prevenido, tomando el rábano por donde no debiera, llegar a conclusiones que se apartaban mucho de las propuestas por los críticos.

Y esto fue lo que ocurrió. La crítica de Clarín —decidieron "las fuerzas vivas" de la literatura de fin de siglo—, llena de violencias, de chistosos ataques que llegaban casi a la injuria personal, era verdadera crítica. El modelo de críticas.

La labor de Valera, por el contrario, risueña casi siempre, favorable en su mayor parte, comedida y sutil, resultaba algo diametralmente opuesto a lo que hacía Clarín. Y si "aquello" era la crítica, "esto" de Valera no podía ser calificado como tal.

Se le acusaba de bondadoso sin tener jamás en cuenta el hecho de que don Juan, intencionadamente, sólo juzgaba en público (veremos cómo en privado es diferente) lo que le parecía digno de ser tenido en cuenta. No "daba palos" porque no había para qué. Lo malo —repitió a lo largo de toda su obra— es mejor dejarlo al margen de nuestro trabajo. El tiempo y el olvido harán su labor definitiva [5].

El "rigor" de Clarín como la "bondad" de don Juan, por otro lado, no son sino elementos más o menos importantes de sus respectivas tareas críticas. Lo que importa, a la hora de estudiar estas tareas, es lo que representaron su trabajo y sus opiniones en el mundo de las letras en su tiempo, y lo que tienen hoy de válido

---

[5] Tal postura la mantiene Valera en la mayor parte de sus críticas. Para no cansar al lector le remitimos solamente a O. C., III, pp. 610 y siguientes, idem, 1146 y 1185.

para nosotros. Los términos "blando" o "duro" son adjetivos que
en sí mismos nos dicen poquísimo. Lo sustantivo es la crítica realizada, adórnese con uno u otro ropaje.

Entiéndase bien que, al enfrentar aquí la violencia clariniana a
la bondadosa actitud valerina, no pretendemos mermar en un ápice
el valor absoluto de los juicios de Clarín ni la categoría de gran
crítico que pueda tener a los ojos de quien nos lea. Nuestra intención es subrayar en lo posible dos actitudes críticas muy diferentes.
Quienes llegaron a las conclusiones que señalábamos más arriba nos
parece que obraron con una ligereza que no quisiéramos imitar.

Si la fama de benévolo le llega a Valera más que nada por contraste con la severidad acostumbrada en Clarín, los historiadores
de la literatura contemporáneos suyos no se tomaron la molestia
de tratar de explicarse, y explicarnos, el por qué de tal actitud. (Ni
uno solo menciona los repetidísimos argumentos del propio Valera
acerca de la poca confianza que le merecía la crítica en general y la
crítica violenta en particular.)

Solamente se preocupan de echar de menos más severidad en
sus apreciaciones y de lamentar que, con las excepcionales dotes de
sensibilidad y buen gusto de que don Juan estaba dotado, no tuviera valor para escribir una crítica más eficaz. ¡Como si crítica eficaz
no quisiera decir más que crítica severa! Y no analizaron, claro
está, lo que de aprovechable tenía aquella "bondadosa" crítica valerina que censuraban.

¿Es posible que ni sospecharan lo que de positivo tenían (y siguen teniendo, después de más de tres cuartos de siglo pasados
desde que se publicaran por primera vez) los ensayos críticos de
Valera?

Nos tememos que no. Que, cegados por sus propios prejuicios,
no vieron más que la decidida intención de don Juan de no hacer
sufrir a nadie abiertamente con sus ensayos. Su voluntad firme de
no atacar.

Véase, para ilustrar con un ejemplo cuanto decimos, la obra del
P. F. Blanco García, *La literatura española en el siglo XIX* [6]. Debió
ser una de las primeras obras en donde se hablaba —no sin gran
respeto y admiración, es cierto— de la bondadosa actitud de Valera
como crítico. A pesar de las diferencias de criterio que separan a
Valera del P. Blanco García, está claro que éste no pretendía dañar
a don Juan. Sin embargo, quienes quieran buscar argumentos en
contra de la crítica valerina, pueden espigarlos en abundancia de
entre aquellas líneas escritas sin malicia.

Otro tanto ocurre con el breve, pero inteligente, análisis de la
crítica del siglo XIX, hecho por don Francisco A. de Icaza y titulado
Examen de críticos [7].

Los historiadores posteriores, en lugar de analizar de primera
mano, como era su obligación, los ensayos de crítica valerina, se li-
mitan a repetir parecidos argumentos cuando hablan de Valera crítico, que en muchas ocasiones no hablan.

Dejemos a un lado, entonces, el consabido argumento. Olvidemos intencionadamente la bondad de la crítica de Valera para preguntarnos por su validez, por su eficacia.

Comencemos por plantearnos estas simples preguntas:

a)   ¿Fue realmente don Juan Valera un crítico literario?

Y si lo fue:

b)   ¿Tuvo su crítica alguna efectividad en nuestra literatura?,
o dicho de otro modo: ¿Cooperó al mejoramiento literario de su
tiempo, o fue, por el contrario, la suya, una obra extraña, tenida
en cuenta únicamente por la gracia y buen estilo con que estaba
escrita, como ocurrió con su novela?

Esperamos, al analizar en detalle la crítica literaria de Valera,
encontrar las respuestas a tan sencillas —pero fundamentales— preguntas.

---

[6]   Vid. Vol. II, pp. 598-600. Ed. Sáenz de Jubera, Madrid, 1909.
[7]   Madrid, 1894, pp. 78 y s.

CAPÍTULO I

DON JUAN VALERA CRÍTICO

Un poco más de los dos tercios de la obra completa de don Juan Valera están dedicados a la crítica. De ésta, una parte no muy extensa, a la política y filosófica. Y el resto, unos 30 volúmenes en la edición de la Imprenta Alemana de 1905, a la puramente literaria.

A lo largo de más de sesenta años de lector infatigable, brotaron de su pluma cientos de artículos y ensayos en los que se propuso unas veces dar a conocer a los hablantes hispánicos temas o libros que él consideraba de cierto interés; otras, discutir, con agudeza inigualable y finísimo ingenio, los principios o teorías con los que no estaba de acuerdo o que le parecían iban a poner en grave peligro "al enfermo" (nuestras letras) que con tanto cuidado había que tratar. Otras, para alabar sin rodeos y denunciar a los cuatro vientos la aparición de un autor novel de talento.

Pero siempre movido por la generosa necesidad de ayudar, con sus consejos y su experiencia, al lector tanto como al autor. Autores y lectores no sólo de España, sino de las diecinueve repúblicas de la América Hispana.

Desde sus primeros pasos como escritor, cuando recién llegado a la capital, con tanta abundancia de ilusiones como escasez de peculio, anunciaba a su padre que estaba componiendo un sistema filosófico, una novela y proyectando diversos dramas [1], vemos manifestarse en Valera un agudo espíritu crítico. Ese espíritu que le llevará a tomar la pluma en cuantas ocasiones encuentre algún tema o punto que llame su atención.

Toda su vida se quejó de "esterilidad creadora". Como él dijera, sufría de "dificultad para expeler las ideas artísticas que le bullían en la cabeza" [2]. Ahora bien: esta premiosidad se refiere siempre a la obra puramente creativa, ya sea verso o prosa, novela o drama.

Cuando hace crítica se deja llevar, pura y simplemente, de su claro talento discursivo y la palabra le fluye sin tanta dificultad. Discurrir, partiendo de la obra ajena, le es tarea muy fácil, más natural que la compleja creación artística. Lo prueba el hecho de que en casi todas sus admirables cartas, incluso en las de mayor intimidad familiar, las menos literarias, lucen destellos críticos surgidos del menor pretexto. Recuérdese la serie de *Cartas desde Rusia,* deliciosa crítica de costumbres que iguala, si no supera, a casi todas nuestras mejores obras costumbristas.

En carta a su padre de 27-III-1850, escrita desde Madrid, cuenta don Juan cómo "días pasados viéndome sin dinero, aburridísimo y sin esperanza de destino, me encerré en mi cuarto, y a pesar de mi rabia y desasosiego me puse a escribir un artículo sobre los frailes para llevárselo a Tassara [3] y empezar así mi carrera pe-

---

[1] Vid. "Correspondencia", O. C., III, pp. 31, 36 y 30, respectivamente.

[2] Véase *Epistolario de Valera y Menéndez Pelayo,* p. 146, Espasa Calpe, Madrid, 1946.

[3] Gabriel García Tassara, director de *El País* y amigo de Valera.

riodística ... me cuesta sudores de muerte el confeccionar trozos de elocuencia periodística" [4].

El artículo a que se refiere (y que Tassara debió prudentemente no aceptar, pues iba más allá de la política que *El País* seguía) desgraciadamente no se conserva. Era el primer trabajo que escribió don Juan para la prensa periódica, en donde había de publicar después la mayor parte de su obra. Y ya en aquel primer artículo, sus quejas; cincuenta años más tarde seguirá doliéndose, en carta a don Marcelino Menéndez Pelayo [5], de la misma dificultad de verter sus ideas a las cuartillas.

Tassara, adivinando sin duda los escondidos valores que tras aquellos balbuceos de principiante se ocultaban, le anima para que escriba crítica literaria. Y el mismo escritor que "vertía sudores de muerte" para confeccionar "trozos de elocuencia periodística", discurría sin dificultad alguna a lo largo de muchas páginas en cuanto se ponía a estudiar las obras de los demás.

El azar diplomático le apartó del mundillo literario activo de Madrid, en el que, de haber continuado, hubiese adquirido muy pronto buen prestigio como crítico, pues ni al mismo Valera se le ocultaba (lo repite frecuentemente en sus cartas de aquellas fechas) que había muy pocos mejor preparados que él mismo para ejercer la tarea de censor y corrector de unas letras que dejaban bastante que desear.

A pesar de su voluntaria separación del mundillo madrileño, no se conforma Valera con vivir apartado de la crítica, y en casi toda la correspondencia que de él se conserva —lo mismo desde Nápoles que desde Lisboa, Brasil, Alemania o Rusia— hay notas que nos descubren al crítico innato que pugna ya por darse a conocer como tal. Estaba seguro de que sus cartas, dirigidas a la familia o

---

4   Apud Edith Fishtine *Juan Valera, the Critic*, Bryn Mawr, 1933, página 12.

5   Obra cit., p. 142.

a sus amistades, verían un día la luz pública. Y no eran, por tanto, tan "privadas" como él simulaba que fueran.

Es más, en algunas de aquellas cartas, tal por ejemplo la escrita al mismo Gabriel García Tassara de quien hablábamos más arriba, desde el Brasil [6], se ve un primer esquema, un esbozo de un ensayo crítico que redactará años más tarde —1856— en defensa de Donoso Cortés [7]. No podemos hablar de autoplagio, pues se da con mucha frecuencia en Valera el hecho de encontrar una idea, en esquema, en sus primeras cartas y verla luego ampliamente desarrollada en escritos posteriores. Valera debió conservar un duplicado de casi toda su correspondencia, pues confesaba que su memoria, si extraordinaria en los últimos años de su vida, era pésima en los de su juventud. Y hay argumentos de esas primeras cartas, escritas a muy diferentes destinatarios, citados textualmente muchos años después de la redacción de aquéllas.

Y en una extensa carta escrita al poeta Heriberto García de Quevedo —también desde el Brasil— pueden encontrarse explanados muchos de los principios a que se atendrá su crítica posterior. Entre ellos, por ejemplo, la idea de que sólo lo que merezca la pena debe ser criticado:

"El criticarlos yo es prueba de que los aprecio, pues a juzgarlos malos no los criticaría" [8].

Palabras en las que nos parece que hay que buscar el origen verdadero de su bondadoso criterio.

Comienza Valera, pues, la tarea crítica de un modo un tanto irregular. Publicando sus primeros ensayos en la prensa de Madrid [9], cuando sus largas ausencias por el extranjero no se lo im-

---

6   Carta de mayo de 1853, O. C., I, p. 63.
7   Cf. "Ensayo sobre el Catolicismo... etc.", O. C., II, pp. 1384-1399.
8   Carta de 1 de mayo de 1853, O. C., III, pp. 54 y s.
9   Fueron muchas las "publicaciones periódicas" en las que Valera presentó sus ensayos críticos. Primero en *Revista de Ambos Mundos* y en la *Revista Peninsular,* que venía a ser un sustituto del antiguo proyecto que

pedían. Sin perder por ello el uso de la palabra en materia literaria,
ya que, aunque no iban destinados al público, no dejaba de escribir
sus juicios a los amigos para analizar el último libro que había caído
en sus manos o para discutir diferentes puntos de vista estéticos.

SUS PROPÓSITOS

Dos son los motivos, a nuestro entender, que empujaron a don
Juan Valera por el camino de la literatura crítica. Uno de tipo
personal: su dificultad para expresarse en el mundo de la pura creación, la novela y el cuento, dificultad a la que ya hemos aludido.
El otro motivo es de índole "nacional": el mal estado de la literatura española a mediados del siglo XIX.

Valera conocía muy bien su propio valer. Desde su llegada a
Madrid se percató de que no había muchos hombres de letras con
una formación comparable a la suya [10]. Y las letras españolas pre-

---

tuviera don Juan en Lisboa de fundar, con Latino Coelho, una revista
bilingüe cuyo título sería *Revista Ibérica*. Dicho proyecto no se llevó nunca
a cabo, pero en cambio logró Valera fundar con Sinibaldo de Mas y Fernando Caldeira dicha *Revista Peninsular*, en 1856. Continuó escribiendo
en *El Estado, La América* y *El Mundo Pintoresco*. Hasta que en 1859
funda, con sus amigos Miguel de los Santos Álvarez, P. A. de Alarcón,
Maldonado y Macanaz el periódico satírico-literario *La Malva*, donde "escribió no poco". El año siguiente funda con A. Segovia (El Estudiante)
otra revista satírico-literaria, *El Cócora*, donde según el propio Valera "en-
cocoramos a todos los literatos ramplones..." (Vid. para más detalles la
"Noticia Autobiográfica de don Juan Valera", publicada en 1914 en el
Boletín de la Real Academia Española, vol. I, páginas 134 y s.). También
escribió en *La Crónica de Ambos Mundos*, revista quincenal primero, y
luego diario político. Por esos mismos años hizo también periodismo político en *El Contemporáneo*.

    [10] Vid. J. F. Montesinos, *Valera o la ficción libre*, p. 20 y s., ed. Gre-
dos, Madrid, 1957.

cisaban de un guía, un espíritu caritativo y generoso que las cuidase con amor y esmero. No arrancando solamente los arbustos menos bellos de nuestro jardín, sino plantando, con el buen ejemplo, otros esquejes que lo hermosearan.

Creo que merece la pena detenerse unos instantes a estudiar estos dos motivos que parecen haber inclinado a don Juan Valera por el camino crítico. El más interesante —por lo que de revelador de una personalidad tan rica tiene— es el de sus dificultades primeras en la literatura de creación.

Son muy conocidas las cartas en las que el ambicioso y elegante joven, recién terminada su carrera de leyes (que no le serviría sino de adorno más tarde en la vida), escribía desde la Villa y Corte madrileña a sus padres y amigos. Contaba en ellas, punto por punto, las terribles angustias y luchas que la pura creación en prosa le proporcionaba. Con una sinceridad que encontramos en muy pocos autores, Valera se nos muestra forcejeando con su propio estilo —¡él, que lo llegaría a hacer tan personal y hermoso!— "sudando tinta", son sus palabras, al intentar los primeros pasos por la novela y el cuento. Confiesa, con sinceridad asombrosa en hombre de tanto orgullo, sus tanteos y sus fracasos.

Se ha dicho no pocas veces que cuando Valera se dio a conocer como escritor de novelas lo hizo con una madurez poco frecuente. Que comenzó como maestro acabado. Lo que no suele tenerse en cuenta es que su primera novela fue escrita cuando contaba don Juan cuarenta y ocho años. Como desde su adolescencia tenía Valera una clara vocación de escritor, el lapso de tiempo transcurrido es bastante elocuente. Trabajó con ahínco, hizo y rehizo sus primeros tanteos con una voluntad autocrítica extraordinaria, abandonó sin acabarlo nunca lo que hubiera debido ser su primer libro en prosa (*Mariquita y Antonio*) y sólo se dio a conocer cuando estuvo seguro de que lo que salía de su pluma era digno de su persona. No antes.

Mas esta premura, esta lentitud que encuentra para verter al papel sus ideas creadoras, no se le presenta cuando Valera se dedica a estudiar y comentar la obra de los demás. Tampoco cuando escribe cartas. (Nos parece que no fue pura coincidencia el que su novela primera *Pepita Jiménez* esté escrita en forma epistolar.)

Cuando escribe para la familia, o para los amigos, su atormentado "espíritu de creador" se libera de prejuicios y temores. Su pensamiento discurría con gracia y galanura inigualables. Pero tan pronto se ponía a llevar al papel el enredo novelístico que "le bullía en la cabeza", don Juan tenía que declararse vencido, inerme ante la dificultad. Como las cartas no iban más allá de una intimidad relativa, su vocación de escritor público no quedaba satisfecha. Sólo le quedaba el recurso de la crítica; y a él se lanza.

Analizando una obra, por muy pobre de valores que ella fuera, se le venían a las mientes multitud de ideas. Brotaban con tal intensidad que, a veces, a él mismo le parecía excesivo. Este girar en torno a la obra, este ir y venir, con mil pretextos, de la obrilla analizada a sus problemas estéticos personales es uno de los encantos mayores de la crítica de Valera, a nuestro entender.

Para muchos, por el contrario, estos "devaneos intelectuales", tan agudos como se quiera —argumentan— son muy poco esclarecedores para la comprensión de la obra que en ellos se analiza. Además de que merman grandemente el valor de la crítica valerina. Entre los que así pensaron figura el gran novelista Ramón Pérez de Ayala. Expuso su sentir en una serie de artículos publicados en *El Sol* y que fueron recogidos mucho más tarde en su libro *Divagaciones literarias* [11]. El título de los artículos nos ahorra comentarios: "Valera o el arte de la distracción".

Es cierto que el crítico, entre otras muchas cosas, debe llegar a una valoración justa de la obra estudiada por él. Pero no es tarea exclusiva de la crítica la valoración. Es, sí, uno de los múltiples

---

[11]   Biblioteca Nueva, Madrid, 1958.

quehaceres, mas no el único. Negar, por tanto, valor crítico a los ensayos de Valera porque "muchas veces nos deja sin un fallo" nos parece francamente injusto. Es cierto que a veces se olvida de señalar la nota final que en un hipotético examen de ingenios don Juan Valera, profesor-crítico, hubiera debido concederle. Pero no se olvida siempre. Y veremos cómo otras muchas veces lo que a primera vista parece una digresión muy valerina, visto con ojos expertos no es sino una elegante manera de decir cosas que otra persona menos fina y sutil hubiera dicho haciendo sangre en la carne de su víctima.

Si constreñimos las tareas de la crítica a un repartir premios y castigos, si la limitamos a tan estrechos vallados como los que establecen quienes le niegan el título de crítico a don Juan, tendremos que confesar con ellos que Valera no fue crítico.

Afortunadamente la verdadera crítica literaria, la que en muchas páginas hiciera don Juan, no consiste sólo en distribuir premios y castigos.

Bien lo sabía Valera. Para él, la verdadera crítica debía de ser, antes que nada, normativa. Su misión, no sólo el derribar las estatuas de los falsos diosecillos, sino el descubrir los verdaderos. Enseñar el evangelio de la belleza literaria. Y esto podía lograrse haciendo una crítica nueva (¡para su tiempo, que afortunadamente no lo es para el nuestro!) personal y ligera, sin enredarse los pies en tareas tan bajas como la concesión de premios o censuras.

A Valera le interesaban, tanto como la obra juzgada, las normas o principios que de su lectura brotaban en su clara inteligencia. Por ello mismo es verdad que, muchas veces, la obrilla en cuestión quedaba relegada a un margen secundario y que "el vuelo portentoso de su imaginación se remontaba como un águila a los espacios del pensamiento" para descubrir nuevos horizontes orientadores. Jugaba con la facilidad y la buena organización de su cerebro a construir principios con los que frecuentemente se divertía y deleitaba a los lectores que no buscaban en sus críticas una mera valoración. Tal actitud irritaba a los lectores acostumbrados a la crítica tradicional.

Así como la novela de Valera fue, según el profesor Montesinos, "novela en libertad" [12] la crítica que, desde los comienzos de su carrera hasta el final de sus días, ejerció don Juan, fue también una "crítica en libertad".

Trataremos de dilucidar si fue —libre o no— verdadera crítica. Lo que está claro, en cuanto el lector se enfrenta con ella, es que se trata de una crítica absolutamente personal. No creía demasiado en la posibilidad de un amplio objetivismo, por lo que las normas a las que se atiene serán tan flexibles como las que rigen su propia personalidad, si bien no dejen de tener bien hincadas sus raíces en la estética tradicional.

El segundo motivo que mencionábamos al señalar las razones por las que don Juan se había inclinado hacia la crítica, era el mal estado de las letras españolas hacia mediados del siglo XIX.

Cuando don Juan llega por primera vez a Madrid y contempla de cerca el panorama que ofrecían las clases superiores del país, los intelectuales y hombres de letras que él se hubiera imaginado como una *élite* ejemplar desde su rincón andaluz, no puede por menos de confesar su enorme desencanto.

La incultura y la vulgaridad de la mayoría de los que pasan por "escritores consagrados", su mediocridad y estrechez de miras y la ramplonería general de la sociedad madrileña ("esto es un presidio rebelado", llegará a decir) le producen una irritación que no se oculta en las indignadas cartas que escribe a sus padres.

El público, por otra parte, falto de obras que merezcan la pena, anda desorientado y "los poquísimos que leen" lo hacen sin el apoyo de una autoridad que les guíe, les abra los ojos y les enseñe —en una palabra— lo que puede tener de bueno o de malo una obra literaria.

---

[12] Vid. J. F. Montesinos, obra cit., p. 26.

La crítica verdadera o no existe [13] o es una serie de ditirambos exageradísimos, bombos ridículos y falsos en su mayoría y un mutuo llamarse "genios y padres de obras geniales".

Valera, que llega con una formación muy superior a la del nivel medio, con un índice de lecturas clásicas y modernas incomparablemente más rico que el de los demás, se percata de que su ayuda puede tener cierta utilidad.

Ve con agudeza clarísima que no es sólo "recriminación y mano dura con los que escriben" lo que se precisa, sino algo mucho más importante y más caritativo: enseñar al que no sabe.

Quiere, antes de nada, adoctrinar al público lector. Preparar a esa pequeña minoría que lee, ampliar su número cuanto fuera posible, porque "... en España no leen más que los que escriben, y nosotros somos el público de nosotros mismos, y toda la literatura es enseñanza mutua" [14].

Don Juan Valera se percató de la dolencia que aquejaba a nuestras letras y de la gravedad del estado de salud de aquéllas. Tan grave, que más que practicar dolorosas operaciones quirúrgicas (para las que no veía ni "instrumental" adecuado ni preparación en los "doctores oficiales", en España) habría que intentar la salvación del enfermo mediante píldoras y reconstituyentes tolerables. (Aún no se habían descubierto ni las vitaminas ni los antibióticos, de que tan frecuentemente se habla en nuestros días. Nos imaginamos que Valera hubiera empleado tales términos con sumo gusto, para sus metáforas, si en sus tiempos hubieran existido.)

Había en primer lugar que reanimar al enfermo (lectores y letras). Una vez conseguida cierta mejoría temporal, podría aplicarse y aún sería aconsejable, un tratamiento más enérgico. Pero antes no.

---

[13] Cf. "Correspondencia", O. C., III, pp. 28 y s. Y "Otras cartas", O. C., III, p. 616.

[14] O. C., III, p. 616.

Con sus artículos de crítica pretendía Valera, sin que nunca lo ocultara, administrar esa especie de reconstituyente que proporcionase una lenta pero eficaz mejoría del estado de nuestras letras.

Y es curioso ver cómo fueron los autores que no se sentían halagados por los artículos de don Juan —don Armando Palacio Valdés y doña Emilia Pardo Bazán, por ejemplo— los que comenzaron a tomar los trabajos de Valera no como las medicinas provechosas que podían ser, sino como "paños calientes" de poca o ninguna utilidad. (Más adelante veremos cómo don Juan deja, deliberadamente, fuera de su crítica a los escritores que él consideraba más capaces. Entre ellos figuran precisamente doña Emilia y Palacio Valdés.)

Las palabras de Valera no dejan lugar a dudas: "el público español no necesita desengaños, sino estímulo y aliciente, y los escritores españoles, que por lo regular alcanzan tan poco provecho de lo que escriben, necesitan como en compensación alguna gloria más de la justa" [15].

Y las afirmaciones del crítico —es curioso observarlo— no van a cambiar mucho con el paso de los años. Encontraremos muy leves correcciones, en lo que respecta a sus conclusiones críticas, si practicamos una serie de calas a lo largo de su obra, tenidas en cuenta las diferentes fechas. En los artículos críticos de sus años mozos vemos las mismas posturas que mantuvo en los que salieron a luz al fin de sus ochenta y un años [16].

Una de las más importantes afirmaciones, en la que, como dijimos, nos parece ver la raíz auténtica de lo que pasa por ser para algunos el defecto principal de la crítica valerina, es la que se refiere a que no deben criticarse más que las obras que merezcan la pena. Que las tareas críticas deben consagrarse solamente a las obras

---

[15] "Poesías de F. Zea", O. C., II, p. 125.

[16] Compárense las afirmaciones de la nota anterior con las que mantiene en 1901 en el artículo "Huellas de Almas", O. C., II, p. 1073.

que tengan algo de positivo. No vale la pena pararse a criticar "las tonterías de los tontos, sino que hay que analizar las de los discretos", puesto que los frutos vanos nacen ya condenados por sí mismos y el tiempo se encargará piadosamente de darles sepultura.

¿Cabe una más grande generosidad de criterio en fecha tan temprana como 1853? [17].

No es el desprecio altivo, ni las veladas reticencias (que semiocultas entre las alabanzas quieren ver otros) las que le hacen hablar así. Sino la pura convicción de que nada se adelanta con gastar tiempo y espacio en las revistas literarias para vapulear a los desdichados padres de aquellos "abortos literarios".

Para don Juan Valera —y la fecha de la siguiente afirmación es 1858, recordémoslo— "la crítica de una producción literaria no se ha de escribir con la intención de favorecer o perjudicar al autor sino con *el más elevado propósito de dilucidar los puntos oscuros de la filosofía del arte...*" [18].

Ésta será la razón que justifique el que muchas veces, partiendo de la obra que analiza, se eleve a otras cuestiones estéticas de más interés para el lector y, ¡bien seguro!, para el mismo Valera. Sin preocuparse luego, más que de pasada, de recomendar o incluso de analizar la obra que motivara el ensayo. Tal hizo repetidamente en los "prólogos críticos" en los que tan generosamente se prodigó.

Quiere sobre todo "enseñar buen gusto al público, y crear público y poner a los autores a cada uno en su lugar 'sine ira et studio' con imparcialidad serena" [19].

Buscar lo mejor de entre aquella producción de tan baja calidad; entretenerse (¡y deleitarse en lo posible!) con ello y mos-

---

[17] Cf. O. C., III, pp. 54 y s. con "Cartas de Madrid", O. C., III, páginas 610 y ss.

[18] "Observaciones sobre el Drama *Baltasar*", O. C., III, pp. 111-112.

[19] Vid. *Epistolario Valera-Menéndez Pelayo*, ed. cit., p. 129.

trarlo luego a los demás, explicando sus virtudes sin dejar de señalar los defectos que hubiere.

Se oponía resueltamente a la "quema total" purificadora, predi-
cada y, lo que es peor, ejercida por los críticos famosos por su severidad con los autores menos afortunados.

Nuestra "haza literaria" —metáfora carísima a Valera— aunque abundaba en "malas hierbas", no dejaba por ello de producir
algunas florecillas de colores delicados y hermosura cierta. El cultivo de estas pocas exquisiteces, de estas florecillas silvestres, era más
importante para él que la siega despiadada de los cardos inútiles [20].

Estas, y no otras, eran las premisas en que se apoyaba la "reconocida suavidad de maneras" de don Juan Valera crítico.

Las florecillas que él descubriera —que él dio a oler a los demás,
para seguir con su metáfora favorita— puede que no fueran siempre de lo más hermoso. Puede que muchas otras pasaran incluso
desapercibidas a su sensibilidad y olfato. Tal le pasará, por desgracia, con una de las más delicadas y tiernas plantas de nuestro jardín
literario: nuestra lírica primitiva. Veremos cómo la ignoró, porque
su olfato —o su gusto— no estaba preparado para captar el áspero
y delicioso aroma de las flores silvestres. Prefirió siempre las rosas
de los jardines versallescos, aunque de vez en cuando, en sus paseos
por su campo andaluz, o en las afueras de su Granada estudiantil,
se agache a recoger un manojito de violetas.

Si Valera no nos presentó "todas" las flores que pueden darse
en el jardín hispánico, tenemos que agradecerle, al menos, descubrimientos tan positivos como los de un Rubén Darío, o un don Marcelino Menéndez Pelayo, para no citar más que dos casos, en fechas
tan tempranas que, puede afirmarse sin temor a error, fue la agudeza valerina la que, anticipándose proféticamente, los descubrió.

---

20 Así lo manifiesta en diversas ocasiones. Véanse, por ejemplo, O. C.,
II, p. 912 y III, pp. 427 y 1146.

SUS ESPERANZAS

En ningún momento se le ocultó a don Juan que la tarea del crítico es uno de los trabajos más penosos e ingratos en todo el campo literario. Vio claramente las dificultades que tal labor llevaba consigo.

Sus lecturas le habían enseñado que es casi imposible fijar cánones, establecer un criterio exacto que permita calibrar sin error notable la calidad de una obra. Desde sus comienzos como crítico lo confiesa sin embarazo [21]. Le preocupaba sinceramente llegar a conclusiones que pudieran estar no ya equivocadas, sino ni siquiera mal justipreciadas.

Y es este temor a errar, más que su amable escepticismo, el que inclina a Valera hacia la alabanza con más facilidad que al castigo. De equivocarse por algo, que sea por exceso, no por defecto, parece pensar.

Desconfía con razón de la infalibilidad de toda crítica. Teme que la crítica excesivamente rigurosa (aplicada a los autores sus contemporáneos en especial) pueda ser muy discutible y que en definitiva sólo la posteridad vendrá a confirmar o negar sus conclusiones [22].

Pensando en la posteridad precisamente llega a afirmar, con modestia que nos parece excesiva, que su crítica no dirá "nada de trascendental a los futuros siglos" [23].

Al ponerse a juzgar una obra ajena tiene siempre en cuenta su propia experiencia, la dolorosa creación, la dificultad de escribir "obras de arte" y teme ser juez severo [24].

Su larga vida, sin embargo, le permitió conocer el triunfo de unos cuantos autores a los que él había pronosticado éxito cierto.

---

[21] "Revista dramática", año 1861, O. C., II, p. 261.
[22] O. C., II, pp. 511, 681 y 1642, y O. C., III, pp. 268, 487 y 491.
[23] O. C., III, p. 540.
[24] O. C., II, p. 681.

Mas también vio cómo otros hombres, a los que su bondad había tratado benignamente, se hundían lenta pero inexorablemente en el olvido.

Valera mantuvo siempre el principio de que si la flor presentada al certamen de los críticos era bella, y su perfume verdadero, llegaría a ser conocida y admirada por todos a pesar de las posibles críticas adversas. Y que si, por el contrario, carecía de aquellos valores era trabajo inútil alabarla o rebajarla apasionadamente, ya que, al fin y al cabo, sólo la belleza de ley es imperecedera.

Para don Juan, que veía más en el fondo de las cosas que la generalidad, la labor del crítico debía consistir, ante todo, en analizar las virtudes de cada obra literaria y enseñar al simple lector a descubrirlas. Crítica positiva. Denigrar las obras mediocres no valía la pena. Además: "¿Cómo cerciorarse de la medianía de ellas? ¿Dónde está el instrumento... que marque los grados hasta donde llega la medianía y por cima de los cuales empieza la bondad, la sublimidad o la belleza que le dan vida inmortal, nombradía e inmarcesible gloria?" [25].

Vemos pues cómo no confiaba enteramente en decisiones finales que tendieran a rebajar o ensalzar el buen nombre de un autor. Y es este afán de no querer llegar a conclusiones terminantes —conclusiones que él afeaba en otros críticos, especialmente en Clarín, como veremos— el que le lleva a realizar una clase de crítica que hoy encontramos en muchos casos enteramente moderna y que en su tiempo debió, por lo desacostumbrada, causar asombro, cuando no descontento.

HACIA UN CONCEPTO DE
LA CRÍTICA EN VALERA

Temeroso siempre don Juan de las posturas tajantes, de los dogmas de cualquier tipo, se cuidó muy bien de no dar nunca una clara definición de lo que él entendía por crítica.

---

25 "Nuevas cartas americanas", O. C., III, p. 501.

Encontramos, entre mil rodeos, salvedades e indirectas, y desparramadas en diversos artículos, afirmaciones que pueden conducirnos, más o menos, a descubrir las normas y criterios a que se atuvo para ejercer esa labor de la que tanto desconfiaba. Pensamos que justamente por esa falta de módulos, esa carencia de principios inmutables con que tropezaba de continuo su mente al analizar un trabajo y tener que fallar en consecuencia, es por lo que sus conclusiones resultaban al lector exigente tan vagas, tan poco terminantes, tan flexibles y, en general, tan benévolas.

Para Valera existen dos especies de trabajos literarios: la primera compuesta por las obras duraderas, las obras inmortales. Por aquellas obras que, por lo general, no suelen alcanzar en los momentos de su aparición ni el favor del público ni la popularidad, salvo en muy raras ocasiones. No son fruto de modas pasajeras, sino eternas como el arte mismo, como la belleza a la cual encarnan. Sólo con el paso de los años van alcanzando un prestigio que no tuvieron al nacer. Van revalorizándose hasta que crítica y público las aclaman unánimemente declarándolas por encima de toda posible interpretación equivocada. Ellas son las joyas mejores de la literatura universal, las que no conocen fronteras lingüísticas ni de otra clase [26].

La segunda especie, compuesta por todas las demás obras, es infinitamente mayor en número. Gran parte de ellas son obras nacidas para la moda y el gusto de un tiempo determinado y, por ende, limitadas. Son obras de tono más superficial. Hasta pueden llegar, en su ligereza, a tener poco o ningún valor para el futuro. Alcanzan, a veces, un éxito fulminante, "hacen furor" para decirlo con el popularismo que le corresponde, entre los lectores de un país, llegando incluso a ser traducidas a otras lenguas. Pero en su ligereza, en su rápido éxito, llevan la condena a muerte; pasada la moda desaparecerán como pompas de jabón sin dejar más huella que la del título, y en muchos casos ni eso.

---

[26] Véase "Revista dramática", O. C., II, pp. 241 y ss.

Así como hay dos clases de obras literarias, así habrá que ejercer dos clases de crítica, o mejor dos tareas diferentes, aun cuando se busque un solo fin en ambos casos.

Para las obras de categoría superior habrá de aplicarse una crítica profunda, erudita, que analice la obra literaria cuidadosamente, ateniéndose para ello a un "elevado ideal de perfección". Ejerciendo esta tarea, el crítico tendrá que emitir su conclusión sin temor, abiertamente y sin rodeos. Será una labor, la de tal crítico, más que difícil, comprometida, puesto que la fama en el mundo de las letras no depende de un solo crítico, sino del conjunto que forman crítica y público unidos. Y los módulos con los que mida habrán de ser buscados tanto en las estéticas clásicas como en las modernas, ya que en estética la evolución es continua.

Conociendo un poco la psicología de Valera no nos extrañamos de que, a renglón seguido, se declare a sí mismo "incapaz" para ejercer tal tarea pretextando nada menos que ¡falta de preparación!

"Esta clase de literatura, que es la de verdad, la sólida y la legítima, merece la crítica sabia, que nosotros, aunque haya ocasión, no podemos ejercer por falta de sabiduría" [27].

La falsa modestia (a la que por cierto no fue muy aficionado, pues más bien prefería ser tenido por presuntuoso, ya que, conociendo la poca calidad del mundillo de las letras que le rodeaba, sin llegar al desprecio total, se consideraba muy por encima del nivel medio), la irónica modestia, repito, convenía aquí a don Juan para ahorrarse otras enojosas explicaciones.

Echándose la culpa, se evitaba la desagradable tarea de tener que decir, por ejemplo, que aquellas obras que constituían lo que él llamaba "joyas eternas" no se daban por aquellas calendas.

Es, ante todo, correctísimo. Afortunadamente para nosotros, sus teorías no van siempre de la mano de sus hechos. O dicho con otras palabras: con sus escritos, a la larga, se desmentirá.

---

27 "Revista dramática" (8-XI-1861), O. C., II, p. 241.

Sus mejores tareas críticas —sin olvidar el sensacional descubrimiento del triunfador del Modernismo— están hechas precisamente sobre obras y autores que en nada verían mermadas sus glorias si el juicio de Valera no se hubiera volcado sobre ellas (*Don Quijote, Fausto,* etc.). Y, sin embargo, contribuyó con su agudísimo ingenio a descubrir muchas de las bellezas que aquellas obras contenían y que otros críticos que le habían precedido en la tarea no habían señalado.

Si Valera no se dedicó siempre a esta clase de trabajos y sí a la crítica que él gustaba de llamar "efímera", no fue por falta de conocimientos o incapacidad personal, como con ironía socarrona dijera. Era simplemente porque, sabiendo la floja condición de la mayoría de las obras que en sus días alcanzaban éxitos resonantes, recelaba que no resistirían tales "criaturas" aquel exacto y completo sistema analítico que preconizaba para las "grandes obras de arte". Que puesto a ejercer la tarea de crítico auténtico —con aquellas obras nacidas en la segunda mitad del siglo XIX— iban a ser muy pocas las que sobrevivieran la dura prueba de ser analizadas al través de un potente microscopio.

Por otra parte, el público no estaba acostumbrado —ni preparado para ello— a leer "pesados artículos de erudición crítica" ni abundaban los lectores de otra cosa que no fueran simples gacetillas o artículos amenos y breves.

Valera no podía dar estas razones que nosotros exponemos aquí más que como lo hizo: con toda delicadeza. Siempre tan correcto, calló los verdaderos motivos y demostró, con la crítica seria, que no hablaba con absoluta sinceridad desde las columnas del periódico.

Puesto que las obras que veían la luz cuando él comienza a ejercer la tarea de crítico eran justamente "la flor de un día que deleita al vulgo y aún a los doctos" y que de todas formas iban a morir muy pronto sin dejar huella, el crítico, en lugar de entrar en ellas "a saco, quemando a hierro y fuego", prefiere ejercer la tarea

de guía y mentor para autores y lectores, más modesta y de menos
relumbrón que la del juez: "Valerse del arma de la crítica elevada,
aunque nosotros supiéramos esgrimirla, a fin de combatir contra
esta literatura, sería lo mismo que empuñar la clava de Hércules
para matar moscas" [28], acaba diciendo con un rasgo de humor que
nunca le abandonará.

Puso todo su empeño en tratar de mejorar cuanto se producía,
no cortando de raíz (no castigando severamente), sino tratando de
"abonar", depurar y obtener la mejor cosecha posible en tan defi-
ciente terreno. Nada se adelanta con sembrarlo de sal. Porque, por
otra parte, el poco público lector en España: "quiere cosas nuevas,
aunque sean malas, y *el crítico mismo debe contentarse con ellas o
escribirlas mejores, que sería el modo más conveniente de criti-
carlas*" [29].

He aquí su sincera y noble solución. La única solución viable
para el autor de *Pepita Jiménez*. Mejorar el jardín ajeno con el
ejemplo del propio. Predicar, dando trigo.

Le enojaba sobremanera ver aquellos catones censorinos, incapaces de escribir dos renglones de pura creación a derechas, esgri-
miéndose en jueces inquisitoriales y administrando injustas —por
lo extremadas— sentencias, en nombre de unos cuantos principios
estéticos mal digeridos, tomados de acá y allá, casi siempre de segunda o tercera mano. No es que desconfiara Valera de los principios estéticos en sí, sino de la aplicación y la libre interpretación
que de ellos hacían los criticuelos de cafetín, que tronaban dicterios
en la prensa diaria.

Aunque la estética, como la moral, tenga un decálogo establecido con normas relativamente fijas, en arte no se puede aplicar
dicho decálogo con la misma seguridad con que lo haría la moral.
Es difícil que en moral haya divergencia de opiniones, por muy di-

---

[28] O. C., II, p. 242.
[29] O. C., II, p. 242.

ferentes que sean los jueces, al discutirse la bondad o malicia de
un acto humano.

En cambio, al juzgar una obra literaria, aun manteniéndose los
mismos principios, para unos sería una joya de las más preciadas
lo que para otros no pasaría de ser un mineral de lo más común.

La explicación a tan extraño hecho la encuentra don Juan en la
complejidad que ofrece el análisis de toda obra de arte. Si a la enorme cantidad de aspectos diferentes que la obra literaria presenta a
quien pretenda analizarla, y al criterio más o menos elevado que
se quiera establecer para con ella, se une la pasión personal, inevitable, de la persona que juzga, rara vez podrá llegarse a un resultado justo, sereno y bien intencionado.

Con cierta habilidad, y sin recta intención, se puede llegar a
demostrar que una obra mediocre es excelente y viceversa. Por
todo esto se apresuró a decir muy pronto don Juan Valera que su
crítica iba a ser "anticientífica, blanda, cariñosa y suave" [30].

Porque para él la crítica que se base solamente en preceptos y
reglas sirve nada más que para medir "las cosas que son de sentido
común, lo que está por debajo del arte, no el arte mismo" [31].

La crítica negativa, a lo sumo, serviría para delatar los defectos
de una obra, lo que no es arte, justamente. Pero no servirá para
descubrir la piedra preciosa que pueda yacer oculta entre pedazos
de carbón.

Tal le pasó a Moratín con el estudio que dedicó al *Hamlet*. No
puede por menos de estar de acuerdo Valera con él, en los defectos que señaló a la obra de Shakespeare. Lo que parecía injusto a
don Juan es que "aquello" fuese toda la crítica literaria que Moratín hiciera de tan importante obra del mejor dramaturgo inglés.
Que no dijera una palabra acerca de las muchas virtudes del drama,
de sus bellezas y valores. Se quedó Moratín —en opinión de Valera— en la mitad menos importante del trabajo, ya que "apenas

---

[30] O. C., II, p. 242.
[31] "Discursos, Libertad en el Arte", O. C., II, p. 1091.

entrevió una belleza de cada ciento en aquel poema dramático" [32].

Y aún irritaba más a Valera el ver cómo muchos de los que se llamaban críticos y ejercían la crítica literaria en periódicos y revistas, sin tener el talento de Moratín, copiaban su manera de hacer crítica. El resultado... latigazos crueles cargados de sarcasmos y ni una sola frase aleccionadora o de aliento artístico.

Para ejercer la crítica negativa son suficientes los "principios de retórica" aprendidos de mala manera. Para ejercer, en cambio, la crítica preconizada por Valera había que poseer no sólo una retórica bien asimilada sino una sensibilidad y un buen gusto capaces de descubrir los más ocultos destellos artísticos.

La retórica, sólo como auxiliar de la crítica negativa, grita con machacona paciencia a quienes no tuvieron oídos para escucharle. A los que se apoyaban en mil principios para castigar sin piedad.

El crítico auténtico, para Valera, debe, como el artista, estar tocado de la gracia especial. Como el artista creador, debe poseer un intuitivo conocimiento de la belleza que le impulse a crear, o buscar, obras bellas. Tiene que poseer en sí "una noción a priori de la belleza".

Y es por medio de esta noción por donde el crítico podrá descubrir lo que los seres normales, menos afortunados, no alcanzan a ver con los ojos solos de la razón, o validos de los fríos artículos del decálogo estético.

La primera cualidad que debe tener el crítico, pues, es la de poder calar en las bellezas, antes que reparar en los errores. Asimilar lo percibido como "sustancia propia" y enseñarlo al mundo, luego, "con orden, luz y sello individual y propio" [33]. Pospone así Valera la erudición que el crítico debe poseer, la formación adquirida por el estudio y las muchas lecturas, a ese "soplo de gracia", ese "juicio luminoso y sereno para rechazar lo feo y amar lo her-

---

[32] *Ibidem.*
[33] Vid. "La España Literaria", O. C., II, p. 1134.

moso", que, como privilegio de escogidos, a muy pocos les ha sido concedido.

El menester de crítico, como tal oficio, era digno de toda consideración a los ojos de Valera. Si bien siempre se negó a sí mismo tal título, debido seguramente a lo discontinuo de su colaboración en periódicos y revistas por sus frecuentes ausencias del terreno patrio, trató por todos los medios de no perder el contacto con sus lectores y con los autores españoles e hispanoamericanos (que para él contaban lo mismo, con tal que fueran de calidad). Desde los más apartados empleos diplomáticos escribió cientos de cartas, para nuestra fortuna muchas de ellas hoy publicadas, y varias docenas de artículos críticos.

En una carta escrita a su amigo Narciso Campillo, desde Bruselas, 22-X-1887, en la que parece responder a frases poco amables de éste para Clarín, afirma Valera que la labor crítica por sí misma da categoría de autor estimado, con tal que la crítica sea buena. Confiesa luego no haber leído aún la famosa novela de aquél, *La Regenta,* que se había publicado dos años y medio antes (1884-85): "pero aunque sea pésima *La Regenta,* la crítica de Leopoldo Alas no pierde por ello" [34].

Resumiendo: El crítico, para don Juan Valera, no es otra cosa que el creador, que sin el soplo momentáneo de la inspiración para dedicarse a la pura creación de la belleza, mas poseyendo siempre ese concepto apriorístico de ella, dedica sus esfuerzos a estudiar y decidir sobre lo que otros han creado, valiéndose para ello de esa especie de ciencia infusa que recibió gratuitamente.

Van apareciéndosenos claras las razones por las cuales la crítica de Valera resultó, y sigue resultando para quienes se empeñan en no estudiarla de cerca, tan distinta a la que solía hacerse en nuestro país hacia el tercer cuarto del siglo pasado.

---

[34]   Carta a Narciso Campillo. Vid. *Revista de la Bibl., Arch. y Museo Municipal,* T. II-III, año 1926, p. 440.

Es una diferencia no sólo de gusto y criterio, sino de simple postura crítica. Aquellos "catones censorinos" —entre los que no podremos por menos de colocar alguna vez a Clarín, como veremos— se empeñaban en hacer crítica mirando hacia atrás, como si dijéramos.

Miopemente se entretenían en deshacer, con el látigo de su castigo, las obras que caían en sus manos. Su mirada —su tarea— no iba más allá de la obra analizada. Y como por desgracia la mayoría de las obras eran de una calidad más bien inferior, sus críticas se limitaban a descuartizarlas con los mejores argumentos y a negar valores que cualquier lector sensato podría fácilmente echar en falta.

Valera, en cambio, con su evidente superioridad de formación (y no sólo de agudeza mental) analizaba las obras con perspectiva de futuro. Su crítica no iba dirigida, las más de las veces, al autor de la obra analizada en cuanto padre de ella, sino en cuanto posible padre de obras futuras.

Consideraba Valera que el crítico no podía hacer mucho en pro de una obra juzgada (a no ser ilustrar o ayudar a los lectores), puesto que, desde el momento de su publicación, toda obra está "terminada", hecha; algo muerto, en definitiva, para su creador en cuanto creador de "aquella" obra en particular [35].

---

[35] Idea tan perfectamente actual que no resistimos a la tentación de reproducirla —esta vez en inglés— como la hemos encontrado en boca de uno de los mayores novelistas contemporáneos, John Steinbeck. El reciente premio Nobel de literatura dijo así en una entrevista publicada en *The Sunday Times* londinense el 16 de diciembre de 1962, p. 30: *I carry nothing conscious over from one book to another. A book is finished; it dies. It's a real death. I couldn't go back. Reviews come after the event —too late to be of any use to me.*

Y más adelante, en la misma entrevista, encontramos otra de las ideas que Valera, con cerca de un siglo de anticipación, había expuesto en más de una ocasión: *Literature grows out of people, not out of criticism.*

Si el crítico —y volvemos a Valera— no puede hacer nada positivo por la obra sino tratar de interpretarla para los lectores menos perspicaces, sí podía hacer, en cambio, bastante por el autor. Aconsejarle para la realización de obras futuras, guiarle, aleccionarle amorosamente. Es decir, mejorar la calidad de las futuras flores de nuestro jardín.

He aquí lo que nos parece otra de las razones por las que Valera muchas veces se dejaba perder en divagaciones que poco o nada tenían que ver con la obrilla por él analizada. Aquellas divagaciones valerinas que irritaban incluso a los que se tenían por entendidos y eruditos, eran, en nuestra opinión, las primeras muestras de una crítica diferente. Una manera de hacer crítica que abría el camino a otra inmediatamente posterior en el tiempo, la del noventa y ocho. Don Juan estaba haciendo el cimiento de lo que sería una crítica perdurable y nueva que, contrariamente a la de gran parte de sus coetáneos, iba a quedar para los lectores del futuro —para nosotros— con una frescura jugosa y un interés cierto que los historiadores de la literatura no se han tomado la molestia en descubrir.

CAPÍTULO II

ESTÉTICA DE VALERA

PRINCIPALES IDEAS ESTÉTICAS

Hemos ido intentando, hasta aquí, perfilar los conceptos de crítica y crítico en nuestro autor. Vamos a tratar ahora de poner al descubierto los cimientos sobre los que se levantó su edificio crítico: sus principios estéticos.

Tampoco en éste, como en casi ninguno de los problemas que don Juan se planteara, dejó trazado un sistema completo que nos ilustre sin peligro de llegar a erróneas conclusiones. No se encuentra en su obra, establecido como un todo sistemático y claro, un credo estético, o una poética, a los que tan aficionado fue el siglo XIX, especialmente en Francia.

Y sin embargo ninguna de sus preocupaciones literarias fue más honda que la de los problemas del arte y la belleza.

En la mayoría de sus artículos de crítica, unas veces tangencialmente y otras concediéndole lugar de preferencia, podemos encontrar principios, pensamientos o digresiones que nos sirven de positivas guías en nuestra búsqueda.

Con todo, hay un cierto número de ensayos dedicados específicamente a esta materia. Entre ellos las tres conferencias —de las que desgraciadamente no se conserva la primera— que bajo el título "Filosofía del Arte" pronunció en el Ateneo madrileño en 1859 [1]; el discurso académico titulado "La libertad en el Arte", pronunciado en 1867 [2]; los artículos que para el *Diccionario Enciclopédico Hispano-Americano* escribiera bajo los epígrafes "Estética" y "Belleza" [3] y los titulados "Qué ha sido, qué es y qué debe ser el Arte en el siglo XIX" y "Fines del Arte fuera del Arte" [4].

Escribió sobre estética y sus problemas en otros muchos artículos de simple crítica (de cuyos títulos hacemos gracia al lector por no hacer la lista interminable, pero a los que nos referiremos en concreto más adelante) al tratar puntos que le sugerían posibles aclaraciones o digresiones de tal índole.

¿Cuáles son los autores citados por don Juan —directa o indirectamente—, a qué filósofos de la estética hace referencia, y en cuáles basa la suya? La lista de nombres que puede ser espigada en sus artículos —o a los que por sus doctrinas se refiere, que tanto da— no es corta tampoco [5].

---

[1] O. C., III, pp. 1439-1453.

[2] Idem, p. 1087.

[3] Vid. *Diccionario Enciclopédico Hispano-Americano,* Vol. III, p. 429 y Vol. VII, p. 1007.

[4] Vid. O. C., II, p. 219 y II, p. 917, respectivamente.

[5] Las citas que siguen tienen un propósito de mera curiosidad estadística, y están sacadas únicamente de los artículos que tratan específicamente de problemas estéticos. No hacemos referencia a las innumerables veces que Valera cita a los mismos autores en otros muchos artículos y ensayos de la más diversa índole. Platón: O. C., III, pp. 1439, 1443, 1458 y 1461. — Aristóteles: II, pp. 923, 924, 939 y III, pp. 1092, 1443 y 1498. — Plotino: III, pp. 1093, 1449 y 1461. — Horacio: III, pp. 1440 y 1452. — Filóstrato: III, p. 1093. — San Agustín: III, pp. 1448 y 1461. — Plutarco: III, p. 1448. — Boecio, Alberto Magno, Santo Tomás de Aquino, Dante: III, pp. 1453 y 1461. — M. Ángel, León Hebreo: III, p. 1443. — Gioberti: II, p. 923 y III, p. 1449. — Goethe y Schiller: III, pp. 1094 y 1443. — Boileau: II, p. 731 y III, p. 1461. — Diderot: III, pp. 1093 y 1461. — Voltaire: III, p. 1461. — Hegel: II, pp. 923,

Los autores a quienes Valera menciona con más frecuencia son: Platón, Aristóteles, Horacio, Plotino y los neoplatónicos, Boileau, Voltaire, Diderot, Batteux, Baumgarten, Winckelmann, Kant, Lessing, Hegel, Pictet y algunos más de menor importancia.

Una simple ojeada a esta lista basta para tener una idea —muy superficial, claro es, pero suficiente por el momento— de las huellas o caminos que siguió Valera para trazar sus propias teorías; ya sea para criticar abiertamente las de los otros, como le sucedió con Batteux, Boileau y el mismo Hegel no pocas veces, cuando su criterio no coincidía con los de aquéllos, ya sea para hacerlos suyos de manera más o menos velada.

Resulta muy extraño el que, en tan abundante lista de nombres, no encontremos ni uno solo de los autores que más sobresalieron en la crítica francesa de la pasada centuria. Sospechosamente extraño.

Sin duda ninguna tales nombres no eran desconocidos para don Juan —por no decir que le eran familiares, puesto que sabemos que leía asiduamente la *Revue des Deux Mondes, Le Mercure de France* y las principales revistas literarias de aquel país, entre las que no faltaría *L'Artiste*. Tenía por fuerza que conocer los ensayos críticos de un Sainte-Beuve, un Fromentin o un Hippolyte Taine.

Vemos figuras de menor importancia (a las cuales cita nominalmente o cuyas teorías analiza para combatirlas o para mostrarlas a sus lectores) cuando nos expone sus propios argumentos. Pero las tres máximas figuras de la época no aparecen una sola vez en los artículos dedicados a los problemas de estética en concreto. Alguna leve referencia en ensayos y artículos. A veces el solo nombre, pero nada más.

---

929 y III, pp. 1090, 1449, 1452 y 1461. — Pictet: II, p. 923 y III, páginas 1090 y 1449. — A. Baumgarten: II, p. 1468 y III, pp. 1094, 1458 y 1461. — Batteux: II, p. 731 y III, p. 1093. — Mendelssohn, Lessing, Herder, Winckelmann, Schelling, Fichte, Krause, Solger y Vischer: III, páginas 1090 y 1094.

Y cuando los encontramos citados (tal por ejemplo en el prólogo dedicado a P. A. de Alarcón, en *Nuevo arte de escribir novelas*) no será sin algo más que unas gotas de ironía, que acusan a unos y otros de seguir demasiado al pie de la letra los preceptos —mal asimilados— de aquéllos. Nos resulta increíble, repetimos, que conociendo don Juan a varios escritores franceses, contando a varios de ellos entre sus amigos, ignorara la existencia de la obra —y su importancia— del historiador de Port-Royal, por ejemplo.

Cabe pensar, más bien, en una especie de "ignorancia consciente". Declara Valera en diversas ocasiones que "sólo cita lo que le agrada".

Es Valera hombre a quien las conclusiones le brotan de sus propios manaderos. Cuando ha llegado a las conclusiones que buscaba, y sólo entonces, contento y satisfecho de ellas, las funda en autoridades. Aquellas que le interesan. O sea: que don Juan suele obrar al revés de como acostumbra a hacer la generalidad; sólo está de acuerdo con los autores que están de acuerdo con él. Otra razón más para que no siempre fuera bien acogido.

Y como los tres "máximos críticos" no estaban siempre en perfecta armonía con sus ideas, el crítico andaluz decide ignorarlos.

El apasionado carácter de don Juan hacía que mirara con desconfianza —celosamente— cuanto entraba en España de más allá de los Pirineos. Y si por azar no era él mismo quien facilitaba el "visado de entrada" —lo que, en otras palabras, quiere decir que no fuera él quien lo daba a conocer— tanto peor: "la mercancía", de mejor o peor calidad, no existía para Valera. Ignorancia celosamente consciente.

El mayor agravio que pudo hacerle doña Emilia Pardo Bazán no fue el escribir *La cuestión palpitante* contra las teorías idealistas que mantenía don Juan. Lo que Valera no le perdonó nunca fue el que ésta leyera —si bien en traducciones francesas— mucho antes que él las obras mejores de los novelistas rusos... o las de los mismos franceses, a quienes Valera no había —terca y obstinadamente— querido conocer, ni tener en cuenta.

Todas sus teorías en contra de la novela naturalista —que analizamos al repasar su crítica— están basadas no tanto en el horror que "la novela experimental" [6] le produce, cuanto en un honesto intento de prestigiar la producción literaria nacional. Aquella "producción nacional" tan flojita, tan criticada por él mismo en otras ocasiones, pero a la que veía amenazada por la enorme avalancha de obras que los amigos del naturalismo en España pretendían hacer entrar en el país, sin la paternal bendición valerina.

El hecho de que tuviera en cuenta a críticos que, como los positivistas, chocaron con sus ideas —tal como Eugène Verron, cuya obra *L'Esthétique* vio la luz en París en 1883, o como el mismo Taine [7], cuyo positivismo no deja de presentar destellos idealistas— no extraña tanto como el que no encontremos citas o alusiones de autores que mantuvieron las mismas o parecidas ideas de Valera. Encontramos muy pocas referencias concretas, como si don Juan hubiera estado siempre preocupado con la idea de la originalidad en lo tocante a teorías que no fueran las de la estética clásica. Solamente hará breves alusiones, de pasada, a nombres, teorías o principios.

Y se da el caso curiosísimo de que muchos de estos principios, mantenidos luego por nuestro autor, habían sido dados a conocer con antelación en Francia, por lo que no será muy arriesgado pensar que Valera no desconocía los más modernos trabajos de aquella crítica que él, curiosamente, no mencionaba como cosa viva.

Veamos un ejemplo que ilustra cuanto vamos diciendo: Era común —y nada nuevo como idea, a través de toda la estética— el pensamiento de que el fin del arte se encontraba en sí mismo, en la mera creación de la belleza. Sin embargo, hasta 1836 no había

---

6 Véase el concepto valerino de "novela experimental" en "Sobre el nuevo arte de escribir novelas", O. C., II, pp. 625 y s.

7 Hippolyte-Adolphe Taine, *Philosophie de l'Art*, Hachette, Paris, 1881.

aparecido lo que llamaríamos hoy la fórmula mágica, la expresión "el arte por el arte" (expresión que sólo se haría popular hacia el último tercio del siglo). Fue pronunciada por primera vez, sin que se le prestara mucha atención, además, por Victor Cousin, en su famoso "Cours d'Esthétique": "*Il faut de la religion pour la religion, de la morale pour la morale, de l'art pour l'art*" [8]. (Éste fue, según don Marcelino Menéndez Pelayo, el único "pasaje históricamente memorable que estas lecciones de Cousin contienen" [9].)

Aunque Valera había defendido idéntica postura desde sus más tempranos ensayos, no se encuentra la famosa fórmula o expresión en su obra hasta el año 1860, en el artículo titulado "Naturaleza y carácter de la Novela": "Yo soy más que nada partidario del arte por el arte" [10].

Ahora bien, desde que en 1836 Cousin creara la afortunada frase —fortuna que llegaría al abuso años más tarde— hasta el momento en que don Juan la emplea en su artículo, en Francia no habían dejado de dar vueltas a lo que iba a ser la principal doctrina de los parnasianos. Primero, una especie de balbuceos teóricos: Théophile Gautier, el mismo año que Cousin, y en el prefacio a su obra *Mademoiselle de Maupin* se declara partidario de que el arte no tenga otros fines que la producción de la belleza, y en 1857, el mismo Gautier, en su famoso poema "L'Art", traza ya una condensada teoría de la doctrina del arte por el arte.

Con idéntico título al poema de Gautier, apareció en París una revista semanal de vida muy efímera, pues solamente duró los dos últimos meses del año 1856, que proclamaba el mismo ideal.

---

[8] Vid. *Oeuvres de Victor Cousin*, Bruxelles, Société Belge de librairie, 1840, vol. II, p. 115. Cf. Albert Cassagne, *La théorie de l'Art pour l'Art en France*, Paris, 1906.

[9] Vid. M. Menéndez Pelayo, *Historia de las ideas estéticas*, Madrid, 1947, Ed. Consejo S. de I. Científicas, vol. V, p. 23.

[10] Vid. O. C., II, p. 200.

Y Leconte de Lisle desde sus *Poèmes Antiques* (1852), después
en sus estudios críticos, y finalmente —en 1861— en un largo artículo publicado en la *Revue Européenne,* extiende, aclara y precisa
lo que será la doctrina del arte por el arte, según su propio genio
poético.

Tal desarrollo de las ideas estéticas en el vecino país no pudo
ser ajeno a Valera. Y, sin embargo, no hemos encontrado alusión
ninguna en sus artículos de por aquellas fechas.

¿Celos? No sería muy extraño.

Lo más probable, pues, es que, al igual que pretendió ignorar
las obras que él no descubriera, trató de quitar importancia (¡intencionadamente!) a los autores que más la tuvieron en la crítica francesa de su siglo. (¡Con qué orgullo superior, por el contrario, habla
de su propio descubrimiento de Leopardi, y su profética adivina-
ción como extraordinario poeta mucho antes de que lo hubiera
hecho la crítica francesa!)

Don Juan Valera no contradice las ideas mantenidas por los
críticos franceses; sería contradecirse él mismo. Pero, como no quiere pagar tributos (¿orgullo nacionalista?), pretende ignorarlos. Lo
que, conociendo las "maneras" valerinas, significa tanto como un
ataque.

Si don Juan simula una ignorancia voluntaria, creemos firmemente que no lo hizo por miopía crítica, como se pudiera pensar.
No hay que olvidar —por otra parte— que fue la generación del
noventa y ocho quien descubrió, para los lectores españoles, al autor
de *La philosophie de l'Art.*

Uno de los defectos importantes que encontramos en la crítica
de Valera es lo mucho que dejó por hacer; teniendo la preparación
y el talento suficientes para haber llevado a cabo en España, y en
fecha muy temprana, una tarea crítica sistemática y consistente,
comparable —cuando no superior— a la mejor crítica europea del
período, se limitó —justo es reconocerlo— a ignorar lo que le parecía complicado o exigía de él un esfuerzo superior.

Para lograr un corpus crítico semejante al que lograra años más tarde su discípulo y entrañable amigo, don Marcelino Menéndez Pelayo, el elegante señorito cordobés hubiera tenido que sacrificar muchas horas, gastadas en fiestas y recepciones mundanas, al estudio y al trabajo erudito. Don Juan escribió siempre por puro placer, por afición. Y el escribir —especialmente ensayos críticos— era uno entre muchos de los placeres que daban satisfacción al *bon vivant* que fue.

Don Juan Valera anduvo siempre por el campo literario como por juego. Tenía, sí, la vocación suficiente del *dilettante* que le permitía escribir sobre cuanto se le venía a las mientes, siempre que ello no llevara consigo una reclusión permanente en su biblioteca y en el estudio. Hizo su labor de manera admirable, casi siempre. Pero le faltaron la fuerza de voluntad y la capacidad de trabajo de un Menéndez Pelayo, por ejemplo, para haber llegado a ser uno de los mayores críticos literarios de todos los tiempos. Dotes tenía para ello.

¿QUÉ ERA EL ARTE
PARA VALERA?

En repetidas ocasiones, y variando ligeramente la expresión, nos lo define del modo siguiente:

"No es la imitación de la Naturaleza, sino la creación de la hermosura y la manifestación de la idea que tenemos de ella en el alma, revistiendo esta idea de forma sensible" [11].

Es decir: creación de la hermosura partiendo de la idea de belleza que toda alma humana lleva consigo.

Para lograr esta "creación artística" no basta con la belleza existente en la naturaleza, en los objetos todos del universo, sino que se requiere como condición indispensable que exista en el alma de todo creador una idea o concepto previo de la belleza ideal para

---

[11] O. C., II, p. 220.

poder más tarde materializarla y darla a conocer a los demás mortales. Ya sea por medio de palabras, sonidos, imágenes o volúmenes
bellos.

Incluso es preciso poseer esta "idea previa" para la recta per-
cepción de las bellezas naturales, no ya sólo para las creadas por
la mano del hombre:

"El alma, sin lo bello inteligible que viene a ella inmediatamente, no comprendería lo bello sensible que viene a ella por los
sentidos" [12].

¿Y qué es para Valera esa "idea previa", qué es la belleza?:

"... el resplandor del Ser... el reflejo de la belleza Divina" [13],
puesto inmediata y gratuitamente por Dios en algunos seres privi-
legiados.

Los seres todos de la creación hacen brotar de sí el resplandor
de esa bondad, de esa belleza suprema. Ahora bien: esta belleza
se nos manifiesta mezclada con impurezas y fealdades en la vida.
¿Cómo se las arregla el hombre para filtrar, para separar la belleza
de cuanto no lo es? Por medio del arte [14].

No imitando, no limitándose a copiar lo externo de lo que le
agrada, ya por su forma, ya por su sonido hermoso, sino plasman-
do en objetos reales —o en sonidos armónicos— la idea personal
de belleza que todo creador lleva en sí.

Teorías, como puede verse, nada nuevas. Don Juan Valera, con
Plotino y los neoplatónicos, se proclama fiel seguidor de las doctrinas idealistas de Platón.

Desde sus años de estudiante de filosofía en el seminario malagueño acepta las teorías clásicas y se mostrará luego reacio a
aceptar las que él llamaba "transformaciones de las ideas clásicas".
Aunque esto no quiera decir que dejara de conocer cuantos intentos de renovación estética se habían hecho en todo tiempo.

---

[12] O. C., III, p. 1140.
[13] Idem, p. 1141.
[14] O. C., III, p. 1462.

Así lo manifiesta en su estudio sobre el Duque de Rivas: "... se podrá decir que aceptamos las reglas de Boileau y de Batteux, que, al cabo, son las de Aristóteles y Horacio algo echadas a perder" [15]. Reglas clásicas, mundo clásico. Pureza de conceptos. Tales fueron las ideas adquiridas desde muy temprano.

Por otro lado, el hecho de ser uno de los pocos intelectuales españoles capaces de leer latín y griego le daba un cierto e infantil complejo de superioridad sobre quienes habían de contentarse con traducciones, no siempre muy afortunadas, de las poéticas grecolatinas. Era don Juan capaz de agacharse a beber con humildad de las fuentes que él consideraba primeras, sin que le inquietase la pureza de sus aguas. Mas cuando se trataba de calmar su sed "en los arroyos modernos" era muy distinto cantar. Desaparecía su humildad acostumbrada para con los clásicos. Desconfiaba tercamente de cualquier fuente moderna, por temor a contaminarse con los malignos gérmenes que el tiempo, la moda o las costumbres habían desarrollado en Literatura.

Esta misma postura intransigente de idealista extremado, que arraigará más y más en su espíritu con el paso de los años, le impedirá el disfrute de otras bellezas que no se atengan primordialmente a los principios del arte por el arte mismo. Postura que le hará enfrentarse con los positivistas, realistas, naturalistas y cuantas escuelas literarias no se atengan a sus propios principios.

El artista, según don Juan —que sigue a Aristóteles—, no debe copiar la vida misma tal cual es, sino que debe tratar, en su creación, de inventar una vida tal como debiera ser, pues ésa es la diferencia entre la simple historia y el arte de la palabra o literatura.

Le parece imposible a Valera que se produzca arte de calidad usando como primeras materias el dolor, el sufrimiento, las más bajas pasiones humanas, los instintos más depravados y bestiales o las criaturas más desdichadas de la creación.

---

[15] O. C., II, p. 731.

Don Juan no acepta, ni podrá aceptarlo nunca, el que ningún autor —ni aun el mismo Zola— haga sus novelas del mismo modo que el investigador realiza sus experiencias: con materia "viva", analizando con la mayor falta de pasión y sentimientos personales cuanto cae ante su mirada. Cortando sin temor con su pluma-escalpelo, d_secando las zonas enfermas —¡las células podridas!— con especial cuidado y como con delectación, y mostrando luego "con arte" los resultados al lector-espectador.

Valera prefiere "operar" de otra manera. (Y no es lo peor esta preferencia suya, sino su terco no querer admitir como buena otra técnica que no sea la que él mismo aconseja.) Prefiere "construirse" su propio material humano, idealizarlo, inventando después de haberse fijado vagamente en los seres que le rodean y, especialmente, en su propia alma. De aquí el que sus criaturas literarias salgan a la luz un tanto faltas de ese vigor, ese aliento de realidad con que están adornadas las de los autores que él criticara. Aunque las de éstos, claro está, tengan mucha menos "salud espiritual" que los valerinos.

Los hijos espirituales de don Juan —¿o sería mejor decir hijas, ya que tanto se deleitó en la creación de almas femeninas?— vieron la luz siempre un poco como producidos a troquel, "sin sangre", según dijera algún crítico.

Es la elegancia espiritual, la tendencia a ser un aristócrata del pensamiento, lo que le mueve a pensar y obrar así.

La primera cualidad que debe poseer el artista, según Valera, es la capacidad de amor. El amor desinteresado y espiritual que conduce —por medio del arte— a Dios, fuente suprema del amor y la hermosura [16].

Amor desinteresado que no deberá caer "en un exceso de misticismo a fuerza de espiritualizarse" [17], lo cual conduciría a terminar con el arte, pues el artista excesivamente místico, temeroso de

---

16   Vid. "Filosofía del Arte", O. C., III, pp. 1439-1454.
17   Idem, pp. 1444 y ss.

profanar la superior belleza, no osaría revestirla de forma sensible. No porque el misticismo sea contrario al arte, sino porque precisamente es el término infinito de su progreso. El artista no intentaría crear la belleza sensible y los demás mortales nos quedaríamos sin arte. Afirmación que volverá a sostener don Juan contra los que sospechaban que el arte, como la religión, iban a morir a manos de la ciencia en constante progreso, ya que —argumentaban los filo-cientifistas— ésta "disiparía cuanto de misteriosamente poético existe".

El poeta —el artista en general— debe ser alma enamorada y virtuosa (el *vir bonus* que quería el poeta latino), si bien, aclara Valera, basta con que el artista "sea noble y bueno en el momento mismo de percibir la idea de lo bello y de realizarla en su obra" [18]. El santo, como el héroe, por sus fines más sublimes, deberá poseer una virtud más elevada y constante que la del simple artista.

El buen gusto —para don Juan— no depende tanto de la claridad y perspicacia de entendimiento como de la exquisita sensibilidad del alma. Razón que explica el que, a veces, personas de entendimiento muy claro sean incapaces de sentir las hermosuras de un poema, y, por el contrario, personas de escaso entendimiento posean cierto gusto para la apreciación artística. Mas el auténtico buen gusto presupone entendimiento claro y despejado y un cierto grado de imaginación estética o de fantasía.

Diferencia —con Hegel, Gioberti y Pictet— la imaginación estética de la imaginación común o vulgar, puesto que aquélla, aun en los casos en que no está creando nada positivo, puede tener un cierto grado creador tal como en la apreciación de la obra artística de los demás.

Afirma con Plotino que no sólo para producirla, sino aun para sentir la belleza, es necesario que el alma humana participe de ella; que sea hermosa [19].

---

[18] O. C., III, p. 1448.
[19] Vid. Carta a Leopoldo Augusto Cueto, de 5-III-1857, O. C., III,

El artista nos transmite su personal idea de la belleza, valiéndose del sonido o la forma sensible, en la creación de su obra artística. Nosotros la percibimos por medio de los sentidos corporales. Estos captan "el objeto" hermoso para cederlo a la imaginación estética, la que, a su vez, "lo ilumina con los rayos de la belleza absoluta y lo presenta a la voluntad para que ésta guste de él y al entendimiento para que lo juzgue y decida sobre él".

Y como los sentidos del espectador —la vista y el oído— captan ante todo ese sostén material de la belleza, ese soporte sobre el que el artista levanta su obra, tal consideración hace caer a don Juan en la tentación de separar fondo y forma. O dicho de otro modo, inspiración, de expresión. Falacia que le va a conducir a conclusiones tan poco convincentes como la de que "la poesía sin la forma es prosa y vuelan y se apartan de ella gran número de esos incomunicables pensamientos de que hemos hablado" [20].

Como si en la prosa —¿tan poquito significaba para don Juan, uno de los más finos prosistas en lengua española?— no pudiera darse la más delicada y alta poesía. O sólo al verso, que es lo que don Juan quiere decir cuando habla de "poesía", le fuera dado manifestar esos "incomunicables pensamientos".

El artista, según él, deberá cuidar especialmente la forma. Pero "la forma", para Valera, es nada más la forma clásica, claro está. Y quien se aparte de ella cometerá un grave pecado estético, como veremos. Peligrosísimo principio que dará origen a conclusiones valerinas muy discutibles. Quiere ajustarse exclusivamente "a una forma clásica". ¡Como si la tan por él venerada forma clásica dichosa no hubiera sido, a su vez, una invención humana, un simple hallazgo feliz! Tan válido o tan erróneo como las nuevas formas que trataban de encontrar las diferentes escuelas o movimientos

---

página 146, donde cita Valera textualmente a Plotino. También en su discurso académico "La Libertad en el Arte", O. C., III, p. 1090 y III, página 1449.

[20]   O C., III, p. 1449.

artísticos que surgían ante los asustados ojos de Valera, que prefieren ingenuamente cerrarse a la luz para no contemplar lo que él creía "lástimas y desaciertos artísticos" y no ¡sufrir con ello!

Y este querer aferrarse al respeto de la "forma clásica" le hará cometer el más grave pecado, a nuestro juicio, de su crítica: El negar, o no tener en cuenta, la transformación, el cambio de esas formas que él idolatraba; cambio que se opera especialmente en la poesía francesa del último cuarto de siglo.

Conocía la lengua francesa suficientemente bien como para leerla y escribirla correctamente, por lo que se nos antoja imperdonable el que se obstinara en no prestar atención a lo que él llamaba irónicamente "las novedades pasajeras del vecino país". Se obstinó también en ignorar no sólo la escuela naturalista —a la que niega tozudamente todo valor—, sino que ni siquiera admite la existencia de movimientos y revoluciones poéticas tan diferentes del concepto —y en especial de la forma— del arte tradicional, como los de realistas, parnasianos, simbolistas o incluso modernistas.

Descubrió con agudeza extraordinaria, y estimó en todo su valor, como veremos, al desconocido y joven poeta nicaragüense Rubén Darío... mas no quiso Valera admitir la posibilidad de que surgieran tras él, heredando y ampliando las novedades, quienes pudieran formar una escuela poética de valor. No sólo niega validez a aquellas formas que le parecían extranjerizantes para los poetas de la América española; casi las prohíbe para los de la misma España. (Afortunadamente no le hicieron mucho caso nuestros jóvenes poetas de fines de siglo.)

¡Negar la libertad modernista, que era nada menos que el nacimiento de la auténtica nueva poesía, la bocanada de aire puro, frente a los más que usados moldes de poetas cuyos nombres yacen hoy bajo una gruesa capa de piadoso olvido! (Remitimos al lector curioso a la misma *Antología de poetas líricos del siglo XIX*, hecha por don Juan, de donde pueden sacarse docenas de nombres hoy piadosamente olvidados.)

Para don Juan la hermosura poética tiene carácter más espiritual que la producida por las demás artes. Para poder gozar, por ejemplo, con la música o la pintura es preciso contar con el apoyo de unos sentidos corporales especialmente bien dotados, mientras que para gozar, percibir o crear las bellezas poéticas son suficientes las facultades del alma, amor, inspiración y entendimiento.

Un ciego no podrá disfrutar del color o la línea de un hermoso cuadro, al igual que un sordo será incapaz de emocionarse con la más bella de las sinfonías. Mas uno y otro podrán leer, o escuchar, un poema, y gozar y sentir lo que el poeta les comunica. Lo cual justifica la mayor abundancia de poetas y expertos en poesía, al compararlos con los cultivadores y "expertos" en las demás bellas artes.

Al igual que hay grados en la creación del arte, es decir, obras y artistas más o menos excelsos, habrá para Valera diferencias en cuanto a la comprensión de la belleza artística. E incluso puede darse que el observador atento de la obra de arte llegue a descubrir bellezas que al mismo creador le hubieran podido pasar inadvertidas [21]. ¿Cómo puede explicarse tal fenómeno? Sencillamente porque para Valera la creación es fruto de una "inspiración ciega", un *quid divinum* que empuja al artista a veces por caminos para él mismo insospechados, por no decir totalmente desconocidos [22].

Contra la opinión de Hegel y de Boileau —*avant donc que d'écrire apprenez à penser*— mantiene don Juan el criterio de que lo más importante en la creación artística no es la técnica —que puede llegar a ser dominada mediante la práctica y el estudio—, sino ese ardor o comunicación divina que dirige la mano del artista para hacerle concebir y llevar a cabo bellezas sublimes, sirviéndose precisamente de los mismos medios con los que un hombre ordinario realizaría vulgaridades mediocres.

---

[21] O. C., III, p. 1449.
[22] O. C., III, p. 1452.

Por lo cual, si bien es necesario conocer la materia de que el artista ha de hacer uso —color, sonido, lengua—, el solo conocimiento de ella no significará gran cosa para la realización de una obra de arte si carecemos de ese "don divino".

Conviene, sí, llamar a la inspiración, tentar la posibilidad de que el soplo nos visite. Y para ello nada mejor que el trabajo asiduo, la práctica constante y el estudio.

Al mismo Valera le "bullían" en la cabeza, en los últimos días de su vida, cientos de ideas, multitud de "embriones" de obras de arte, a los que no logró dar forma bella sobre el papel, por lo que sufrió grandemente, según contaba a su amigo entrañable D. Marcelino Menéndez Pelayo. Luchaba Valera por lograr esa inspiración que no siempre le fue propicia. Pero cuando le llega, escribe —y en poquísimo tiempo— la juvenil *Juanita la larga*, una de sus obras más "pimpantes", menos trabajadas —según su propia expresión— y, sin embargo, más llena de encanto.

De todo ello, parece deducir don Juan, la crítica: ¿precede o sigue inmediatamente a la creación?

Para el verdadero artista, el juicio crítico acompaña inconscientemente, pero de modo positivo, al acto de la creación; el juicio crítico será quien le haga desechar lo menos valioso y utilizar sólo los elementos más nobles para alcanzar la más pura belleza.

Cuando el artista se pone a medir, a calibrar conscientemente los valores de sus propias obras, en la mayoría de los casos sufre lamentables equivocaciones y nos demuestra que su capacidad crítica "consciente" es muy inferior a la que por intuición posee en los momentos de la creación. Cita el caso de Cervantes, con sus mejores esperanzas puestas en el *Persiles*, una obra más bien mediana, y no en su más grande novela.

Ilustrando con otro ejemplo su afirmación, cae don Juan en su propia trampa, declarándosenos incapaz de descubrir "consciente o inconscientemente" las bellezas del *Polifemo* o *Las Soledades* de Góngora, que pone como ejemplo de fruto malogrado (¡...!), producto de la reflexión y del estudio, frente a los "deliciosos romances del mismo autor nacidos espontáneamente" [23]. Afirmaciones ambas que no precisan discusión ni comentario.

Nada dice de su propio problema, ya fuera por modestia (cosa que dudamos, pues no fue ésta una de sus "virtudes"), ya porque a él mismo, como le pasó al autor del *Quijote,* se le ocultaba la verdad. Valera se creyó siempre poeta, por encima de toda otra cosa. Poeta en verso, claro es, que si hubiera dicho "poeta de la prosa" nada hubiéramos tenido que añadir. Pero poeta, autor de versos de la calidad que él creyera... sí que no lo fue. Ni en vida, ni mucho menos hoy, fueron sus versos —artísticos, trabajados, cerebrales, clásicamente fríos— excesivamente apreciados. Poco le importó, sin embargo, para considerarse a sí mismo "poeta antes que otra cosa".

La teoría de Valera, con todo, y aunque tengamos que decir repetidamente que él mismo no la sigue siempre a pies juntillas, no invita al artista al *dolce far niente,* mientras el soplo divino no le visite. No. Conviene trabajar, esforzarse, estudiar y ejercitarse continuamente hasta que esa fuerza superior llegue. Lo afirma en repetidas ocasiones [24].

Quejándose, otra vez, del desdén que por los autores manifestaba el público —lo que había conducido a un abandono del estudio serio por parte de aquéllos y a una prosa descuidadísima— aconseja el estudio como remedio del mal: "Cuando no se estudia, o se estudia poquísimo, nadie, a no ser un ingenio portentoso, acierta a escribir algo que sea de gusto o de provecho" [25].

---

[23] "Filosofía del Arte", O. C., III, p. 1453. Juicios similares se encuentran repetidamente en los trabajos críticos de Valera. Véase, por ejemplo, O. C., II, p. 8 y III, p. 215.

[24] Vid. "Novelas recientes", O. C., II, p. 1097 y "Elogio de Santa Teresa", III, p. 1146.

[25] "Sobre la duración del habla castellana", O. C., II, p. 1045.

Creemos sinceramente que a Valera le fue mucho más fácil concebir la teoría de sus principios que poner éstos en práctica. Pero no se olvide tampoco que "el vivir" era para él una posible obra de arte. El buen vivir, naturalmente. De aquí el cuidado que por embellecer ese su vivir, por gozar de la vida como del mejor regalo que los cielos concedieron al hombre, pusiera siempre.

Citemos, para terminar con este punto, la carta que escribió a su amigo el Dr. Thebussem el 7 de enero de 1896. Confiesa seguir "... dando más importancia a la inspiración que al estudio... yo me digo: D. J. Ruiz de la Vega sabía gramática, retórica, poética, historia, latín, algo de griego y otra multitud de cosas, y escribió el poema *Pelayo* que nadie, sino él y el corrector de las pruebas de imprenta, han podido leer hasta ahora; y en cambio Zorrilla, que no sabía gramática, ni retórica, ni nada, escribió *Margarita la tornera*, *El zapatero y el rey*, *Don Juan Tenorio* y otras obras inmortales que, a pesar de sus defectos, se leen y se oyen todavía con extraordinario placer y admiración a veces" [26].

FINES DEL ARTE

Valera, ya se ha dicho, fue hombre de principios rara vez cambiables. Antes de darse a conocer como escritor, había madurado casi todas sus ideas artísticas estudiando la estética clásica, a la vez que se creaba una propia. A ninguno de entre sus principios estéticos se aferró tanto y tan profundamente, estudiándolo y dedicándole tanto espacio, como al de los fines del arte.

El fin del arte, para don Juan, no era otro que el de la pura creación de la belleza. Y como en él basó su crítica, lo convertirá en castillo defensivo y en arma de combate para emplearla contra quienes no piensan como él. Por lo que lo vamos a encontrar no sólo en los trabajos dedicados específicamente a la estética y sus

---

[26] Vid. "Carta inédita al Doctor Thebussem", apud Edith Fishtine, obra citada, p. 33.

problemas, sino también en cuantos artículos críticos o discusiones literarias le proporcionaban los defensores de las doctrinas naturalistas, de las que muy pronto se había declarado abierto enemigo.

El arte, prosigue, debe simplemente proporcionar diversión y alegría, elevar al hombre —mediante el milagro artístico— a esferas superiores. Mejorarle, si cabe, no mediante la prédica de moralidades más o menos disfrazadas (el arte auténtico va siempre de acuerdo con la moral, para don Juan, según veremos), sino por la simple contemplación de esa superior belleza de la que el arte humano no es más que un débil reflejo. Que el amor —el apetito de belleza neoplatónico— nos haga buscar el arte. Y del arte, como por una escala ideal, ascendamos al Artista supremo, a Dios.

En fecha tan temprana como la carta, ya mencionada, desde el Brasil a su amigo Heriberto García de Quevedo, lo había declarado por primera vez. Y es curioso —y nada casual, por otra parte— que sea el primer brote de novela realista española del siglo XIX, la prematura *Gaviota* publicada en 1847, el que haga volver a Valera a extenderse más en su afirmación.

El naturalismo como escuela literaria en España aún está muy lejos y sus futuros apóstoles, si habían nacido, contaban muy pocos años de edad. Mas la novela de doña Cecilia Böhl de Faber (criticada por don Juan en la *Revista de Madrid* de 31 de julio de 1856) le hace afirmar categóricamente, como el anuncio de lo que treinta años más tarde volverán a sugerirle las novelas naturalistas:

"El único fin y objeto de la poesía, y poesía son las novelas, es la realización de lo bello, escaso, confuso y fugitivo de la naturaleza en el arte permanente, rico y depurado. Lo bueno y lo verdadero no son el fin de la poesía; pero al realizar lo bello se encuentra en él la verdad y la bondad como sus atributos esenciales. *Al arte, que tiene en sí mismo su fin,* se le rebaja y desdora al hacerlo instrumento de estas o aquellas ideas y armas de partido" [27].

---

[27]   Véase artículo citado, O. C., II, p. 86.

La belleza como primer fin. Y como atributos inseparables lo bueno y lo verdadero. No es sino la famosa tríada clásica de Platón que, como vemos, don Juan adoptara desde muy temprano.

Pero no critica el que todo artista se proponga un fin, ya sea moral, cultural o político, en el momento de ponerse a crear una obra [28]. Admitirá que tal propósito no tiene malicia en sí. Que incluso puede ser el motor que impulse al artista hacia la consecución de sus fines.

Lo que a Valera no le agrada es que el artista, consciente de ese "propósito secundario", posponga para su mejor logro lo que don Juan considera primer y más importante fin del arte: la pura creación de la belleza.

No niega que toda obra de arte pueda desprender cierta enseñanza —junto al puro goce o placer intelectual— a quien la contempla. Que nos mejore, incluso, en nuestro íntimo ser, con lo cual la obra de arte alcanzará una enseñanza de mucho valor. Lo que niega categóricamente don Juan es que toda obra artística tenga por obligación que llevar en sí una enseñanza, una consecuencia o una "moraleja". La sola belleza lograda en la obra de arte puede mejorar nuestra personalidad, no las enseñanzas que se nos dan bajo forma de ese arte que Valera, dejándose llevar de la irritación, llama bastardo e impuro.

(Resulta curioso señalar cómo, transcurrido casi un siglo desde que don Juan empleara estos argumentos, muchos de ellos son todavía válidos frente a muchas de las ideas existencialistas de Jean-Paul Sartre y su "Littérature engagée".)

---

[28] En efecto, para Valera, el escritor "se pone" en todo cuanto escribe. Y ahora que se habla con frecuencia de "literatura comprometida" o "de tendencia", será bueno recordar lo que decía don Juan a este respecto: "Toda literatura, siempre, y más aún en nuestros días, tiene que ser literatura de tendencia. Es falso que el autor se eclipse. Su personalidad informa siempre el libro que escribe". "Sobre el arte de escribir novelas", O. C., II, pp. 689-690.

Ni Virgilio (ejemplo tan prodigado por D. Juan) se propuso enseñar nada de cuanto se relaciona con la agricultura y el campo en *Las Geórgicas*, ni las enseñanzas que en ellas se nos dan a este respecto ocuparían algo más de unas pocas páginas en una elemental cartilla de agricultura. Y, sin embargo, qué alta poesía, qué arte divino hay en los versos del poeta latino para don Juan, a quien la agricultura y el campo en sí mismo le causaban tan poca impresión. Por otro lado, los grandes maestros de la humanidad, los que más enseñaron —Cristo, Buda y Confucio— no se propusieron hacer arte, sino enseñar. Nada escribieron y, sin embargo, hoy seguimos aprendiendo de sus enseñanzas. Resume así nuestro autor:

Nada debe, pues, enseñar la obra artística; y si por azar se desprende alguna enseñanza de la contemplación o disfrute de una obra de arte, que sea esta enseñanza la del optimismo, la felicidad y el mejoramiento de la vida.

Para enseñar, no es necesario tener siempre que mostrar las lacras, las heridas, llagas y dolores de los seres desgraciados a los que tienen la fortuna inmensa de no soportarlas, ¡como era el caso de Valera mismo!

No es que a don Juan se le ocultaran los sufrimientos y las desgracias amargas que tanto abundaban en los tiempos en que le tocó vivir. La miseria y el dolor se daban, desgraciadamente, con más frecuencia que las arcadias felices y doradas con que él pretendía entretener y animar a sus lectores.

Mas al escritor exquisito, al hedonista que él era, le molestaba sobremanera el empleo de tan poco "nobles materiales". El hambre, el dolor, la miseria y el sufrimiento eran feos en sí, cuando no "de pésimo gusto", para ser elevados a obra de arte.

Y no solamente porque el arte no deba enseñar nada (¡ni siquiera la realidad cotidiana!), sino porque el uso de tales "materiales" como elementos de una obra de arte es antiartístico, la negación del arte mismo.

Pero no crea el lector que Valera sea hombre que llegue a conclusiones tan francas como la que acabamos de exponer. Hablar de esta manera, para don Juan, hubiera sido muy peligroso. Aclaremos que, si bien pensó siempre como decimos, no se atrevió a decirlo nunca más que como él acostumbraba a decir las cosas, entre líneas. Insinuando, o como él gustaba de decir, "hablando de costado".

Años más tarde, criticando una obra de Carlos Reyles —a quien reconoce virtudes de gran escritor, por otra parte— afirma que una novela "debe ser un libro de pasatiempo y solaz, debe elevar y no consternar el ánimo; debe, como decía Aristóteles, purificar las pasiones... serenar y elevar el espíritu y no perturbarle, humillarle o deprimirle". Le parece cosa endiablada que un autor inteligente "se proponga escribir novelas no para darnos buenos ratos, sino malos". Llega a una conclusión don Juan que no nos coge, a estas alturas, de sorpresa:

"Tales cosas me parecen enormidades, y no sólo *pugnan con toda la estética que yo había estudiado o que me había forjado, sino también con mi condición apacible, suave y algo inclinada al optimismo*" [29].

En sus novelas todas, las únicas miserias que se notan son la falta de amor, el amor imposible, la escasez de bienes materiales, o problemas de conciencia de toda índole. Pero jamás ninguna de sus criaturas literarias sufre realmente padecimientos ordinarios, como los que suele padecer cada hijo de vecino. No. Tampoco pinta Valera, en sus novelas y cuentos, una sociedad como la que, sin ninguna duda, le rodeaba en su Andalucía natal o en el poblachón madrileño de la segunda mitad del siglo. ¡Dejaría de ser don Juan Valera si tal cosa hubiera hecho!

No pinta nunca una sociedad, o un personaje, que no sea "ideal". Porque don Juan predica con el ejemplo: busca la belleza idealizando la realidad. Sus personajes femeninos, acusados tantas veces

---

[29] Vid. "Nuevas cartas americanas", O. C., III, p. 484.

de tener un "alma libresca", de ser "puro intelecto", "marisabidillas", y hasta de ser "verdaderos tratados de sabiduría", no se parecen mucho (por no decir nada) a las mujeres con que don Juan se tropieza a diario en calles y salones. Las traza así deliberadamente. Incluso cuando están vagamente fundadas en personajes reales, como el caso de *Pepita Jiménez*. Las traza así no porque trate de enseñar a sus lectoras femeninas cómo deben comportarse en situaciones parecidas, sino por creer que, obrando así, se acerca más y mejor al logro de esa belleza ideal y superior, por la que todo artista debe luchar al ponerse a realizar toda obra de arte.

El profesor Montesinos ha estudiado en su magnífico libro —probablemente el mejor estudio que sobre la novela de Valera se haya hecho nunca— el proceso creativo de la novela valerina. Del personaje de Valera, por mejor decir. Valera no se atenía —resumimos las palabras del Prof. Montesinos— a las superficies externas, como operaban los realistas. Recogía datos que armonizaban y los combinaba en un canon más bello que el de la generalidad de los seres que vemos. Se atenía sobre todo "a la idea". Su idea de belleza, ya fuera física, ya moral. Hace así, con su método personal, una novela experimental, la única que, a su juicio, merecía la pena de ser hecha [30].

Resumiendo, pues, vemos cómo ni en la teoría ni en la práctica de sus principios admite don Juan otros fines en el arte que los del arte mismo. Si alguna enseñanza se desprende, que sea positiva. Es decir: ensalzando los valores humanos, no negándolos. Y si hay enseñanza, que sea un alto ideal para el alma humana, que nos conduzca "a esferas superiores por la contemplación de lo ideal y de lo que se acerca a lo perfecto" [31].

Sólo podrán obtenerse resultados positivos, es decir, mejorar la situación moral del pueblo español (en un intento de paliar las calamidades de todo tipo que se abatían sobre él), ayudándole a le-

---

[30]   J. F. Montesinos, obra citada, pp. 193 y 194.
[31]   "Nuevas cartas americanas", O. C., III, p. 917.

vantar su ánimo. Poniéndole ejemplos optimistas, no demoledores. La contemplación de lo desagradable no puede sino entristecer —cuando no embrutecer, o despertar las pasiones menos nobles a quienes lo contemplan. Afirma Valera que, así como los escultores griegos del siglo de Pericles lograron, uniendo rasgos y líneas tomados de seres vivos, figuras bellísimas, estas obras, a su vez, tuvieron más tarde un efecto positivo: contribuyeron a mejorar el grado de belleza del pueblo griego, ya que las damas griegas, por la contemplación de las obras hermosas de la escultura y de la pintura, vinieron a ser mucho más bellas que las mujeres de los siglos anteriores [32].

Afirmación que no debe ser tomada muy en serio, aunque nos tememos que don Juan, a fuerza de sostenerla, llegó a creerla verdadera. En cartas particulares, en otras ocasiones, dice que visitando, en sus años mozos, el Capitolio romano, se admiró del parecido que encontraba entre las mujeres romanas y las estatuas de la antigüedad. Y no porque las estatuas hubieran sido hechas copiando los rasgos más sobresalientes de las doncellas más hermosas de la localidad, sino porque "debido a la contemplación de dichas bellas estatuas, la mujer romana había ido perfeccionándose de líneas al paso de los tiempos".

Exageración burlesca típicamente valerina —¡íbamos a decir... andaluza!— que le sirvió para apoyar su postura de fe ciega en las posibilidades "mejoradoras" del arte sobre la naturaleza humana.

ARTE Y MORAL.
¿VALERA PURITANO?

El arte auténtico de superior belleza está íntimamente ligado con la moral; no hay, no puede haber, según esta concepción va-

---

[32] Vid. "Teatro libre", O. C., II, pp. 982 y s.

lerina, solución de continuidad entre la estética y la moral porque
ambas son "como ramas de la misma raíz" [33].

Moral universal y belleza artística coinciden sin posibilidad de
separación, y cuando "se ataca o se ofende de modo grave a la
moral, toda belleza artística desaparece avergonzada", dice al criticar, con severidad en él desacostumbrada, el libro de poemas de
Salvador Rueda titulado *Himno a la carne* [34].

A primera vista puede parecer un tanto paradójico el que don
Juan sea tan tajante respecto a los problemas morales; él, que tan
benévolo fuera siempre con toda clase de pecados y de pecadores,
que tan dispuesto al perdón del pecado artístico —el más grave
ante el tribunal de la belleza— estuviera siempre, sea tan intransigente con los pecados morales.

Es claro que en hombre de pensamiento tan libre no debemos
esperar que rinda culto a una moral limitada a una fe concreta, ya
sea la moral natural, católica, protestante, budista o mahometana.
Valera rinde culto a la "moral universal". Cualquier ataque a cualquier moral es pecado tan grave que oculta, que destruye toda
belleza.

No pone trabas al pensamiento, por libre, por ilimitado que éste
sea, con tal de estar bella, delicadamente expuesto. Su propio pensamiento rozó muchas veces, y los sobrepasó no pocas, los límites
de la ortodoxia cristiana. No le importa que Leopardi sea ateo,
Manzoni progresista católico y Carducci celebre a Satanás, aborre-
ciendo a Cristo. Los tres le entusiasman.

En lo que don Juan no hace concesiones es en la manera de
decir. Que cuanto se diga esté dicho siempre con elegancia y brío.
No es menester comulgar con la idea que se desprenda de la obra
de arte para gozar con ella. Si ambas cosas se dan juntas, el placer

---

[33]   "Sobre el nuevo arte de escribir novelas", O. C., II, p. 704.
[34]   Véanse los artículos "Disonancias y armonías de la Moral y de la
Estética", O. C., II, pp. 838-848.

será completo. Mas se puede aplaudir una obra, reconociendo la manera bella en que está realizada, sin tener que estar de acuerdo con el pensamiento o las intenciones del autor. (El ejemplo de tomar a varios autores, de ideales muy diferentes, se va a repetir frecuentemente, no sólo con poetas extranjeros, como los citados, sino también con nombres españoles, como por ejemplo el Duque de Almenara, Gustavo Adolfo Bécquer y Quintana [35].)

Lo que no puede tolerar, lo que rechaza con todas las fuerzas de su alma Valera es que determinadas materias sean objeto del arte. Nadie en su tiempo, mejor que él, estudió en España el amor humano en sus más variados matices. Puede decirse, con el profesor Montesinos, que "todas sus novelas son novelas de amor" [36]. Y aun cuando en ellas se den, como se dan en la vida misma, los llamados "pecados de amor" que la moral cristiana condena, don Juan se cuidó muy bien de no trazar un solo rasgo que pudiera escandalizar a la más púdica de las recatadas lectoras. Bastaba una leve insinuación, un "hacer comprender sin decirlo todo", y escribir "veladamente" para que, sin ocultar hipócritamente los hechos, no sean estos mismos hechos, o su escabrosidad, mejor dicho, el motivo del deleite artístico.

Tal deleite, en todo caso, se dirige a las facultades menos nobles del espíritu. A los sentidos, más bien.

Su idealismo, en esto como en todo, le impide asociar belleza pura con lo que él consideraba la parte menos noble —la carne—, si bien necesaria, del amor. De aquí sus repetidas condenas a los autores que, amparándose en las doctrinas realistas o naturalistas, dan a conocer, en verso y en prosa, interioridades humanas que no son para puestas a la vista de nadie, ya que, según Valera, "no es artístico el describir prolijamente los placeres de la alcoba" [37].

---

[35] "Sobre el arte de escribir novelas", O. C., II, p. 685.
[36] J. F. Montesinos, obra citada, p. 204.
[37] O. C., II, p. 840.

Ahora bien: si lo que don Juan prohibe no es el que encontremos tales escenas o descripciones en las obras de arte, como inevitablemente se dan en la vida misma, sino el que "se describan con todo detalle", ¿no podríamos acusar a nuestro autor de un excesivo celo puritanista? Se nos aparece cuidadoso, no de la moral en sí, sino de las apariencias de una moral a la que importa, más que respetar, dar la impresión externa de que se respeta.

Pero tal acusación —si hay quien se atreve a hacerla— nos parecería, amén de excesiva, injusta. Porque la prohibición de don Juan está desligada totalmente de la idea moral de pecado. Su "no" tajante se dirige más al detalle, a la explicación morosa —con intenciones artísticas— de la que usan y abusan los escritores naturalistas, que a la transgresión moral en sí misma.

Si como autor de novelas Valera fue un moralista [38], como crítico literario transige con que el arte vuele "por cima de todo límite", incluida la moral más ortodoxa. Y por ello mismo rechaza la idea de que el autor se detenga en los pormenores menos elegantes. Pormenores que, como el dolor, el sufrimiento o las miserias corporales, producen horror a su alma de hombre exquisito. No son materia digna de la atención del artista ni de las personas de buen gusto.

El acto amoroso, privado de lo que de ideal le envuelve, no queda más que en la pura animalidad, y es a esto justamente a lo que dedican páginas y estrofas los escritores naturalistas. Don Juan no se lo perdona; no puede perdonarles. Sin embargo, es muy tolerante con el pecado de pensamiento, ya que no con el de obra.

Cuando sus criaturas pecan, las vemos luchando más con la idea de pecado que con el pecado mismo. Vemos a la piadosa Pepita, durante páginas y páginas, debatirse con ese amor que la inclina hacia el seminarista de un modo más "humano" de lo que ella misma deseara. Pero Valera nos cuenta en unas pocas líneas, y del

---

[38]   José F. Montesinos, obra citada, pp. 190 y ss.

modo más discreto, la caída, el acto pecador, la auténtica transgresión de la moral que Pepita acataba. Sospechamos que un autor realista —y no digamos uno de la escuela naturalista— en lugar de Valera hubiera aprovechado esa especie de "clímax" que alcanzan las luchas interiores de los dos protagonistas para pintarnos una escena final —el triunfo y apoteosis del amor humano— con los más atractivos colores de su paleta y las líneas más atrevidas. Valera, como es de rigor, prefirió lo contrario. Se deleita con los procesos mentales, los problemas de conciencia. Pasa rápidamente sobre el lado práctico de la cuestión [39].

No es, pues, un auténtico freno moral el que Valera predica, sino sencillamente una dosis de buen gusto, de elegancia elemental.

Si los sonetos de Salvador Rueda hubieran cantado más espiritualmente, con menos lujo de detalles, los mismos placeres que describen, Valera no tendría que reprocharle nada y hasta puede que los hubiera aplaudido. No lo hizo porque eran demasiado atrevidos: ¡glorificar, nada menos, un tema que don Juan consideraba "tabú"! No porque tal materia fuera siempre inmoral, sino por "glorificar" cosas que, al entender valerino, debían permanecer "veladas y como en sombras", si no en secreto total. Pero nunca ser materia artística.

Importaba a don Juan, sobre todo, el tono en que se dijeran las cosas, puesto que así lo confiesa en la referida crítica. Si los sonetos de Rueda hubieran sido escritos "de broma", por alegrar las pajarillas, nada hubiera tenido que objetar. Pero estaban escritos seriamente, con un título que debió escandalizar no poco a Valera [40].

Que esto es bien cierto lo demuestra el hecho de que publicó don Juan, sin ningún reparo —aunque no sin muchos miedos—, en 1896 una colección de cuentos y chascarrillos andaluces que no se distinguen por el buen gusto precisamente y a los que él mismo calificó de "harto subidillos de color".

---

[39] Vid. *Pepita Jiménez*, O. C., I, pp. 178-179.
[40] Vid. "La Moral y la Estética", O. C., II, p. 843.

Habían colaborado con Valera en la recogida de materiales el doctor Thebussem (Mariano Pardo de Figueroa), el Conde de las Navas y el poeta Narciso Campillo, bajo los seudónimos de Fulano, Zutano, Mengano y Perengano. La crítica acogió el librillo con bastante dureza, pese a ser buen negocio de venta. Tenían material para un segundo volumen y, temerosos de levantar más protestas, no lo dieron a la imprenta. Don Juan se apresuró a declarar que la intención que les había llevado a recoger tales cuentos populares no era otra que la de "distraer y alegrar las pajarillas" de los lectores con la chispa y gracejo de sus paisanos. Ni por un momento ninguno de los autores había pensado en ser tomado en serio ni mucho menos pretendieron hacer arte. Esto les disculpaba, pues, del tono poco serio y de las libertades de gusto dudoso y subido color que se habían permitido [41].

La moral de Valera, como vemos, es también peculiar, muy personal: es el *dandy* que no soporta el pecado, no por el pecado en sí, sino por lo que de bajo placer tiene. No es la suya una auténtica moral —tal y como la vemos sin las agudezas a que Valera quiso someterla—, sino sencillamente una prédica de buen gusto. Es la moral hedonista del personaje principal de *Genio y figura*, que se entrega a sus amantes por caridad, por hacerles felices.

Todo depende del tono con que se diga. Y cambiando ligeramente la frase —que es de don Juan— depende de la manera como se haga. No dice "no matarás" porque las leyes divinas y humanas así lo ordenan, sino porque el derramamiento de sangre le parece espectáculo poco grato. Tampoco su moral nos prohibe pecar contra determinado mandamiento, con tal que lo hagamos discretamente. Lo que don Juan no permite es que con ello se haga materia de arte. Don Juan se desentiende de la moralidad, pues, para predicar buen gusto.

---

[41] Vid. Santiago Montoto, *Valera al natural*, Madrid, 1962, Cap. titulado "Las amarguras de Don Juan", pp. 35 y 54. Hubo una segunda edición de los *Cuentos y chascarrillos andaluces* en 1898.

Le vemos así enfrentándose una vez más —por su especial postura— a los escritores de su tiempo. A los unos —realistas y naturalistas extremados— porque les afea esa especie de delectación que sienten describiendo "materiales de baja calidad" [42]. A los otros, los que cultivaban un realismo digamos más comedido, los que se alejan menos de las normas idealistas, porque en el fondo don Juan no predica moral ninguna con su "moral especial". Lo que él llamaba "moral universal" no era sino una pura elegancia de forma por la que abogó siempre. Don Juan Valera, pues, nadando involuntaria pero fatalmente entre dos difíciles aguas, sin sentirse a gusto en ninguna de ellas.

---

[42] "Sobre el arte nuevo de escribir novelas", O. C., II, pp. 637 y s.

CAPÍTULO III

LOS GÉNEROS LITERARIOS

¡ "COSAS DE VALERA" !

La dureza de los juicios críticos de Clarín era tradicional, como lo era la benevolencia de los de don Juan. Para todos los autores —salvo raras excepciones— las conclusiones del profesor de Oviedo no eran sino una sarta de varapalos que, con frase de Valera, "levantaban túrdigas de piel a quienes los recibían". Especialmente en sus publicaciones *Solos de Clarín* y *Paliques.*

Sin embargo, ni uno sólo de los críticos del siglo XIX —y casi podríamos asegurar que ninguno de los posteriores— llegó a alabarle tan sin reservas, tan de buena intención, y a calar tan hondo en las bellezas de Valera, como lo hizo él para otros terrible y temido Clarín.

Admirador de buena fe, poniéndole los reparos —breves, sinceros, justos— que a él se le alcanzaban, desde los primeros artículos que le dedica, confiesa Clarín que don Juan es, en su tiempo, "el primer literato español". Y resulta un tantico extraño —en pluma tan impregnada de acidez como era la de Leopoldo Alas— no encontrar una muestra de ironía o dureza a la hora de juzgar las producciones valerinas. Por el contrario, vemos en él mucho cariño, frases de aliento para consolar a don Juan del poco aprecio que el público y un sector de la crítica oficial demostraban ante la aparición de sus últimas obras; palabras en las que encontramos no alabanzas exageradas, sino acotaciones inteligentes. No un incensar continuo y ridículo, como por desgracia era de costumbre entre críticos y escritores amigos. En cuantos artículos le dedicó —varios y de no escasa importancia— se trasluce una admiración sincera y un profundo respeto por parte de Alas.

Conviene que nos detengamos unos instantes, no a comparar las dos tareas críticas —por el momento—, sino para dejar bien sentado que la frase "¡cosas de Valera!" que el ingenio del crítico de Oviedo inventara con la mejor buena fe, no nació con ánimo de causar el menor daño a don Juan ni con intención de reproche, sino más bien de todo lo contrario.

Críticos de "suavidad" más reconocida que la de Clarín, pero también con más incapacidad que aquél para ver en el fondo verdadero de las cosas, críticos como Armando Palacio Valdés o doña Emilia Pardo Bazán, se aprovecharon de la sin duda ingeniosa y (en boca de Clarín) verdadera frase, para rebajar aquel mérito que, a decir verdad, ni una ni otro descubrían. Porque ambos estaban muy lejos de las delicadezas y la finura intelectual que requerían aquellas "cosas de Valera"; de aquello que para Clarín tenía el mérito innegable de ser el fruto de un talento privilegiado.

Doña Emilia por enemistad de partido, principalmente, y don Armando porque "habiendo dado las novelas de Valera a leer a su novia las encontró aburridas"[1]. Humorística razón que, si carece de consistencia, le evitaba más profundas explicaciones.

Lo cierto fue que la frase de Clarín, originalmente una alabanza, se convirtió con el tiempo en motivo de desengaño para Valera, si no de disgusto. Claro que las palabras del mismo Clarín en un

---

[1] A. Palacio Valdés, "Novelistas españoles: Valera", en *Revista Europea*, Madrid, abril-mayo, 1878, p. 523.

artículo de fecha anterior, dedicado a comentar la segunda edición
de las poesías de don Juan, servirían de explicación para comprender esa incapacidad en una España "donde los más claros ingenios
de ahora son ignorantes en grado inverosímil" [2].

No le parece mal a Clarín el que don Juan pinte "cien frailes,
cien toreros, que en el fondo no sean más que otros tantos Valeras.
¿Qué importa? Mejor" [3]. Porque a Clarín crítico, en los personajes
de don Juan, se le aparecen las bellezas del alma de su autor, mientras que al lector superficial —¡la novia de Palacio Valdés!— se le
escapan matices hermosos, colores delicadísimos que hacen muy diferentes, aunque sean homogéneos, los personajes de una familia en
la cual todos los hijos llevan como impreso el sello familiar.

Nació la expresión, tantas veces ya citada, en el artículo de *Solos*
dedicado a revisar las *Tentativas dramáticas* de Valera. Encabezando dichas tentativas iba una carta prólogo del autor en donde se
disculpa de no ser autor dramático, pese a sus mejores intenciones.
A don Juan le zumbaban aún en los oídos las poco amables indirectas que de unos y otros habían logrado sus últimas novelas y se
cura en salud anunciando que lo que esta vez daba al público no
eran "dramas en el más estricto sentido de la palabra". Se quedaban en meras "tentativas".

Gustaron, con todo, a Clarín, quien, después de alabarlas sin
escatimar los méritos, termina diciendo: "Podrán no ser dramas,
pero son joyas literarias. ¿Cómo las llamaremos? Ustedes dirán. Yo,
entretanto, las llamo 'cosas de Valera'" [4].

Clarín, el crítico que había visto con agudeza certera que en
Las ilusiones del doctor Faustino hay "un género de gracia que no
se había visto en España después del Quijote, y el público no lo

---

[2] Leopoldo Alas, *Obras Selectas*, Biblioteca Nueva, Madrid, 1947, página 523.

[3] *Ibidem.*

[4] L. Alas, Clarín, *Solos de Clarín*, IV, Fernando Fe, Madrid, 1891, página 326.

había notado" [5], no tenía mala intención al escribir tales palabras. Porque para él, como para cualquier lector objetivo de la obra de Valera, lo primero que salta a la vista es el autor, ya sea aquélla un ensayo crítico, una carta de burlas o veras, o un capítulo de novela.

Valera había visto como nadie que en la inmortal obra de Cervantes lo más hermoso que podía encontrarse era el alma del autor, derramándose en páginas que nos hablan de las andanzas y desventuras de un personaje loco y un escudero rústico. Precisamente la originalidad de tales personajes no descansaba en ellos mismos, sino en la gracia con que, sobre ellos, iba depositándose la hermosura del alma de Cervantes. Sí. Se descubría al Cervantes burlón tras la socarronería de Sancho, al igual que Cervantes el bueno se retrataba en la grandeza de alma de don Alonso Quijano. Mas aquello poca importancia tenía. ¿Restaba ello valor alguno a la inmortal obra, o acaso el lector dejaba de disfrutar por tales causas con la lectura de las peregrinas aventuras del caballero de la Mancha?

Tal era, pues, el punto de vista de Valera. Nunca se le ocultó que toda su obra rezumaba autobiografía. Nada hizo para que no fuera así. No se proponía tampoco encasillar todos sus escritos en un determinado género literario. Don Juan Valera —y volvemos a tomar el hilo que abandonamos al escribir el título del presente apartado tras un rodeo que se nos antojaba necesario— no tenía ningún inconveniente en que le motejaran de "demasiado personales", "poco ortodoxos", o incluso de "inclasificables", los géneros que él cultivaba indiferentemente. Porque —digámoslo ya— lo que el artista buscaba no era la novela, el poema, o el drama en sí mismos, sino la belleza que podía obtenerse por medio de la palabra, bajo cualquiera de sus formas poéticas.

¿Drama, novela, cuento, poema...? Todo ello no es, en su opinión, más que la misma y eterna especie: poesía. Poesía que reviste formas que difieren levemente, mas en lo sustancial son idénticas;

---

[5] *Ibidem.*

que se separan en cuanto al ropaje exterior con que las reviste el artista, pero que tienen siempre el mismo y único objetivo: creación de la belleza literaria.

De aquí lo poco ortodoxo del cultivo de los géneros en Valera. Lo que don Juan pretendía —ya fuera teóricamente, cuando hacía crítica, como en la práctica, cuando escribía novelas o cuentos— no era enseñar nada. Quería simplemente divertir, intentando crear belleza para unos pocos lectores "que tienen el buen o mal gusto de entretenerse leyendo las novelas y los cuentos que escribimos" [6].

El autor está en cuanto escribe. Podrá a lo sumo disimularse (y don Juan se disimulaba mal porque no se tomaba la molestia de esconderse tras sus personajes), pero "es falso que el autor se eclipse. Su personalidad informa siempre el libro que escribe... se infunde en la obra de cada autor aunque él no lo pretenda, aunque no lo quiera, aunque procure evitarlo" [7].

Es posible que don Juan, tras los ataques que le dirigiera parte de la crítica por "ponerse demasiado" en su don Juan Fresco, el Comendador o el Doctor Faustino, tratara de "eclipsarse" al máximo en las obras que siguieron. Y nótese que hemos dicho "eclipsarse", no desaparecer, cosa imposible para él, dados sus principios; esconderse detrás de sus criaturas; pero muy pronto debió abandonar tales propósitos. Prefirió alzarse contra la opinión común. Ir contra el precepto naturalista que propugnaba la objetividad absoluta en la narración, copiando fielmente de la realidad, lo cual parecía a Valera "una monstruosidad" siempre que la realidad no sea hermosísima, como no suele serlo en la mayoría de los casos. Prefirió seguir fiel a su principio de que "en todo escrito está el alma del que lo hiciera".

---

6   O. C., II, p. 947. La misma idea puede encontrarse en muchos otros artículos de Valera, por ejemplo en O. C., III, p. 690 y en el *Epistolario Valera-Menéndez Pelayo*, ed. citada, p. 373.

7   "Sobre el nuevo arte de escribir novelas", O. C., II, p. 690.

Si el autor "está" en cuanto escribe —deduce Valera— lo menos importante será el apartado especial en que coloque sus obras, la forma material de su creación. Esa forma que no consistía, según él, en "este o aquél pensamiento" ni en "tal descripción o sentencia" o frases "de que tal vez otros autores se han servido". La forma, en resumen, no es sino "el alma del poeta que pasa a su obra y vive allí como encantada" [8].

Tal es la única forma esencial que a don Juan le preocupaba. La otra, la externa (pese a que alguna vez, obligado a ello por el giro especial de la polémica, se vio obligado a separar forma de fondo, como ya se dijo) apenas tenía importancia. El artista deberá cuidarla en tanto en cuanto ella es la representación sensible de su pensamiento. Mas no es un cuido externo puramente el que requiere, de adorno y de afeites más o menos artificiales, sino una perfecta disposición interna, cuidando de que la expresión sea siempre "pura y transparente". Porque "ningún pensamiento bello será comunicado al lector si no está bien expresado" [9].

VALERA Y LA
POESÍA LÍRICA

De todos los géneros literarios, o apartados en que pueda subdividirse el arte de la palabra, como quería don Juan, es la poesía lírica el que exige un más delicado cultivo de lo que tradicionalmente se entiende por "forma".

Para Valera poesía lírica es sinónimo de pureza de idea y de aspecto formal: "siendo sincera, como debe de ser para ser buena, es autobiografía del corazón y de la mente: es exhibir el alma al público en su desnudez" [10].

---

[8] "Sobre los discursos académicos de Segovia y Cañete", O. C., II, página 137.

[9] "Filosofía del Arte", O. C., III, p. 1451.

[10] "El Parnaso Colombiano", O. C., III, p. 275.

Y exhibir el alma propia, sin otro pretexto que el de sus propios valores, le parece a Valera lícito, siempre que se exhiba con mérito auténtico y hermosura de forma.

Lo que don Juan no admite son las libertades —libertinajes, decía él— de metro y rima, y a veces hasta de tema, con que hacían poesía las nuevas escuelas, que se apartaban irrespetuosamente de la norma tradicional. Prefirió negar tozudamente todo valor a semejante poesía, cerrando sus ojos a ella con manifiesta injusticia. Sin hacer el menor esfuerzo por comprender que cabe el mismo grado de honradez de expresión en el artista que se atenía a las normas clásicas como en el que deliberadamente las abandona en busca de nuevos horizontes.

La forma —piensa don Juan— es el todo en poesía (en poesía lírica, naturalmente). Imaginarse una poesía sin forma bella sería algo así como el ver a una mujer "hermosa de cuerpo que, si no se viste con aseo y con primor, empaña y turba la natural hermosura" [11]. Es el vestido, en la mujer hermosa, el encargado de realzar sus encantos naturales. Si el poeta en prosa —dramaturgo o novelista— puede descuidar hasta cierto punto el aspecto externo, es porque en su menester u oficio entran por mucho "la pintura briosa de los caracteres o la fecundidad ingeniosa de los argumentos o enredos" [12] de cuanto escribe. Mas el poeta lírico debe exponer, ante todo, su propia alma. Esa hermosura interior que se hace patente sólo mediante la perfección de la forma; por la belleza del ropaje, como si dijéramos [13].

No se percata Valera del sofisma en que cae partiendo de la falsa premisa de que sólo la forma clásica es valedera para el logro de la belleza. Es tan ingenuo como asegurar que no hay más ves-

---

11 "Obras poéticas", O. C., II, p. 103. Semejantes afirmaciones abundan en otros muchos artículos.

12 Vid. O. C., II, p. 512.

13 "Sobre los discursos de Cañete y Segovia", O. C., II, p. 137. Valera repitió tales conceptos en muchas otras ocasiones.

tidos hermosos —para emplear su metáfora— que los de la antigüedad clásica, vueltos a poner en uso con mucha fortuna por los autores del Renacimiento. Se empeñó don Juan tercamente en negar la belleza de "nuevo corte". Prefiere las togas y clámides de la antigüedad, antes que los vestidos de Worth y otros sastres elegantes a los que tantas veces cita.

Las libertades románticas, como las "modas naturalistas" y las extrañas nuevas formas que parnasianos, modernistas y simbolistas estaban llevando al campo poético, parecían a don Juan no solamente verdaderos crímenes de lesa poesía, sino adornos de muy mal gusto. Un amante reconocido del progreso, como él decía ser, liberal de pensamiento (aunque conservador de la *old fashion,* para decirlo en inglés, como él gustaba decir) no pudo ser más retrógrado en lo que se refiere a "nuevas formas poéticas".

Y es una verdadera lástima —justo es reconocerlo— que por su intransigente postura nos privase de crítica y consejos que hubieran sido de un valor incalculable. No porque hubieran podido adelantar el brillante momento de la poesía que comenzaba a florecer ante sus cerrados ojos (desgraciadamente en los dos sentidos de la frase), sino porque, de haber sido más comprensivo —¡él que lo fue tanto en otras ocasiones!—, hubiera ayudado a escardar el haza de nuestras letras de cuanto no eran flores de superior belleza.

Con su aplauso a las viejas formas y su menosprecio de las nuevas, es cierto que no llegó a segar en flor las creaciones de mérito de muchos jóvenes escritores del último cuarto del siglo XIX, pues tuvo el suficiente talento como para guardar un prudente silencio ante las obras que no le gustaban, como se verá al analizar las críticas de los primeros escritos de quienes iban a formar "la generación del noventayocho"; mas, con su actitud, don Juan contribuyó a mantener aquella medianía general de los poetas que preceden cronológicamente al grupo mencionado.

Digamos en descargo de Valera que no era (el aplaudir de preferencia las viejas formas tradicionales) un mal que solamente le

aquejaba a él. Los otros dos grandes críticos del xix, don Marcelino Menéndez Pelayo y Leopoldo Alas, Clarín, no anduvieron mucho más afortunados al juzgar a varios de los poetas contemporáneos. Ambos alabaron, entusiásticamente en algunos casos, producciones que, pocos años después, quedarían como valores puramente
arqueológicos, o poco más. Ambos también dejaron escapar bellezas
verdaderamente nuevas, si no por los mismos prejuicios que mer-
maban la capacidad crítica de Valera, por otras razones que les impedían ver con ojos diferentes. Las alabanzas que dedicaron a
Núñez de Arce, Grilo o Campoamor son muy superiores a las que
dedican —cuando lo hacen— a Bécquer y Rubén, por no citar nombres más modernos. (Suele olvidarse con frecuencia que la mayoría
de los autores del 98 habían publicado no poco al comenzar nuestro siglo, y que la "nueva crítica" que la poesía, especialmente, ha
logrado en nuestros días nació al mismo tiempo que la nueva lírica.)
El mismo sentido crítico del poeta, que hizo abrir nuevos horizontes para la poesía, fue el que hizo surgir una crítica distinta de la
tradicional, abandonando en ambos casos fórmulas y formas ca-
ducas.

Quizá el haber visto claramente que la lengua española —como
la italiana— se presta más que las lenguas de origen germánico a
la vana palabrería, al sonsonete [14], es lo que hiciera ser a Valera
más cauto, más receloso de lo nuevo. Había hecho traducciones del
alemán y del inglés, y ante la concisión, la forzada estructura sin-
táctica de ambas lenguas, las de origen latino le parecían, si más
ricas en posibilidades, también mucho más peligrosamente inclina-
das —por su riqueza— a degenerar en cataratas de fácil musicalidad.

Por otro lado, no debe olvidarse que don Juan no llegó a descubrir —ni mucho menos a disfrutar con ellas— las bellezas retó-
ricas de Góngora y Quevedo, mientras por el contrario se entusias-

---

[14]   Vid. "Rimas de W. Querol", O. C., II, p. 517.

maba con la "sin igual pureza de lengua de un Garcilaso o un Fray Luis".

No sólo cuando escribe para el público, sino también cuando lo hace en privado, en una de sus cartas a su amigo Campillo, vuelve a exponer su punto de vista personal con toda claridad: "Sin metro y sin lenguaje poético no hay poesía, o bien la poesía es un empalagoso delirio" [15].

Llama luego nada menos que "nauseabunda" a la prosa lírica (a esa delicada prosa que iba a producir muy pocos años más tarde las *Sonatas,* los inimitables paseos de Sigüenza o las deliciosas y tiernas andanzas de Platero, el burrito juan-ramoniano).

Era la primera prosa modernista, la de Rubén Darío y Salvador Rueda, la que don Juan menospreciaba. (Haciéndolo, claro está, muy "valerinamente": de costado, sin atreverse a citar nombres.)

Y termina: "por lo mismo que mucha poesía, como novelas, comedias y cuentos, se escribe hoy en prosa, lo que se escribe en verso debe ser más *primoroso,* más *atildado,* más *sublime* y más *limpio* que nunca", añadiendo en un arrebato de cólera, rarísimo en hombre de tan comedidos modales: "Así que los versos ramplones que hoy se usan, me revientan sobremanera" [16].

Obsérvense los adjetivos que hemos subrayado: primoroso, atildado, sublime y limpio. Tales tenían que ser los versos que a don Juan le parecían el colmo de la posible hermosura. Así puede que sean los suyos; primorosos y atildados en grado sumo. Pero fríos.

NOVELA SIN LÍMITES

Para don Juan, en verso se puede no decir nada y encantar al auditorio, aunque lo que se haga esté muy lejos de la auténtica

---

[15] Carta de 1887 a Narciso Campillo, *Revista de Archivos, Bibliotecas y Museos,* 1926, T. III, p. 434.

[16] Carta citada.

poesía. Basta para lograr ese éxito fácil "habilidad de hallar consonantes difíciles y de hacer versos sonoros y rotundos". En cambio, para la prosa el quehacer no es tan sencillo: "El escribir en prosa, aunque sea mala y vulgar, requiere otros preparativos, exige que se diga algo, aunque sea insulso" [17].

Si bien se nos antoja que hay no poca ironía en ambas afirmaciones, era cierto lo que decía a Campillo: escribir en prosa, para don Juan, tiene más exigencia de fondo, de argumento o enredo. Lo importante es decir, contar cosas de interés, sea cualquiera el género que el escritor adopte dentro de la prosa. Y, como siempre, don Juan predicó con el ejemplo: en muchas de sus obras las barreras que separan algunos géneros o no existen (novela-cuento, cuento-novela) o si existen (drama-diálogo moralizador) se interpenetran con suma facilidad. Incluso en el género epistolar, en sus deliciosas cartas privadas a la familia y a los amigos, abandonará, en ciertos casos, las formas tradicionales para convertirlas en ingeniosísimos artículos críticos o esbozos de ensayo, cuando no verdaderos ensayos en el moderno sentido de la palabra.

Se sorprendió a sí mismo como novelista cuando intentaba hacer, en su ánimo de apoyar a la escuela krausista, un ensayo filosófico literario en forma epistolar. Nada más lejos de su imaginación —nos dice el propio autor— que el intento de escribir una novela, si aceptamos las palabras que puso como prólogo a la edición en lengua inglesa de su más famosa novela.

En dicho prólogo, Valera nos da la razón en cuanto llevamos dicho hasta aquí a este respecto: llama novela a su obra seis veces. En tres ocasiones más se refiere a ella llamándola cuento. Si esto hizo en un prólogo de poco más de seis páginas, no deberá extrañar el que, a lo largo de su obra completa, encontremos muchas veces más la confusión o, para ser más exactos, la indiferenciación entre ambos géneros.

---

[17] "Poetas líricos españoles del siglo XVIII", O. C., II, p. 391.

Desde sus escritos primeros siente una tendencia a llamar cuento "a todo lo que se cuenta", a toda narración, sea cualquiera el medio empleado, prosa o verso; así, casi siempre que se refiere a su traducción de la leyenda oriental "El paraíso y la Peri", de Thomas Moore, hecha en 1846, la llama "cuento en verso"[18] o simplemente "cuento"[19], lo mismo que otras traducciones en verso, tales como el episodio del Mahabárata que tituló "Santa", el poema del poeta americano James Russell Lowell "Las hojas que cantan", etc. El estar escritas en verso no es inconveniente para que las llame "cuentos"; en ellas "se cuenta algo", y esto es lo importante.

Si con tanta facilidad hace caso omiso de los límites que hay entre verso y prosa, vamos a ver en seguida cómo los que existen entre otros géneros (especialmente entre cuento y novela) desaparecen para nuestro autor a medida que la necesidad, o las prisas en alguna ocasión, le empujen a ello.

No nos parece que Valera rompa tales fronteras —dejémoslo bien sentado aquí— porque ello le conviniera para su modo de escribir. No. No fija tales límites porque con su personal concepto del campo literario ni podía ni quería verlos. No rompe: cultiva sus campos sin los linderos a que estamos habituados. Verso y prosa, narración o diálogo se confundirán en Valera a la hora de separar.

Veamos uno de los múltiples ejemplos que se pueden espigar. Escribe a don Juan Moreno Güeto, desde Madrid, el 14 de diciembre de 1847. Y entre otras cosas le comunica estar escribiendo "Garuda o la cigüeña blanca":

"Ahora estoy escribiendo otra *novelita* que me parece mejor [había hablado de otro cuento suyo, "El cautivo de doña Mencía"] y de la que estoy bastante contento. Pasa la acción en Viena y en

---

[18] Cuatro veces en carta a su padre de 16-I-1847, Vid. O. C., III, página 14.

[19] Vid. *Epistolario Valera-Menéndez Pelayo*, carta de 21-I-1878, página 21.

los Estados Unidos, aunque al fin no he podido resistir el amor de
la patria, y mi ciudad natal, Cabra, figura también en la *novela*...
Yo espero que el nuevo *cuento* mío que está en el telar y que se
titula 'Garuda...' " [20].

Primero la llama novelita, lo que sería sinónimo de novela
corta; más tarde la llama novela, y por último cuento. En cita de
tan pocas líneas encontramos tres calificaciones que, en otro autor,
dejarían al lector un tanto confuso, sin saber muy exactamente de
qué se trataba. Claro que la confusión no se disiparía luego de
haber leído la obra, pues responde perfectamente a esa especie de
novela condensada que son casi todos los cuentos de Valera, al igual
que —por otra parte— algunas de sus novelas pudieran ser clasifi-
cadas como cuentos largos.

La indiferenciación poema-cuento-novela no es cosa pasajera, de
una época determinada. Se da a lo largo de toda su obra, como
hemos dicho. La actitud de Valera —como en tantas otras materias— es de una constancia que causa asombro.

En la indiferenciación leyenda en verso-cuento cabría pensar que
la motivó un cierto influjo romántico, pues la equiparación era frecuente entre autores a quienes don Juan alcanzó a conocer cuando
era muy joven; pero la otra confusión, novela-cuento, es cosa más
personal.

De todos es sabido que don Juan, muchos años antes de soñar
con ser novelista (cosa que en el fondo le parecía un arte menor
si comparaba la poesía lírica, para él "arte por excelencia", con la
novela, especie de arte de segunda categoría), antes, repetimos, de
ponerse a pensar sus propias novelas, había teorizado suficientemente sobre el género en un largo ensayo titulado *Naturaleza y carácter de la novela,* publicado en 1860. (Su primera y más famosa
novela vio la luz en 1874.)

---

[20]   *Correspondencia de don Juan Valera,* edit. por Cyrus C. de Coster,
Castalia, 1959, pág. 257.

Teorías que —inmutables en sustancia— fue ampliando en multitud de artículos íntegra o parcialmente a ello dedicados; los más importantes fueron: el famoso libro *Nuevo arte de escribir novelas,* escrito en contra de las teorías de doña Emilia Pardo Bazán [21]; un largo artículo en el que glosa el comentario que la *Revista de Edimburgo* dedicó a las novelas de Fernán Caballero [22]; una carta a doña Emilia sobre las novelas rusas [23]; otro artículo sobre "La novela de nuestros días" (1897) [24] y los dos discursos académicos en contestación a los de Jacinto Octavio Picón y José Ortega Munilla [25]. Aparte, claro está, de las innumerables ocasiones en que, de pasada, vuelve a repetir afirmaciones parciales que antes hubiera expuesto con todo detalle. Y no deberán olvidarse, por lo que de interesantes puntos de vista de autor-crítico tienen, los prólogos con que solía presentar sus propias novelas o cuentos, o las innumerables cartas en que de novelas y cuentos trata.

A estos últimos también les dedicó buena cantidad de escritos. De los más destacables —por no hacer esta relación fatigosa— son: el artículo escrito para el *Diccionario Enciclopédico* de Montaner y Simón (1890) bajo el epígrafe "Cuento"; el prólogo que precede a la citada colección de *Cuentos y chascarrillos andaluces,* escrito en 1896, y el prólogo a su traducción de *Las pastorales,* de Longo, *Dafnis y Cloe,* en su versión (Madrid, 1880).

Apoyándonos en tan abundante material, trataremos de llegar a esas definiciones de las que don Juan siempre se mostró tan enemigo. (Definir era poner límites, y para él ninguno de los dos géneros que vamos a estudiar ahora los tenía.)

Separemos, por el momento, ambos conceptos. Preguntémonos en primer lugar cuanto se refiere a la novela.

---

[21] O. C., II, pp. 622-710.
[22] O. C., II, pp. 232-236.
[23] O. C., II, pp. 715-723.
[24] O. C., II, pp. 933-936.
[25] O. C., II, pp. 1197-1217.

Con una calificación más que vaga, la llama "poesía libre de metro", con la pos.bilidad de ocuparse de temas menos encumbrados que los que generalmente toca la "poesía propiamente dicha". Es un género tan sin límites que todo cabe en él, siempre que sea historia fingida. La novela admite dentro de sí todo lo extraordinario, lo ideal, lo peregrino. De aquí proviene el adjetivo "novelesco", lo que no sucede comúnmente [26].

Advirtamos que el artículo [27] de donde tomamos los anteriores puntos es el destinado a impugnar las teorías de Cándido Nocedal, el cual, valiéndose de la definición que la Academia daba de la novela, quiso limitar el campo de tal género. Va don Juan contra las ideas de Nocedal, por lo que no tendrá inconveniente —con tal de rebatirlas— en dejarse llegar a extremos de los que retornará más tarde por sí mismo, cuando no se le argumente con las mismas razones de Nocedal.

Cuando disputa con doña Emilia Pardo Bazán y las teorías naturalistas (que pretendían nada menos que fijar los modelos, trazar, como si dijéramos, el patrón por el que habían de cortarse las novelas del futuro) reduce, para que sus terrenos de campaña no resulten absurdamente grandes al lado de los de doña Emilia, la extensión que tan generosamente le había asignado.

Señala a la novela como: "espejo de la vida y representación artística de la sociedad toda" [28].

La novela debe representar "los actos y las pasiones de los hombres". Mas no limitarse a contar lo cotidiano, "lo que comúnmente sucede", por lo general muy prosaico. El autor que tal hiciera se limitaría a hacer historia "baja y rastrera". Y la ventaja del arte sobre la historia estriba en que ésta cuenta las cosas como son,

---

[26] "De la naturaleza y carácter de la novela", O. C., II, pp. 189 y 193.
[27] *Ibidem.*
[28] "Arte nuevo de escribir novelas", O. C., II, p. 671.

mientras el arte las pinta "como debieran ser". La historia narra hechos. La poesía debe pintar ideales [29].

El primer y más noble objetivo que el novelista debe trazarse es el de escribir un libro con el cual divierta, dé solaz a los lectores. Antes que nada, divertir, repite incansablemente en casi todos sus artículos. El novelista que no divierte pierde lastimosamente el tiempo. Contar sucesos de la vida cotidiana no es tarea ni artística ni entretenida. Valen más las aventuras ficticias —pero artísticamente verosímiles— del manchego desequilibrado de Cervantes, que todas las miserias y mediocridades que se nos cuentan con todo lujo de detalles en las novelas de Zola y sus seguidores, por muy realistas que ellas sean.

El lector de una buena novela deberá elevar su espíritu con su lectura, no entristecerse con ella, perturbarse o deprimirse. Y esto era, más o menos, lo que parecía a don Juan que buscaban los naturalistas con sus principios y reglas para "copiar la realidad". (Adviértase cómo se encierra don Juan en otro sofisma que le va a impedir ver la realidad clara del asunto: pide al arte, especialmente, que divierta, que deleite y que alegre. Y esto no se consigue más que con fábulas alegres o sanas de espíritu. Como los naturalistas utilizan materiales poco nobles, materias que no eran ni alegres ni sanas, según su personal criterio, los naturalistas no pueden hacer arte, concluye tercamente.)

No le hizo falta leer mucha novela naturalista para saber que no podían gustarle y para negarles toda posibilidad artística. Fue otra de sus ideas *a priori*. Diversión, deleite y alegría eran solamente posibles de un modo: el suyo. No se percataba de que, proscribiendo de la novela "los materiales" que utilizaban los autores naturalistas, también limitaba, "ponía barreras", cosa que tanto afeaba en los otros.

---

[29] "Naturaleza y carácter de la novela", O. C., II, pp. 188-201.

Conocía muy bien las teorías literarias más de moda en Francia (sabemos que leía regularmente la *Revue des Deux Mondes,* en la que Brunetière y Bigot habían publicado los artículos dedicados a estudiar los orígenes de la estética naturalista). Mas prefería divertirse y tomar partido leyendo tales teorías en lugar de leer las obras que le ponían de mal humor. Cuando Valera impugna aquellas obras que él mismo confiesa no haber leído, Clarín le recordará su falta de experiencia práctica en la materia. Y sólo entonces, sin negar la veracidad de cuanto decía Clarín, se pondrá a remediar la falta, leyendo lo que le parecía insufrible de leer: unas pocas novelas de Zola y de los hermanos Goncourt. Obras que —nos dice— se le caen literalmente de las manos y que sólo mediante un acto de voluntad logrará terminar.

Vemos ya claramente que don Juan no iba contra "los frutos naturalistas", las novelas, sino contra las mismas teorías. Afortunadamente podemos seguir el proceso de creación de los artículos que componen el libro *Nuevo arte de escribir novelas* leyendo las cartas que desde Bélgica escribe don Juan a don Marcelino Menéndez Pelayo. En ellas cuenta a su amigo cómo leyendo *El Naturalismo* de doña Emilia Pardo Bazán "su lectura me ha excitado. Estoy escribiendo otro libro también de naturalismo". Le dice que su intención no es otra que "combatir la barbarie", ir no contra lo obsceno, "sino contra lo irreligioso, lo horrible, lo pesimista, lo calumniador del linaje humano y de la naturaleza que hay en el Naturalismo" [30].

Años más tarde (las cartas fueron escritas entre el 2 de agosto de 1886 y julio de 1887) volverá a decirnos en sus *Nuevas cartas americanas* (1891) "... ataqué eso que llaman el naturalismo, el cual venía de mano armada contra nosotros a desacreditar nuestro gusto, a poner fuera de moda nuestros escritos y a relegarnos al olvido más hondo" [31].

---

[30] Vid. *Epistolario de Valera y Menéndez Pelayo,* pp. 284 y 392.
[31] Correspondencia, "Nuevas cartas americanas", O. C., III, p. 420.

Pero volvamos otra vez a sus teorías: Si es cierto, admite, que para lograr la creación de la belleza por medio de la palabra escrita hay que tomar como modelo la realidad de las cosas así naturales como artificiales, no es menos cierto que se puede copiar embelleciendo, no pintando lo triste o lo sucio por puro deleite. Hay una considerable diferencia entre el conocimiento indispensable para la imitación artística y el conocimiento "fatigoso y científico" que los paladines de las nuevas teorías pedían. Para los experimentos, para el logro científico, están los laboratorios, los libros y revistas de investigación, no la novela.

Asignar el papel de auxiliar de la ciencia al arte del entretenimiento le parece empresa descabellada al autor de *Pepita Jiménez:* "La novela es un campo por donde se echa a volar la fantasía. ¿Quién ha de poner puertas o límites a este campo?" [32].

Tal plan le parecía absurdo a Valera. Los naturalistas querían delimitar, fijar estrechos límites a un género artístico en el que no cabía más *non plus ultra* que el del buen sentido. Valera es el apóstol de la total libertad frente a lo que él llamaba "las estrecheces realistas": "Una novela puede ser todo lo disparatada que se quiera (en este punto tengo yo la manga muy ancha) con tal de que el disparate sea ingenioso" [33].

Si el autor es capaz de hacernos creer que un hombre puede, por sus propios medios naturales, llegar a surcar los aires, y gracias al estilo y buen arte del narrador nos trasladamos a regiones en donde tal hecho no sea absurdo, entonces tal autor logra lo que don Juan llama "verosimilitud artística": no lo realmente verdadero, sino lo que es artísticamente verosímil. Es la fe del lector —continúa— conquistada por la gracia del escritor "como lo fuera la de los cristianos que lucharon en el Clavijo cuando vieron ante sus ojos al Apóstol Santiago segando cabezas de infieles" para darles ánimos:

---

[32] "Terapéutica social y novela profética", O. C., II, p. 1127.
[33] O. C., II, p. 1127.

"En el mundo de la fantasía, que es el mundo de la novela, debemos admitir no ya como verosímiles, sino como verdaderos, todos los legítimos engendros de la fantasía" [34].

Basta para ello que la varita mágica de la mente creadora, el estilo del novelista, sea capaz de llevarnos a regiones donde lo estéticamente verosímil sea posible. El hecho de que deforme la realidad para conseguir belleza no es —en sí mismo— pecado de estética. El artista no está obligado a rendir culto a la verdad, a supeditar su oficio a la "verosimilitud real".

El ejemplo de novela perfecta para Valera es el *Quijote*. Y no quiso descubrir en el inmortal libro otros fines que los de entretener y divertir a los lectores, no con verdades científicas o enseñanzas profundas, sino con las peregrinas andanzas de dos personajes que encarnan el espíritu del autor que les dio vida. Cuando en diferentes ocasiones alguien creyó encontrar verdades esotéricas en la genial obra cervantina, protesta don Juan indignado diciendo que las tales verdades más estaban en la imaginación de quienes creían descubrirlas que en la intención de quien lo escribió.

El *Quijote*, como *Dafnis y Cloe* —ejemplo también, diferente, de "novela libre"—, son obras en las que las imaginaciones creadoras anduvieron "más libres que el aire", sin atenerse a más normas, preceptos o reglas que las que dictaba el buen sentido; y las calidades artísticas están patentes en ambas. Sus autores no buscaron sino el entretenimiento propio y el de sus lectores. Pero la verdad artística reside en ambas obras con tanta fuerza que las hace brillar incomparablemente a lo largo de los siglos.

En cuanto a los personajes, el hecho de escogerlos seres vulgares u obscenos, como proclamaba con el ejemplo la escuela naturalista, ponía un serio freno a las posibilidades del autor. Para Valera valía más, artísticamente hablando, el indómito bandido de la serranía que hacía su voluntad más completa, que el pobre minero

---

[34] "Naturaleza y carácter de la novela", O. C., II, p. 191.

que no tenía otro remedio sino acatar la de casi toda la sociedad. Exponiéndonos este punto de vista, grabó una de las frases más verdaderas, graciosas y auténticamente valerinas: "Los contrabandistas son más poéticos y novelescos que los carabineros y que los vistas de aduanas" [35].

Lo que en ningún momento quiere decir que deban copiarse de la realidad misma esos personajes —contrabandistas—, que, si en teoría están cargados de posibilidades poéticas, en la realidad pueden ser de una vulgaridad y una rudeza antiartísticas. Su independencia, más el estilo y la gracia del autor, se conjugarán para el logro poético. Muy raramente los seres vivos tienen suficientes méritos o atractivos como para salir airosos en una aventura novelesca en la que se les pintase "al natural", sin adornos de la fantasía del autor.

Don Juan repetirá incansablemente, en artículos críticos, tanto al frente como al fin de sus novelas, que es mejor la mezcla de realidad y fantasía. Que hay que lograr un ser vivo que, sin ser copia exacta de la realidad, sea como la destilación de las cualidades más interesantes de otros; el fruto conseguido mediante acertados injertos será, a sus ojos, más hermoso que las mismas realidades de donde procedían:

"Nada me ha repugnado más toda mi vida que tomar exactamente de la realidad a mis seres novelescos. Lo que sí hago y no puedo menos de hacer para crearlos es tomar algo de acá y de allá, amasarlo y barajarlo todo y formar así un compuesto que a nada ni a nadie se parezca" [36].

Son los recuerdos vivos los que nutren esa especie de almacén necesario para que el autor de novelas pueda servirse cuando sienta la necesidad de hacerlo.

Sabemos que el episodio amoroso de su juventud, la aventura erótico-sentimental con la cantante Margarita Brohan, en Rusia,

---

[35] "De la nat. y carácter de la nov.", O. C., II, p. 194.
[36] *Correspondencia de Juan Valera*, ed. Coster, obra cit., p. 294.

sirvió al escritor para una de sus novelas, *Mariquita y Antonio,* desgraciadamente inconclusa, pero de la que se conserva la parte que nos interesa. En otra novela (*Genio y figura*) en la que se proponía demostrar que, pese a lo que asegura el conocido refrán español, el ser humano es más libre que el mismo aire para decidir su conducta en la vida, volverá a echar mano de sus recuerdos de juventud.

Muchos de los personajes valerinos están basados en seres vivos (don Juan tuvo que disculparse ante el don Juan Fresco real, de quien tomó poco más que el nombre). Se ha dicho que el sucedido de su más popular novela se dio en unos familiares del propio Valera [37]; el Doctor Faustino es la encarnación de una etapa de la "atolondrada juventud del autor"; el don Paco de *Juanita la Larga,* como el héroe del *Comendador Mendoza,* tienen algo más que unos pocos puntos comunes con el carácter de los años de madurez de don Juan.

Podemos concluir, pues, que Valera, en la práctica como en la teoría, es partidario de la mezcla de realidad con imaginación; no por el placer de mistificar, sino por embellecer, por engrandecer a sus personajes. Tenía Valera instintiva la facultad embellecedora; se pone a contarnos sus recuerdos y, sin el menor ánimo de engañar, los transforma para que adquieran mayor belleza. La memoria como almacén, la imaginación embelleciendo siempre la realidad, y el estilo —el hombre que quería Buffon— poniendo el encanto necesario para que los caracteres pintados resulten vivos a la vez que hermosos.

Hay que observar en el fondo mismo de la vida; saber ver en la naturaleza y desprenderse de lo accesorio. A veces una buena novela puede malograrse —en opinión de Valera— por la cantidad de datos acumulados, de hechos o descripciones innecesarias que

---

[37]   Manuel Azaña, *La invención del Quijote y otros ensayos,* Espasa Calpe, Madrid, 1934, p. 227.

interfieren y hasta ahogan el argumento principal. Conviene la descripción artística, no la minuciosidad fatigante. En esto se adelanta con mucho a los escritores de su tiempo; si no llega al paisaje impresionista no nos da el detallismo, a veces exasperante, de un Pereda, por ejemplo, que acaba por cansar, con tanta minucia acumulada para lograr mayor "realismo en la descripción". El paisaje de don Juan —el recuerdo del paisaje, más bien— no era el tradicional entre los escritores de su tiempo; su técnica (su incapacidad para hacer paisajes que no fueran los de su recuerdo) le separa grandemente del modo de hacer del realismo. No logra, es cierto, un paisaje noventayochista, pero podríamos decir que está más cerca de la interpretación que del paisaje van a darnos los del 98 que de la de sus coetáneos, si se exceptúan Galdós y Clarín.

Aconseja, para alcanzar originalidad, el estudio directo de la naturaleza así como los "usos y costumbres, los lances y sucesos de la vida..." en la naturaleza, en la tierra y en el mismo seno de la sociedad en que vivimos en vez de servirse de libros escritos en otros países. A mayor localismo más universalidad [38].

Recomienda la lectura de los grandes maestros de la literatura universal, pero no para remedarlos sin talento, sino para asimilarlos y escribir "con criterio propio y *castizo* y con imaginación libre, despojada y serena" [39].

No prohíbe la lectura de los autores europeos (la europeización de España, que pedirán los escritores del 98), antes la recomienda. Aconseja casticismo hondo (años antes de que Unamuno lo pidiera en sus ensayos) en todo cuanto se escriba para remediar los males que aquejaban a nuestra literatura. Lo que sí prohíbe es la imitación servil de la literatura francesa —de Zola especialmente—, que, según él, se dejaba sentir en las letras hispánicas.

Afirma el profesor Montesinos entre las conclusiones de su valiosa obra que "la mayor parte de las novelas de Valera son novelas

---

[38] Discursos Académicos: "La novela en España", O. C., II, p. 1204.
[39] "De la naturaleza y carácter de la novela", O. C., II, p. 641.

de amores" [40], demostrándolo con sagaces análisis. Para abundar en su afirmación, nos parece interesante entresacar un texto del propio Valera al que Montesinos no hace referencia y en donde encontramos nosotros la clave explicativa del por qué Valera fue sobre todo autor de "novelas de amores". Lo tomamos de su discurso académico de 1900 titulado "La novela en España":

"El amor, o dígase la unión afectuosa de la mujer y el hombre, es el principal y perpetuo asunto de toda narración deleitable; es fuente que jamás se agota y de donde cada cual saca algo diverso en colorido, sabor y perfume, según la amplitud y la forma del vaso en que recoge la bebida inspiradora" [41].

De tal fuente bebió Valera en repetidas ocasiones y nos ofreció, con mejor o peor fortuna, los frutos obtenidos.

Defendían los naturalistas el empleo de una lengua llana, sencilla, copiada también de la realidad. Don Juan, que conocía lo que de vulgar y falto de gracia puede haber en boca del pueblo, prefiere, como siempre, emplear la selección. No cabe duda que la mayor parte, por no decir todas, de las frases graciosas que don Ramón de la Cruz hace decir a sus majas y chisperos pudo haberlas dicho el pueblo. Pero qué cantidad de frases pedestres, mal sonantes o carentes de gracia no desecharía su talento de artista: "Desengáñese, doña Emilia: el lenguaje realmente natural sería inaguantable" [42].

Como inaguantables eran aquellas conversaciones que don Juan escuchaba de boca del pueblo cuando éste se empeñaba en limitar su expresión a los consabidos moldes de una mediocre vulgaridad. Hay que seleccionar con tino; "no se puede representar servilmente con la fatigosa pesadez que la realidad tiene a menudo". Es el talento artístico el que sabe, siendo fiel a la realidad, combinar con lo ideal. Desechar lo impertinente.

---

[40] J. F. Montesinos, obra citada, pág. 204.
[41] O. C., III, p. 1206.
[42] O. C., II, p. 641.

No es Valera, por cuanto llevamos dicho, enemigo de tomar del pueblo las expresiones castizas, la magnífica riqueza de la lengua popular. Don Serafín Estébanez Calderón le había bañado en las aguas de lo castizo, de lo más genuinamente español, tanto de nuestras letras como en el vivir de nuestro pueblo. (Nunca llegó don Juan, justo es decirlo, a la manía purista del autor de las *Escenas andaluzas*.) La amistad que mantuvo con El Solitario había brotado en los años alegres de Nápoles, duraría muchos más y sirvió siempre a Valera como de filtro purificador en su prosa. Don Serafín había adivinado muy temprano las posibilidades que para la prosa tenía el joven diplomático y le había vaticinado un triunfo en nuestras letras:

"... como llegará a ser un buen hablista castellano porque le hago saber yo, que soy buen arúspice para esta laya de acertijos. Usted ha de descollar en el condimento sazonado de nuestra sabrosísima lengua" [43].

La carta de Estébanez Calderón lleva fecha 16-IV-1851. Trece años más tarde, en el prólogo que don Juan puso a sus estudios críticos (primera selección), publicados en Madrid, reconocerá:

"Quien me bautizó en literatura, sumergiéndome hasta la coronilla en las aguas del Tajo y del Guadalquivir, quien me preparó sólida y macizamente para ser escritor castellano, en prosa y en verso, fue el famoso don Serafín Estébanez Calderón, cuyo ingenio, cuyo saber y cuya manera de sentir y expresar lo que siente son dechado, mapa y cifra del españolismo" [44].

Precisamente ensalzando y defendiendo con ardorosa pasión las *Escenas andaluzas,* obra que había sido muy criticada por estar escrita en "lenguaje anticuado, extraño y artificioso", dice Valera textualmente: "Es necesario escribir consultando a los autores antiguos y al pueblo que también conserva la hermosura y abundancia

---

[43] Apud M. Azaña, *Valera en Italia*, Páez, Madrid, 1929, p. 161.
[44] Prólogo a *Estudios críticos*, 1.ª ed., Madrid, 1864. (No reproducido en las Obras Completas.)

de la lengua" [45]. No copiando el habla popular con todos sus defectos, sino tomando de ella lo que tiene de hermoso, sencillo y naturalmente artístico.

Cuando doña Emilia Pardo Bazán le ataca diciendo que sus personajes más populares (Respetilla, Antoñona, Juanita, el Dientes, etcétera) hablan como él mismo, se defiende don Juan diciendo que tal vez sea aquello más disculpable que el tratar de "imitar de memoria el lenguaje diverso de cada individuo", como hacían los escritores realistas. No sólo no lograban reproducir artísticamente la lengua que imitaban, sino que producían unos modos de hablar falsos, a la vez que inartísticos.

No le parece a Valera precepto naturalista, sino de todos los tiempos y estéticas, el que cada personaje hable con el estilo que le es propio, el acomodado a su categoría social, educación y capacidad intelectual.

No es necesario alterar la ortografía para acercarse más a lo real, a la viciosa pronunciación de ciertas personas o regiones en donde se pronuncia incorrectamente el español. Ni Cervantes, ni Estébanez Calderón —ni él mismo— habían tenido necesidad de alterar la grafía de las palabras para dar un "trasunto ideal" del alma popular de Andalucía. Repite en varias ocasiones la anécdota del maestro de escuela andaluz que decía a sus alumnos: "Sordado se escribe con 'l' y caznero con 'r' ".

Ni la tal servil imitación da chiste al diálogo, ni lo hace más ameno o le imprime carácter. Y en este punto sí que fue maestro: copió artística, maravillosamente, en sus narraciones de ambiente andaluz, la gracia interna, la chispa y vivacidad del estilo de los andaluces sin tener que llegar al torpe recurso de alterar la ortografía. La riqueza, la vivacidad de las metáforas que emplean sus personajes más populares, las expresiones y dichos de muchos de ellos sí que son andaluces hasta los tuétanos.

---

45 "Escenas andaluzas", O. C., II, p. 49.

No se queda Valera en lo externo de la cuestión, en la forma de palabras y expresiones. Va más lejos; penetra en la entraña espiritual misma del habla de su pueblo. Sabe captar como nadie la mejor "gracia andaluza", porque su propia alma estaba adornada con lo mejor de ella. No toma lo que de chocarrero o burdo, lo que de mal gusto y patosería pueden tener ciertos "andaluces a ultranza" o quienes tratan de remedarlos, como los malos cómicos de sainete que "hablan andaluz".

Don Juan es andaluz de los selectos. Cala en las bellezas del habla de sus paisanos e instintivamente separa las fealdades o groserías que pueden dañar a su hermosa lengua. Lograr que todo escritor consiga idénticos resultados a los suyos es lo que no nos parece tan sencillo. Porque, repetimos, él estaba adornado de esa gracia verbal que muchos de los escritores de su tiempo no poseían; Pereda, Palacio Valdés, la misma doña Emilia, muchas veces, al tratar de escribir "lengua popular", se quedan en la copia de la realidad más externa. Pocas veces llegan —cuando lo consiguen— a la profundidad de la imitación artística (a la creación, por mejor decir) a que llegara don Juan.

NOVELA-CUENTO, CUENTO-NOVELA

Si muy difícil resultó a don Juan trazar los límites de la novela, al referirnos a los cuentos veremos cómo la dificultad se le convierte casi en imposibilidad. Cuento y novela no sólo se interpenetrarán sino que en muchos momentos se confundirán en el concepto y en la práctica.

Como le fuese encargado el artículo "Cuento" para el *Diccionario Enciclopédico Hispano-Americano* [46] tuvo que hacer un tre-

---

[46] Vid. *Diccionario Enciclopédico Hispano-Americano*, Barcelona, ed. Montaner y Simón, 1890. Publicado también el artículo en las O. C. de Valera bajo el título "Breve definición del cuento", O. C., I, p. 1046.

mendo esfuerzo para llegar a una definición clara, sin que ello le obligara a poner barreras al género.

Vemos a Valera luchar con la dificultad y escribiendo uno de sus artículos más flojos en cuanto a la disposición de sus ideas y a la claridad se refiere. Definir es para don Juan limitar, encerrar los conceptos, como el entomólogo sus insectos, en cajitas de cristal, por lo que rehuye tan enojoso trabajo; se limita a darnos a conocer el concepto de cuento a través de toda la historia, lo que en cierto modo estaba justificado, pues pretendía llegar a encuadrar todo un género literario.

En un principio era cuento "la narración de lo sucedido o de lo que se supone sucedido".

Como mucha de esta materia formará la epopeya y la historia, más tarde sólo será cuento "el desecho de la historia religiosa, de la historia profana y de la poesía épica".

Surgió el cuento como "ficción involuntaria", como fruto de la fantasía humana puesta a manifestar su admiración o su temor hacia los dominadores de cualquier índole. El cuento con moraleja nacerá después, con la narración escrita, reduciéndose en muchos casos a la simple fábula, al apólogo o alegoría.

Viene después algo que "se funda en el cuento", pero que no es el cuento: es la novela.

Y en este punto se declara Valera incapaz de trazar las barreras que separan a ambos géneros. La única diferencia que él cree ver estriba en que la novela está más cerca de los hechos de la realidad natural, de "los caracteres de los hombres", que el cuento. Y añade: "Salvo la mayor extensión y reposo con que la novela está escrita, la novela se parece al cuento hasta confundirse con él" [47].

(No deja de parecernos curioso que el profesor Montesinos, que había publicado como anticipo de su libro sobre las novelas de Valera un largo ensayo sobre este problema concreto de la indife-

---

[47] "Breve definición del cuento", O. C., I, p. 1046.

renciación de géneros, ni entonces ni más tarde hiciera uso de este texto tan revelador. Tal vez justifique el olvido el hecho de que el profesor español quisiera llegar con sus propias deducciones —y valiéndose de cotejos inteligentes de obras y teorías valerinas— a la demostración que en la cita que copiamos más arriba postulaba Valera.)

¿Y cuáles eran, de preferencia, los cuentos que, según don Juan, se parecían a la novela hasta confundirse con ella? Precisamente "... los cuentos de amor, sobre todo cuando no hay en ellos elemento sobrenatural, son novelas en compendio, novelas en germen" [48].

He aquí una vez más (escrito por el mismo Valera) una explicación a dos de las afirmaciones del profesor Montesinos:

a) Que Valera escribió siempre "novelas de amores", y que

b) dichas novelas no eran sino cuentos largos, al igual que sus cuentos no son sino esquemas o embriones de novelas. Tal es el concepto de "novela libre" de que nos habla don Juan.

El cuento se exime de reglas aún más que los otros géneros; bastará —según don Juan— con que esté escrito "en estilo llano y sencillo; que tenga el narrador candidez o que acierte a fingirla; que sea puro y castizo en la lengua que escribe y, sobre todo, que interese o que divierta" [49]. Los mismos o parecidos preceptos que señalaba a la novela, como se recordará.

En una de sus cartas americanas, en 1900, lo llama "el más primitivo y el menos artificioso de todos los géneros literarios" [50].

VALERA Y EL TEATRO

Analicemos ahora lo que Valera mantenía acerca de los orígenes, concepto y realización personal de la literatura dramática.

---

[48] O. C., I, p. 1047.

[49] "Breve definición del cuento", O. C., II, p. 1049.

[50] "Nuevas cartas americanas", O. C., III, p. 558.

Respecto a los orígenes del teatro, muy temprano (1862) dio a conocer su sentir, enfrentando sus ideas —¡cosas de Valera!—a las que don Manuel Cañete había expuesto en un discurso académico [51]. Con las que don Juan no estaba de acuerdo, claro está. Valera estaba más interesado en contradecir a Cañete que en exponer sus propias ideas. Cañete defendía el origen litúrgico del drama y quería demostrar la superioridad artística del teatro religioso español sobre el profano. Mas lo que movió a escribir los tres conocidos artículos a don Juan, lo que según él era el error fundamental de Cañete, era el intento de separación entre lo que llamaban "arte cristiano" y "arte pagano"; pecado en el que iban a caer más tarde personalidades de la talla de don Marcelino Menéndez Pelayo.

Don Juan no quería discutir si el arte pagano es superior al cristiano, o viceversa, no. Sería ponerse en la misma situación —en el mismo error— que su contrario. Pretendía Valera demostrar que el arte simplemente es bueno o malo, sin que tenga nada que ver la calidad con la filiación religiosa o política que lo anime, así como tampoco depende de las modas pasajeras que de cuando en cuando está teñido. Le molestaba a Valera el que autores como Cañete quisieran levantar unos valladares valorativos que, según él, no podían ni debían existir. Y especialmente molestaba a Valera la idea mantenida —velada, pero firmemente— en todo el discurso de Cañete de que "quien no se admira de los tales dramas es un impío, o por lo menos un hereje" [52].

Según don Juan, uno puede encontrar los dramas a lo divino "absurdos, ridículos y hasta bárbaros" y seguir siendo buen católico, ya que la apreciación de un drama debe ser problema literario, no de religión.

---

[51] "Sobre el discurso acerca del drama religioso español, antes y después de Lope de Vega", O. C., II, pp. 331-342.

[52] O. C., II, p. 332.

Para Cañete —que se apoyaba en la *Introducción a la historia de nuestro Teatro* de A. Schack— el teatro había comenzado como una manifestación de ritos litúrgicos. Valera le da la razón en esto, pero limita tales orígenes a los dramas de las primitivas civilizaciones, cuando poesía y religión eran una misma cosa. Otro caso era el de las civilizaciones modernas, pues que, habiéndose separado muy pronto arte y religión, el teatro que producen es totalmente de origen pagano. No cabe comparar el despertar de la civilización entre los griegos con el renacer de la civilización en la moderna Europa. A lo largo de toda la Edad Media, el teatro se paganiza, ha tenido autonomía propia y sólo volverá a formar parte de las festividades religiosas "después de no corta y tenaz resistencia por parte de la Iglesia", justamente porque veía en el teatro ·demasiadas ideas paganas, demasiado peligro de corrupción. Fue solamente en los albores del Renacimiento cuando la Iglesia decidió incorporar los festivales dramáticos para sus fines de divulgación, no sin gran escándalo de algunos de sus miembros (cita Valera los nombres de San Agustín, el Papa Inocencio III y el P. Mariana).

También encuentra Valera exagerado el valor moral que Cañete, y los que con él piensan, conceden al teatro. Éste no es una escuela de buenas costumbres, sino una diversión más, que puede degenerar con facilidad en "voluptuosa o provocante a los vicios". Más que ninguna otra creación literaria, el teatro, que nace con y para el vulgo, puesto que con él cuenta para subsistir, está supeditado a la moda y gusto del público.

Señala Valera que el criterio de Cañete era preconcebido; pero no se da cuenta de que el suyo propio no lo es menos, y hasta olvida basar su teoría —orígenes paganos del teatro— en pruebas concluyentes. Tenemos la impresión de que, en desacuerdo con los orígenes religiosos del teatro moderno, surgió en él instintivamente la defensa del criterio contrario. Lo prueba el hecho de que en el artículo que sigue dice textualmente que "si quisiera demostrar con mayor claridad [tales teorías] nos sería fácil lucir erudición de segunda mano y acumular cita sobre cita..." [53], y nos da los nombres de autores que "coinciden" con sus ideas.

Trata en este artículo, y en el que cierra la serie, de demostrar que en los llamados "dramas religiosos" abundan las libertades, los malos ejemplos y hasta irreverencias que rayan en el mal gusto, cuando no en la descubierta grosería. No ve, como veía Cañete, en ello "el resplandor de esas santas virtudes", sino que descubre en los dramas —especialmente en los del XVII español— un reflejo de la perversión moral de la época. Las ferocidades que el concepto del honor y su idea llevaban consigo. No encuentra Valera aquella ejemplaridad ni religiosidad auténticas de que hablaba Cañete.

Sirviéndose del estudio de Schack va luego analizando algunas de las comedias de Lope, Tirso y Calderón, para llegar a la conclusión de negar de raíz el argumento de la superioridad moral del teatro religioso del Siglo de Oro español sobre el teatro no religioso de los días en que la polémica tiene lugar. Habla —conviene recordarlo— de valor moral, no del literario, que jamás fue puesto en tela de juicio.

Años más tarde volverá a repetir idénticos argumentos en un artículo dedicado a la publicación que hizo Cañete de la *Tragedia Josefina*. Pero esta vez, acusado por Cañete en artículos anteriores de carecer de suficiente erudición, se justifica don Juan diciendo: "De sobra reconozco la poca o ninguna solidez de mis estudios; y declaro asimismo que escribo con ligereza, sin acudir a muchos libros, y sin hacer largas investigaciones" [54].

Pocas líneas más abajo se contradice, pues en un corto artículo como era aquél, cita nada menos que a Ticknor, Wolf, Schack, Magnin, Germond de Lavigne, Bülow y Gervinus, para apoyar sus propias teorías o hacer suyas las de aquellos que le convenían, como

---

[53] "Sobre el discurso acerca del drama religioso español", O. C., II, página 334.

[54] Vid. "Tragedia llamada Josefina", O. C., II, p. 414.

en el caso de Charles Magnin, cuyo libro [55] había leído muy cuidadosamente, y de donde tomaría la clasificación de teatro "hierá-
tico, aristocrático y popular" [56].

Con mucho más cuidado que ocho años antes, volverá Valera
a negar que el teatro moderno tenga sus orígenes en la liturgia.
Afirma que hubo, sí, una re-cristianización del teatro, al valerse de
él la Iglesia "para dar ornato a sus funciones populares". Pero que
influyó más, a su modo de ver, en el nacimiento del teatro moderno, *La Celestina* que todas las obras "a lo divino" anteriores a Lope
de Vega. (Acababa don Juan de leer los prólogos de las ediciones
que a la magistral obra habían hecho, respectivamente, Lavigne y
Bülow, así como el estudio de Gervinus a ella dedicado.)

Ciñéndose a la obra que provocó la discusión, la *Tragedia llamada Josefina* de Miguel de Carvajal, dice Valera que estima, como
bibliófilo, la edición y no tiene inconveniente en confesar que no
encuentra en ella las hermosuras y el arte de que Cañete hablaba
y que causaban su admiración:

"El que yo tenga el mal gusto o la desgracia o la insensibilidad
y la frialdad paganas de no reconocer esas bellezas... no me impide
el estimar y celebrar que dicha tragedia haya sido publicada" [57].

Cuando nos planteábamos el problema del concepto que del
teatro tuviera don Juan nos vino a la imaginación otra cuestión no
menos interesante: cómo y por qué un hombre que ensayó casi
todos los géneros, que anduvo toda su vida tan preocupado con los
problemas económicos, no prestó más atención, no trató por todos
los medios de cultivar de lleno el único género literario que pro-
porciona riqueza y fama a la vez.

---

[55] *Les origines du Théâtre antique et du Théâtre moderne, ou His-
toire du génie dramatique depuis le I.er jusqu'au XVIe. siècle*, Paris, A.
Eudes, 1868.

[56] O. C., II, p. 415 y comp. con Magnin, obra citada, pp. IV, X, 61.

[57] O. C., II, p. 417.

Cinco años después de la publicación de su novela *Pepita Jiménez* dio a conocer, reunidas en un tomito, bajo el modesto título
de *Tentativas dramáticas,* la letra de una zarzuela y lo que él llamaba "otros dos como cuentos dialogados", *Asclepigenia* y *La ven-
ganza de Atahualpa.* Pero lo que más llama la atención del lector
es el estupendo prólogo-dedicatoria que puso al frente del conjunto.
Allí contesta don Juan a la pregunta que nos hacíamos más arriba:
no cultivó más seriamente el teatro porque se supo absolutamente
negado, incapacitado para ello; para sentir "aquella virtud magné-
tica por la cual el poeta comprende el sentir y el pensar del público
en un momento dado y se pone en consonancia simpática con dicho
pensar y dicho sentir" [58].

Explica con mucha gracia, aunque no sin ironía, cómo le había
tentado la idea de ganar fama y dinero por medio del teatro. Cómo
se las prometió muy felices con los "bien concertados disparates",
los versos tan lindos y la "jocosa ironía" de que tanto abundaba la
zarzuela que había escrito y cuánta fue su desilusión al leerla a
"hombres peritos en la materia" que estuvieron muy lejos de reir
con tales chistes y descubrir las delicadas bellezas. Entre burlas y
veras se adivina el herido amor propio de Valera sintiendo, en lo
más íntimo, el fracaso de sus vanos esfuerzos. No hay ya la protesta
abierta que encontramos cuando la publicación de su primer libro
de versos. Sino la amarga resignación de quien se sabe, por una
vez, incapaz de vencer el obstáculo.

Los chistes que aquellos "peritos" esperaban eran las "salidas"
u ocurrencias pedestres, los contrasentidos insípidos y los juegos
fáciles de palabras, de dudoso gusto, que jamás podrían salir de
pluma tan delicada y fina. La gracia subterránea que él había puesto
en su obra resultaba incomprensible para aquella clase de espectadores. Y Valera no podía descender hasta ellos —ese fue el problema que entendió desde el principio— para ganarse las simpatías

---

[58] Prólogo dedicatoria a *Tentativas dramáticas,* O. C., I, p. 1244.

generales: "Me llené de temor. Al maestro que me había prometido poner música a mi obra le relevé de la promesa, y yo desistí para siempre de mi fugitiva pretensión de ser poeta dramático" [59].

Aun cuando debamos admitir que Valera exagera un tanto al tomar tal decisión por el juicio de unos pocos lectores u oyentes de su libreto, no se puede negar que en dicho prólogo hay mucho de verdad. Abunda en la idea que apuntábamos antes: su incapacidad dramática; el reconocer que, aunque sus obritas son buenas en sí, tal vez lo fueran mejor para ser leídas que representadas. Dice que es irrepresentable, por lo que la da a conocer al público. De *Asclepigenia* piensa que es "de lo menos malo que he escrito en mi vida".

El teatro, para Valera, no es escuela de moral y buenas costumbres, como querían los neo-católicos. Como las demás artes, tiene su propio fin en sí mismo: divertir al pueblo y crear belleza. Y, cuando los críticos de opinión diferente le llaman defensor de la inmoralidad reinante, contesta que no hay por qué exigirle precisamente al teatro más moralidad o más ejemplo que el que debe encontrarse y exigirse a las gentes en la vía pública, las tabernas y cafetines.

No debe estar el teatro protegido especialmente por los gobiernos, ya que, siendo arte popular y para el pueblo, deberá ser éste quien —pagando por verlo— lo proteja. Refleja mejor que las demás artes a la sociedad de su tiempo, por lo que el autor dramático no puede crear o vivir independientemente de su época. El autor dramático tiene que compenetrarse con el espíritu de su pueblo:

"Sólo de esta suerte puede haber autores dramáticos. Los que de otra suerte escriban, podrán ser todo lo que quieran menos tales autores.

Infiérese de todo lo expuesto que la libertad del teatro tiene por límite la voluntad y el entendimiento del vulgo" [60].

---

[59] Dedicatoria a *Tentativas dramáticas*, O. C., I, p. 1244.
[60] "Teatro libre", O. C., II, p. 887.

Lo que extraña, luego de conocidos estos reveladores textos, es el por qué don Juan se asombraba de que sus *Tentativas dramáticas* no fueran bien acogidas por los "entendidos". Con aquel público que le rodeaba, "zafio, tosco y de gusto pervertido", don Juan no tenía nada en común. Y él no podía hacer nada por acortar la distancia que le separaba de aquellas masas.

Se dio perfecta cuenta —a pesar de aquella fingida extrañeza de que da muestra en el citado prólogo— de que él era incapaz de "hablar en necio para darle gusto". Y de que sus tentativas estaban muy lejos de ser lo que ordinariamente se entiende por teatro.

Analicemos someramente lo que para él (y para nuestro gusto) era la joya de su más que limitada producción. La divertida *Asclepigenia:* Su forma dramática se reduce a estar escrita en diálogo y dividida en escenas. Como su autor dice en el prólogo, el hecho de querer encerrarlo todo en breve cuadro dejando hablar a los personajes le hace "ser sobrio, no divagar [e] ir al grano siempre, como vulgarmente se dice". La acción es casi nula. Podría hasta decirse que el argumento —mejor dicho: la tesis— es el mismo que habíamos visto en *Pepita Jiménez,* sólo que escrito esta vez "por lo cómico". Su intención es burlarse de los que pretenden separar, radicalmente, el espíritu de la carne, menospreciando a esta última. El falso misticismo del curita, vencido por el instinto amoroso de Pepita, lo vemos de nuevo, en este delicioso diálogo, en el "desprendimiento terreno del sabio metafísico", sometido finalmente y humillado a las martingalas amorosas de la despreocupada Asclepigenia, mucho más con los pies en la tierra, menos mística, que su admirador filósofo. Es una burla divertidísima y llena de alusiones —no siempre bien intencionadas— a la vida de las altas esferas de la sociedad madrileña; las filosofías de moda —el krausismo y sus defensores fervorosos— puestas un tanto en solfa por el ingenio chispeante de don Juan.

Si llena de bellezas, si muy tersa y bien escrita y con gracia suficiente como para que la admiremos sin reservas, no es sin embargo obra que califique a su autor de dramaturgo. Como él mismo confesara "no hay esa corriente entre autor y público".

Escribió don Juan este diálogo para un público muy especial. Para el mismo público de quien se burlaba. Pretender que los espectadores rieran su propia caricatura, o que el gran público, la masa, entendiera las "pleguerías", veladuras irónico-filosóficas en que la obra abundaba, era pedir poco menos que el milagro.

No, no es auténtico teatro, a pesar de su forma. Son diálogos muy valerinos, muy personales, y por lo mismo muy llenos de chiste para leídos o escuchados de labios del autor. Pero no son representables ante el gran público. Y teatro sin espectadores será todo lo que se quiera, pero no es teatro. En todo caso, será el suyo teatro de salón, que no de sala. De reunión elegante y culta, o de lector solitario. Nunca teatro de gran público.

Más extraña aún (y de menos valor literario) es la letra que don Juan escribiera para una zarzuela. Pretendía haber hecho lo que en Italia hiciera Carlo Gozzi con sus *fiabe* o cuentos de hadas escenificados: una especie de fantasía lírico-musical más cerca de la moderna revista cinematográfica que de la pretenciosa zarzuela decimonónica.

En carta de julio de 1877 al músico don Francisco A. Barbieri [61] cuenta don Juan muy graciosamente cómo, habiéndole pedido la zarzuela el músico vasco Arrieta, la había tenido en su poder algo más de un año y se la había devuelto sin "ponerla en solfa":

"Yo sigo empeñado en creer que está en castellano, que no es logogrifo, y que no es tampoco una obra seria... sino una bufonada un poco menos chocarrera y tabernaria de lo que generalmente se estila".

Este fue el mayor defecto de la zarzuela: no era tabernaria para ser popular, y aunque con posibilidades de lucimiento de "encan-

---

[61] "Centenario del autor de *Pepita Jiménez*. Cartas inéditas", *Revista de la Biblioteca, Archivo y Museo Municipal*, T. II y III, pp. 135-137.

tos femeninos" que suelen atraer al espectador varón en tal clase de espectáculos, los chistes de Valera están muy "bajo la superficie" para hacer gracia o ser captados por el público que tales obras suelen necesitar. Lo cierto es que ni Arrieta, primero, ni Barbieri, después, encontraron las gracias que don Juan se empeñaba en haber depositado en el libreto. Que la zarzuela se quedó nonnata, para decepción de su autor [62].

Toda su vida mantuvo Valera el criterio de que en el género dramático no cabe la distinción cuantitativa: el género chico o el género no chico. Tal distinción le parece absurda. Lo bueno no es chico nunca, por muy breve que sea. Mantiene que hay "no pocos sainetes que valen más que multitud de dramas y de tragedias en cinco actos". Sólo cabe la diferencia de calidad. Le parecía mal que calificaran de "chico" al género cultivado por don Ramón de la Cruz: "Para mí no hay género chico ni género grande: no hay más que género discreto y género tonto" [63].

El fracaso como autor dramático probablemente fue el que menos hirió a la sensibilidad valerina. Así lo confiesa en el ya mencionado prólogo a sus *Tentativas:* "¿Qué le hemos de hacer? Dios no me llama por ese camino".

Esta vez las "cosas de Valera" no tuvieron salida. Allá quedaron, como estancadas, formando un libro, al que más tarde añadiría otros ensayos escénicos —nos resistimos a llamarlos "dramáticos"— que no tuvieron mejor fortuna que los tres de que hemos hablado.

VALERA Y EL ENSAYO

Si bien el cultivo del ensayo (aunque en forma muy primitiva y distinta a la que hoy tiene) se remonta en nuestro país a épocas

---

[62] Véanse más detalles referentes a la zarzuela de Valera en los artículos de Fermín de Iruña en *Semana* de 8 y 29 de noviembre de 1942.

[63] "Nuevas cartas americanas", O. C., III, p. 488.

muy lejanas, la preocupación por el estudio del ensayo como género literario, como ser con independencia propia dentro del mundo de la literatura, es cosa muy reciente. Podría afirmarse que hasta mucho después de la generación del 98 nadie se había molestado en rastrear sus orígenes, trazar sus límites o estudiar su importancia. No obstante, la influencia del máximo cultivador francés del *essai* —Michel de Montaigne, de orígenes y mentalidad peninsulares, conviene recordarlo— fue considerable en casi todos los cultivadores del ensayo en nuestra patria. Más tarde la escuela inglesa de ensayistas (entre los que sobresalen Bacon, Addison y Macaulay) conformarán el modo de ser de la moderna ensayística española [64].

Don Juan Valera ha sido considerado por la mayoría de los estudiosos de este tema como un claro precedente de los cultivadores del ensayo, que tanto iba a popularizarse entre los del 98.

Valera y Ganivet, con Menéndez Pelayo y Clarín, forman el grupo de precursores de los grandes cultivadores que iban a florecer en nuestras letras durante los años finales del siglo pasado y los primeros del xx: Unamuno, Azorín y Ortega, sobre todos.

Sin que pretendamos extendernos demasiado ni hacer un estudio exhaustivo de lo que realmente aportó don Juan al ensayo, analizando para ello cuanto para nuestra opinión es en Valera literatura de ensayo —lo que se saldría del plan de nuestro trabajo— nos parece, sin embargo, útil considerar este aspecto de nuestro autor con un poco más de sosiego y atención de los que nos parece encontrar en quienes, a veces, hablan un poco por boca de ganso o, todo lo más, por simple intuición, no demostrada con pruebas fehacientes.

---

[64] Vid. Ángel del Río y M. J. Benardete, *El concepto contemporáneo de España*, Losada, Buenos Aires, 1946, pp. 14 y s.

Enfoquemos el problema con la aparente paradoja de comenzar por donde se debiera terminar: detenernos primero en el concepto moderno de ensayo, sus límites si los hay, y sus posibilidades. E ir analizando luego lo que, con tales resultados a la vista, podemos deducir de la obra ensayística de Valera. Tal modo de operar, creemos, nos conducirá más claramente y con mayor rapidez al fin que nos interesa: ver lo que de ensayista moderno hay en don Juan Valera.

La definición que del género "ensayo" nos da la Academia es demasiado amplia ("escrito, generalmente breve, sin el aparato y sin la extensión que requiere un tratado completo sobre la misma materia"). Según esto, cabrían dentro del género muchos escritos que están lejos del concepto que nos hemos ido formando a través de nuestros años de lecturas de ensayos.

Consideremos lo que de la cuestión dijo el primero que de ella se ocupó con cierto detenimiento en nuestro país: Eduardo Gómez de Baquero, Andrenio, en su obra *El renacimiento de la novela en el siglo XIX*, capítulos dedicados al ensayo y sus cultivadores:

"El ensayo es la didáctica hecha literatura, es un género que le pone alas a la didáctica y que reemplaza la sistematización científica por una ordenación estética, acaso sentimental, que en muchos casos puede parecer desorden artístico" [65].

Aunque don Juan Valera se pasó la vida diciendo que nada quería enseñarnos, lo repitió tan machaconamente que suena un poco como a falsa justificación; puede que lo que no quisiera hacer fuera dogmatizar, hablar ex-cátedra, cosa a la que no sucumbió nunca; mas enseñar al público menos favorecido intelectualmente, sí que lo deseó. Si no enseñaba nada en sus novelas —ya vimos cómo atacaba a los autores que pretendían hacer tribuna de ense-

---

[65]   Madrid, Mundo Latino, 1924. Reproducidos en *Antología de ensayos*, Ed. de Antonio Alonso, New York, 1936. D. C. Heath & Co., páginas 12-13.

ñanza desde tan popular género— no era el mismo caso cuando escribía trabajos de crítica sobre cualquier materia para el periódico, y no se olvide que todos sus artículos nacieron para la hoja volandera. Los artículos de don Juan eran, pues, didácticos.

En cuanto a la última parte de la definición de Andrenio, nos parece haber sido escrita teniendo en cuenta ese "aparente desorden artístico" que podemos descubrir en algunos escritos de don Juan. Ese alejarse del tema principal intencionadamente, en vuelos poderosos de su inteligencia, para caer sobre él, como en picado, en el momento oportuno, cuando menos lo esperábamos y como haciendo alarde de sus brillantes posibilidades.

Para Andrenio el carácter específico del ensayo lo da esa "estilización artística de lo didáctico" que lo convierte en disertación, que encontramos en todos los escritos críticos de Valera.

Y continúa: "El ensayo es la interpretación personal, es exteriorización del espectáculo interior". Don Juan, por cuanto llevamos dicho, no dio otra cosa que sus puntos de vista, su "espectáculo interno", en todo cuanto escribió. Se le atacó continuamente porque era "demasiado personal"; le decían que sus criaturas literarias no eran auténticas, sino solamente versiones diferentes de la personalidad del propio autor. Su obra era lo que llamaban sus enemigos "cosa poco objetiva", pues sobraba en ella mucha nota personal.

Tenemos la convicción de que don Juan Valera se hubiera encontrado mucho más a gusto, por su manera de ver y de hacer, en compañía de personalidades como las de un Unamuno o un Azorín, que en compañía de quienes fueron sus coetáneos. Y fue probablemente ese estar a caballo entre ambas mentalidades lo que valió a don Juan más de un disgusto. Demasiado "avanzado" para los antiguos y demasiado "tradicional" para los renovadores.

Decididos los del 98 a romper con lo que no les interesaba, a derribar los falsos genios del siglo que les había visto nacer, negaron —cuando no enterraron entre el cascote de los templos derribados— muchos nombres de los que les habían precedido, algunos de los cuales, incluso, les habían hecho posibles. De aquí el que no mirasen con el respeto que se merecían a figuras de la talla y personalidad de Valera. Pero cuando se analizan someramente los temas de muchos de sus escritos vemos que precedió a la generación del 98 escribiendo no sin pasión acerca del que sería más tarde caballo de batalla de aquellos escritores: España y sus problemas.

Don Juan, como los escritores mencionados harían finalmente, contemplaba el triste espectáculo que daba el país. Movido por aquella contemplación, se plantea la búsqueda de las causas que le hundían desde muy atrás en la historia. Las analiza y si bien no aporta soluciones por temor, escepticismo o mera incapacidad, para enmendar tal situación, no se puede negar que denuncia abiertamente los males en sus escritos políticos o de historia. Denunciar es una de las tareas del ensayista. La incapacidad para la acción (recordemos que Baroja, Azorín, el mismo Unamuno se refugiarán al fin en la soledad de su creación), aquella incapacidad que le había separado de la política activa en tantas ocasiones haciéndose ver a sí mismo más como hombre teórico que práctico, es otro lazo común de Valera con los ensayistas del 98. Y esta incapacidad para la acción, este escepticismo que se convertirá más tarde en amargo pesimismo en aquéllos, le impide hallar soluciones. Denuncia situaciones, plantea problemas, pero es incapaz, como lo serán los otros, de acción directa y positiva para mejorar lo que a sus ojos no tenía solución inmediata. Prefiere contemplar el triste espectáculo del acontecer patrio refugiado en una postura de amable ironía, que le sirvió de escudo para encubrir tal vez su hondo escepticismo.

Por la personalísima manera de tratar tales temas, repetimos, está más cerca de los ensayistas que llamamos "de hoy" que de los artículos-acusación de Larra o Mesonero Romanos.

Encontramos aún otro lazo que le une a la generación del 98: su admiración sin tasa por el padre de los ensayos modernos, por Montaigne.

Valera leyó desde muy pronto, y reposadamente, los escritos del "señor de Montaigne", como respetuosamente le llamará siempre. Quizá fuera este autor uno de los que más influyeron en la educación juvenil de Valera. Hay siempre en él una especie de respetuoso cariño en las frecuentes citas que del autor francés podemos encontrar en la obra valerina: "Excelentísimo y amabilísimo señor de Montaigne", dice en otra ocasión. Admiración que tal vez hiciera nacer en Azorín el título que puso a don Juan: "Montaigne amable y moderno".

Precisamente el que a más altas bellezas conducirá el ensayo entre los cultivadores modernos, quien le dio sus formas más hermosas, el autor que mejor y más libremente dejará correr su pensamiento sirviéndose de este género, don José Ortega y Gasset, fue quien más contribuyó, con sus agudas (y muchas veces injustas) críticas, a la minusvaloración de don Juan Valera como crítico.

Es a todas luces evidente la distancia que hay entre los dos escritores. Que los ensayos de Ortega son, por muchos conceptos, superiores a los valerinos, tampoco es discutible. Pero no acertamos a comprender el por qué de las acerbas críticas de Ortega contra la obra de Valera [66].

En cuanto a la conocida definición orteguiana del ensayo ("la ciencia menos la prueba explícita") creemos que abarca casi todos los trabajos críticos de Valera. Hemos dicho antes que una de las características más señaladas era su poco o ningún amor a la erudición. Perderse entre el mundo de notas, fichas y datos, libros de consulta y acotaciones al margen, eran cosas que le asustaban. Lo que el mismo Ortega dirá después —"no escribo rodeado de libros ni de notas"—, el mismo sistema de aludir vagamente a las fuentes que le hicieron brotar sus personales sugerencias, es idéntico al seguido por don Juan.

---

[66] Véanse los tres artículos titulados "La crítica de Valera", "De la dignidad del hombre" y "Valera como celtíbero", en *Obras Completas de Ortega*, vol. I, pp. 159-163, Revista de Occidente, Madrid, 1946.

Leyendo los ensayos de Ortega, viendo su manera peculiar de tratar los temas, es justamente cuando el lector atento de ambos escritores puede ver cómo lo que don Juan había hecho antes no fue sino el anticipo, el embrión si se quiere, de lo que Ortega elevará más tarde a la categoría del ensayo magistral.

No somos nosotros los primeros que creemos ver en Valera un claro antecedente de la manera orteguiana. Giménez Caballero, en un trabajo dedicado a Valera el año 1924, precisamente publicado en la *Revista de Occidente,* así lo sostiene: "Discurre con talento y gracia sobre cuanto lee... Es el predecesor, bajo este aspecto, de Ortega" [67].

Don Juan, con gran finura y perspicacia se había separado intencionadamente de la "manera de hacer" de cuantos le rodean. Precisamente se quejó no poco en varias ocasiones de que uno de los males de la crítica española de su tiempo era el excesivo "amor al análisis meticuloso". Método, a su entender, peligroso y con el cual se podría demostrar que cualquier obra o autor de mérito presentan defectos mucho mayores de los que realmente presentan. O viceversa.

Don Juan prefiere la crítica sintética, el análisis amplio, a la moderna. Un poco a la manera como los autores del 98 escribieron sus "divagaciones", sus ensayos a propósito de una obra, más que la vana pretensión de los irascibles seudocríticos del xix, que colocaban las obras literarias sobre sus mesas de operaciones y gozaban deshaciéndolas punto por punto.

Al analizar el "modo de operar" de Valera, cuando hacía crítica, vimos cómo aquello era algo que había surgido "a propósito de una obra", con el pretexto de una obra, mejor que el artículo de crítica al uso. Llega, incluso, en ocasiones a olvidarse de la obra que diera origen a su ensayo. (De lo cual será acusado por Pérez

---

67   *Revista de Occidente,* octubre, 1924, T. VI, p. 148.

de Ayala en los tres ensayos que le dedicó el año de su centenario [68].)

Cuanto llevamos expuesto creemos que nos autoriza a llegar a la conclusión de que don Juan no fue solamente un claro antecedente de la literatura de ensayo moderna, sino uno de los primeros cultivadores en el tiempo.

Si en sus ensayos no se encuentra la perfección de forma que le darían los ensayistas que vinieron tras él, conviene tener en cuenta que don Juan se enfrentó con campos literarios apenas roturados. Que él fue uno de los primeros en abrir vallados y trazar nuevos surcos y que por ello mismo es más disculpable la imperfección del trazado. Los ensayistas de nuestros días, los maestros del ensayo de que empezábamos hablando, se encontraron ya una labor consistente mucho más lograda y en desarrollo de lo que ellos mismos confesarían. Su preocupación por la renovación de formas, por la lengua, por tomar ejemplo de las nuevas corrientes europeas no era cosa tan nueva en nuestras letras.

Precisamente debió adoptar Valera el ensayo (él no se atrevió a llamarlo así) porque era el género que mejor se prestaba para hacer aquellas "cosas de Valera" de que ya hemos hablado. Y es que, valiéndose de tal modo de escribir, sus "cosas" no parecían tan fuera de lugar.

A los otros géneros les había derribado las barreras de contención, deshaciendo aquellos límites absurdos que estrechaban las posibilidades del artista creador. En el ilimitado campo del ensayo (¡qué distancia entre los artículos valerinos y los de un Velarde, un Revilla o el mismo Palacio Valdés!) se sintió siempre Valera más libre, más seguro que en los otros géneros. Aquel su "teatro irrepresentable" (y por tanto no auténtico teatro), aquellas novelas que él quería "más libres que el aire", o los cuentos largos hechos novelas, aquellos cuentos en verso que llegaron a ser muchos de sus

---

[68] Ramón Pérez de Ayala, "Don Juan Valera o el arte de la distracción", en *El Sol*, 16, 17 y 18 de abril de 1925.

poemas, escandalizaban a los lectores del siglo pasado que no estaban preparados para dar aquellos "saltos espectaculares" de género a género.

Como ellos mismos decían, con peor fe que el autor de la frase, todo era muy valerino, todo eran "¡cosas de Valera!".

Pero lo más curioso es que donde más brilla su capacidad renovadora y donde más libre vemos volar la expresión de su pensamiento, en los ensayos, es en donde pocos quieren ver esas buenas "cosas de Valera".

Podemos decir con Edith Fishtine: *Valera's fantasy flits freely and irresponsibly from one theme to another, touching upon all, exhausting none* [69].

Con todo, terminemos esta parte de nuestro estudio diciendo lo que ya insinuamos: que le debemos una obra crítica exquisita, certera y sagaz, brotada de su mente como por juego.

Que don Juan Valera no fue lo que hoy entendemos por un profesional de la pluma, sino un diplomático, un hombre elegante de su siglo. Y que, no obstante ello, pese a haber disfrutado del vivir como el que más, tuvo la gentileza de hacernos el regalo de lo mejor de su espíritu en forma de una prosa admirable en sus novelas, y una tarea crítica comparable sólo a lo mejor de nuestro mayor crítico, su querido amigo y discípulo, don Marcelino Menéndez y Pelayo.

---

[69] Vid. Edith Fishtine, obra citada, p. 30.

LA CRÍTICA

CAPÍTULO IV

LITERATURA MEDIEVAL

Si bien es frecuente encontrar las mismas o parecidas posturas defendidas por Valera con ardor a lo largo de su obra, pocas veces veremos una idea tan invariablemente fija como sus opiniones y juicios sobre la literatura medieval.

Hemos dicho ya que en el Valera crítico ha de tenerse en cuenta una especie de incapacidad para alterar sus modos de ver. Su dificultad para reconocer abiertamente que sus ideas no son más que eso, ideas personales. Incluso, a veces, no las verdaderas, y que la flexibilidad mental es absolutamente necesaria para la tarea crítica. En cuanto se refiere a sus trabajos sobre literatura medieval, hemos de tener todo esto muy presente si no queremos llegar a conclusiones poco favorables para don Juan.

Fijada su actitud frente a la literatura primitiva en la que manifiesta bien pronto su falta de interés (su incomprensión, digámoslo ya) por cuanto huele a primitivo, a popular, mantendrá Valera, contra todos los pareceres, su posición y admitirá ligeros cambios en muy contadas ocasiones.

Ni la admiración y amistad verdadera que sentía por su querido amigo Menéndez Pelayo, quien, enamorado de tal parcela de nuestras letras, intentó, con tacto y cariño, hacerle ver lo injusto de sus apreciaciones, ni los ataques de los críticos adversos, lograron no ya derribar sino ni siquiera agrietar el muro de su incomprensión.

De avanzada edad, ciego ya, rectificó muy ligeramente sus antiguas opiniones. En ninguna otra materia, repetimos, el espíritu apasionadísimo de Valera se mostró tan obstinado defendiendo sus convicciones; utilizando los mismos argumentos, citándose a sí mismo sin reparo. Desde sus ensayos primeros hasta los que precedieron a su muerte, el gráfico de su pensamiento respecto a la literatura medieval podría representarse como una constante línea recta con ligerísimas ondulaciones producidas por los ataques de quienes no pensaban como él. Y, a lo largo de tales juicios, el lector encuentra casi a flor de piel la radical incomprensión valerina, su falta de olfato especial para gozar con el sencillo perfume y la belleza de lo primitivo. De aquí sus teorías, sus justificaciones; incluso sus esfuerzos por tratar de comprender —de gustar— lo que otros comprendían claramente. Su buena voluntad chocaba siempre con una realidad áspera y llena de fuertes —por primitivos— sabores. Su delicado paladar (el mismo que se negó a saborear las amarguras de la novela naturalista), hecho para apreciar las quintaesencias clásicas, no supo, ni pudo, muchas veces, bien a pesar suyo, paladear tan sencillo manjar espiritual.

SU POSTURA PERSONAL

Fue en contestación a Cañete y Segovia —cuyo discurso académico leído en 1859 versaba sobre la poesía de Garcilaso, Fray Luis y Rioja— donde por primera vez dejó ver Valera, de pasada, sus dudas respecto al valor de la lírica medieval.

Defiende contra Cañete y los neocatólicos el valor de la mitología, de la naturaleza, de los grandes temas renacentistas como elementos poéticos de importancia, sin tener en cuenta si habían sido purificados o no por el agua bendita del catolicismo. No nos importa tal diatriba. Lo que sí nos importa es la siguiente afirmación en boca de Valera:

"Y merced a la revolución poética de Garcilaso y Boscán se desarrolló y empezó a florecer la gran poesía castellana, antes apenas digna de este nombre, si se exceptúan las célebres *Coplas* de Jorge Manrique, algunas de las *Trescientas* de J. de Mena, y los romances populares, aunque de los que quedan han de ser pocos y no de los mejores, los que se escribieron antes de la revolución mencionada" [1].

Encontramos dos afirmaciones interesantes; la primera, que para Valera la auténtica poesía no nace exactamente hasta la revolución mencionada, salvados los casos que especifica. La segunda —ciñéndose ya a los romances— la de que fueron pocos y no de los mejores los que antecedieron a tal momento.

Sigue diciendo en el artículo que, pese a las afirmaciones de los investigadores, las obras líricas primitivas tienen un valor muy relativo; ni Berceo, ni el Arcipreste, ni los poetas del *Cancionero de Baena*, etc., son verdadera poesía. Tienen puro interés arqueológico o todo lo más filológico, pero poco o ningún mérito como obras de arte. Al menos nada comparable a la belleza de las obras en prosa, tales como *Las Partidas,* el *Amadís* o *La Celestina.* No admite en la lírica primitiva nada comparable a la del xvi. Y la prosa sólo "para manjares delicados".

Al año siguiente, y con más detalle, volverá a mostrar su opinión en un artículo dedicado al libro de Wolf sobre la literatura española en la Edad Media [2]. La teoría, que va haciéndose lentamente en la cabeza de Valera, comienza ya a esbozarse. Sin atreverse aún a negar todo valor a las producciones medievales, confiesa "no enco-

---

[1] "Reflexiones críticas sobre los discursos de Cañete y Segovia", O. C., II, p.131.

[2] F. Wolf, *Studien zur Geschichte der spanischen und portugiesischen national Literatur,* Berlín, 1859. El artículo de Valera se titula "Sobre la Historia de la Literatura Española en la Edad Media", O. C., II, p. 150.

miarlas tampoco con entusiasmo" y se atreve, sin rodeos esta vez,
a juzgar el *Poema del Cid*. Lo llama "trabajo artificial"... "dificul-
toso y tan sin numen y cadencia". Si tal le parecía lo que asegura-
ban ser la joya del tesoro medieval, bien poco estimaba la poesía
restante. En cambio, la prosa "vale diez veces más que todo lo restante" [3]. En opinión de don Juan, fueron los prosistas doctos quienes despertaron, con su estudio y ejemplo, los afanes creadores del
pueblo, hasta entonces sin impulso propio para cantar y hablar.

Glosando al año siguiente el libro de Milá y Fontanals dedicado
a la poesía medieval, e intentando dar a conocer al público una
materia que consideraba de interés, las ideas que había expuesto
Valera anteriormente van a madurar, a tomar cuerpo de teorías [4].

En donde Valera está de acuerdo con Milá hará suyas las afirmaciones del erudito catalán y nos amplía las ideas que tenía acerca
de la lírica en general y la popular castellana en particular. (Hemos
de decir, por parecernos detalle interesante, ya que nos revela el
poco interés que sentía don Juan por la poesía popular y las investigaciones que en España se estaban llevando a cabo, que solamente cuatro años antes —1856— supo de la existencia del sabio catalán. Hablando en Moscú con el erudito ruso Serge Sobolefski,
quien al parecer conocía perfectamente, y estimaba en mucho, el
libro de Milá, al preguntar a Valera sobre el valor que en España
se le concedía, tuvo éste que confesar —sospechamos que no de
muy buen grado, pues era admisión de su ignorancia— que no conocía ni el libro ni a su autor [5]. Poco después estudió Valera con
atención los trabajos de Milá y firmó la propuesta para hacerle
académico.)

---

[3] Idem, p. 152.

[4] *Observaciones sobre la poesía popular*, M. Milá y Fontanals, Bar-
celona, 1853. Los tres artículos que Valera dedicó a estudiar la obra de
Milá figuran bajo el título "La poesía popular de M. Milá y Fontanals",
O. C., II, pp. 201-211.

[5] Vid. "El regionalismo literario en Andalucía", O. C., II, p. 1047.

Vemos en estos tres largos artículos, repetimos, la formación de sus teorías. Necesitado de argumentos para negar valor al "manjar" que le servían, necesitado sobre todo de justificaciones, eleva sus intuiciones a teorías; nos explicamos tal hecho pensando en la formación archiclásica que desde sus primeros años había recibido don Juan. La perfección y la exquisitez de lo clásico impedían a Valera encontrar bellezas en lo que él consideraba obras rudas, cuando no vulgares.

No estaba preparado para descubrir con humildad los tres hermosos versos que, de pronto, entre fárragos enormes "pedantescos y prosaicos", como maliciosamente los llamará otra vez, saltan a los ojos de quien estudia y busca sin prejuicio, compensándole de la paciencia y el esfuerzo que ha tenido que poner para llegar al descubrimiento de tal joya. (Pensamos en un texto de don Ramón Menéndez Pidal encomiando la finura de Menéndez Pelayo, que supo descubrir la delicada perla de la célebre estrofa del Marqués de Astorga: "... vida de la vida mía, / ¿a quién contaré mis quejas / si a ti no...?" hallada "entre una balumba de versos insignificantes" [6].) Don Juan no tuvo la paciencia de aquéllos. Hombre de jardines versallescos, modales distinguidos y plantas cultivadas, fue incapaz de encontrar, ¡ni siquiera de buscar!, la humilde florecilla serrana nacida entre peñascos o yerbas poco vistosas. Hombre de perfumes exquisitos, se empeñará en negar que de plantas rústicas puedan extraerse olores aprovechables. De aquí su menosprecio por cuanto fuera primitivo.

SUS TEORÍAS, SU JUSTIFICACIÓN

¿Qué es para Valera la poesía popular? Valiéndose de la definición de Milá, ampliando y aclarando convenientemente, nos lo

---

[6] R. Menéndez Pidal, *Estudios literarios,* Buenos Aires, 1938, p. 202.

explica por extenso. Es la que para su uso compone o modifica ya el pueblo, ya los poetas que a él se dirigen. Con el mismo amor inflamando sus corazones, idéntico pensamiento iluminando su mente, el poeta compone lo que el pueblo le dicta y le inspira; y el pueblo recibe la composición como obra propia.

Tales circunstancias, afirma Valera, se dan muy raramente, y por tanto muy rara será la poesía popular auténtica. Si en el pueblo decae el espíritu poético o se desmaya o muere la gran idea nacional que le animaba, la poesía que el pueblo compone, pese a parecer linda e ingeniosa, no llegará a ser verdaderamente popular, y se limitará a ser vulgar.

¿Cuándo se da esta compenetración entre pueblo y creador? Solamente en los momentos de coincidencia del esplendor de la lengua con la inspiración; en momentos de gran civilización o, paradójicamente, en las civilizaciones primitivas. En la India y, entre los occidentales, en Grecia, quien "o no tuvo poesía popular o fue popular toda su poesía, desde Homero hasta Píndaro". Los demás pueblos de civilizaciones derivadas no pueden comenzar su historia literaria con esos vagidos poéticos que serían la poesía popular, sino reviviendo los poemas eruditos de las civilizaciones que les precedieron; la poesía de los países latinos no tendrá la originalidad de la griega ni su sencillez; será sin duda más rica en ideas, más elevada de pensamiento, de más dilatados horizontes, pero no saldrá de todo ello nada comparable a la Ilíada. Cuando un idioma llega a la perfección, la llama de la inspiración popular se ha extinguido.

Para los países de "civilización derivada", los grandes poemas épicos no serán la suma, la perfección de una poesía popular "imaginaria", sino el comienzo, el embrión, el origen de tal poesía. De los romances en España.

No pretendemos nosotros criticar la crítica de Valera, puesto que nuestro trabajo tiene por objeto exponer —más que discutir— los criterios de que se valía don Juan para hacerla, hallar éstos y juzgar su validez. Ahora bien, se nos ocurre preguntarnos cómo hubiera reaccionado nuestro autor si, en lugar de discutirle con diferentes argumentos, como hicieron los que en su tiempo se le enfrentaron, lo hubieran hecho no dando por válida tanta teoría, tanto principio. ¿Por qué admitir que solamente Grecia —civilización primitiva por excelencia, según don Juan, lo cual no deja de ser muy discutible— fue capaz de una poesía popular? ¿Es que antes de los poemas homéricos, ejemplo supremo para él de poesía popular, donde pueblo y poeta coincidían en sentimientos y anhelos, no pudo haber otros muchos poemas de los que no quedaron huellas ni rastros...? ¿Es que realmente antes de la gran civilización helénica no hubo un gran período de ebullición de cultura latente, de preparación para etapas posteriores de esplendor, como lo fue la Edad Media en los países latinos...? ¿O tal vez es que en Grecia y la India, según don Juan, habían nacido estas brillantes civilizaciones primitivas por milagrosa generación espontánea...?

RAÍZ DE SU INCOMPRENSIÓN

Contemplando el problema en la distancia, nos parece encontrar el origen de esta incapacidad de Valera para apreciar en su justo valor la poesía primitiva, en una especie de orgullo mezclado con simple falta de sencillez. Lo primitivo, como lo popular, le parecía inartístico. Sin embargo, sabios de la categoría de Milá y Fontanals, de Menéndez Pelayo y de muchos otros, ponen por las nubes "aquello" que a Valera no le parecían sino balbuceos torpes de una literatura de segunda categoría. Incapaz, por otro lado, de contemporizar saliéndose por una tangente fácil de alabanzas no sinceras, se aferró a sus negativas. Creó principios y reglas para justificar su falta de interés.

Por otro lado, el hecho de no conocer, o conocer tarde, los trabajos de los eruditos españoles y extranjeros en dicho campo, y el haber llegado a ellos movido un tanto por lo que él consideraba "alabanzas excesivas", hace que el espíritu de contradicción que llevaba en sí don Juan le lance, irremediablemente, a combatir las teorías de los otros, inventándose las propias. No olvidemos que, cuando, impugnadas sus ideas primeras desde las páginas de la *Revista Ibérica* (15 de abril de 1862) por don Francisco de Paula Canalejas, don Federico de Castro, desde Sevilla, y un anónimo "Sr. X", con el que más agriamente disputará Valera, desde Granada, y al contestar en dos largas cartas dirigidas al primero, molesto hasta el enfado por lo que él consideraba "intromisión", se disculpa del "poco orden y mal concertadas razones que la carta lleva" y dice, confirmando nuestras sospechas: "Yo no presumo ni quiero que nadie crea que yo presumo de pedagogo; pero cuando piensa alguien serlo conmigo, prefiero serlo yo con él, a trueque de no someterme a su férula" [7].

En su discurso de ingreso en la Academia —leído el 16 de marzo de 1862— ratifica sus opiniones y él mismo confiesa que no es tal trabajo "un ensayo volandero", sino que desea escribir algo que si breve sea duradero, no como otros muchos escritos suyos "perdidos en el inmenso fárrago de los periódicos, y condenados al olvido para siempre". Consciente de la responsabilidad de sus afirmaciones, va a tratar de aquilatarlas al máximo.

Comienza su discurso [8] alabándose como español de que nuestro país sea el que represente más riqueza, en cantidad y en calidad, de cantos populares en el romancero; lo que molesta a Valera es el afán de todos por ensalzar tal poesía enfrentándola con la erudita: "Muchas personas han acabado por preferir los aullidos poéticos de los caribes a las *Odas* de Horacio; los himnos latinos bárbaros de la Edad Media a la *Cristiada* de Vida, y una canción de gesta a la *Eneida* o a la *Jerusalén*" [9].

---

[7] "Carta a don Francisco de Paula Canalejas", O. C., II, p. 325.

[8] "La poesía popular. Ejemplo del punto en que deberían coincidir la idea vulgar y la idea académica sobre la lengua castellana", O. C., III, página 1049.

[9] "La poesía popular", O. C., III, p. 1050.

Irritado por la tendencia del momento a ensalzar —exageradamente, según su criterio— la poesía primitiva, adoptó la postura de intransigencia que él afeaba en los demás, sólo que con argumentos contrarios. Por lo cual no se entendieron.

Mantiene que las grandes y primitivas poesías populares no pueden ser obra del vulgo, tener origen plebeyo. Son creaciones de una aristocracia sacerdotal o guerrera. Le molesta incluso el hecho de que un poeta como Berceo descienda a hablar el habla grosera del "bajo pueblo": "en la fabla que el vulgo le fabla a su vecino", remeda el exquisito Valera, casi con un gesto de repulsa ante tanta barbarie que transforma la poesía en "una antigualla o en mala prosa".

No tuvo paciencia para un estudio penetrante, amoroso, de lo verdaderamente sencillo y popular, para encontrar aquel "fondo nacional" que viera don Marcelino Menéndez Pelayo [10]. Para Valera "nuestra literatura medieval se puede demostrar que es menos original y hasta menos católica que la posterior al Renacimiento" [11].

Niega que hubiera un despertar poético medieval, puesto que entonces no nació la civilización, sino que renació gracias a los doctos y a la erudición de entonces. Repite la valoración que había hecho años antes y sigue dando "diez veces más importancia a las *Partidas, El Conde Lucanor, las Crónicas* y la *Celestina* que a todos los poemas y canciones anteriores al siglo XVI".

Hablando del *Poema del Cid,* confiesa abiertamente sus pocas simpatías hacia él, a pesar de las buenas intenciones de Wolf, don Pedro José Pidal y Durán, "parecerá siempre a los más de sus lectores un trabajo artificial y erudito, donde se nota el esfuerzo para expresarse en una lengua ruda y apenas formada, y donde se imita la versificación francesa de las Canciones de Gesta" [12].

---

[10] Vid. Ramón Menéndez Pidal, *Estudios literarios,* Buenos Aires, 1938, p. 200.

[11] "La poesía popular y la lengua castellana", O. C., III, p. 1060.

[12] O. C., III, p. 1060.

Estamos por pensar que don Juan no pudo nunca concluir la lectura del poema, por mucho que lo intentara. Más adelante rectificará muy levemente sus opiniones. Reconocerá valores que había negado antes ("verdadero espíritu poético y nobilísima inspiración nacional", por ejemplo). No sin cierta ironía sonríe al decirnos: "Hasta los negros de Angola y los hotentotes tienen cantares, coplas y refranes bonitos. ¿Pero acaso merece esto llamarse poesía popular?" [13].

No molestaba a Valera el género en sí mismo; era lo que él consideraba la tontería de las gentes que, en su alabanza por lo popular, llegaba a negar y desprestigiar lo erudito. Confundiendo lamentablemente "lo popular con lo doméstico o lo rastrero o lo pueril y lo anacrónico" [14].

En otro discurso académico, leído el 12 de febrero de 1873, y en el que estudió las *Cantigas* del Rey Sabio, con más detenimiento, cariño e interés del que solía poner en obras de lírica primitiva, vemos entre las conocidas afirmaciones de siempre un cierto espíritu de buena voluntad. Es un ensayo con verdadero sentido moderno de crítica y en el que, si se descuenta el fallo excesivamente parco en alabanzas, como más adelante veremos, se trasluce el excelente y agudo sentido crítico, el mucho conocimiento del oficio y la mejor gracia valerina al servicio de una crítica que se hace amena, ilustra al lector y que, incluso hoy, puede servir como ejemplo de crítica literaria de la mejor calidad. Estudia fuentes, compara fechas y datos, hace un ligero estudio de estilística y, en una palabra, analiza como no se había hecho antes en nuestro país la obra lírica del Rey Sabio. Lástima que a la hora final, la valorativa, Valera, fiel a sus principios, se queda corto en el encomio. Parece un contrasentido que él, un hombre tan dado a "bendecir", tan

---

[13]   Cartas citadas, a don Francisco de Paula Canalejas, O. C., II, página 325.
[14]   *Ibidem.*

lleno siempre de bondad, de transigencia para las obras que analizó, solamente se mostrara realmente duro, áspero, con la parcela de nuestras letras que más cariño y benevolencia requiere para poder ser saboreada.

En 1896, y con motivo de la publicación de la *Antología de poetas líricos*, de Menéndez Pelayo, volverá don Juan *publice et privatim* a recordar su postura. En un artículo publicado en *El Liberal* [15] y en carta a su amigo y discípulo [16].

Alaba encarecidamente el esfuerzo que en pro de la historia de las letras españolas está llevando a cabo su gran amigo; alaba al investigador... y resta importancia al material investigado.

Le contesta don Marcelino y, con todos los respetos, se atreve a decirle: "no podemos estar de completo acuerdo ... hallo en estos versos más cosas dignas de alabanza de las que Ud. admite. ... Pero todo esto puede ser cuestión de gusto individual, y yo sobre estas cosas nunca disputo" [17].

Ya no es el anónimo "Señor X", de Granada, al que Valera había pulverizado con sus frases ingeniosas, su erudición y su ironía, quien le contradice; ahora es persona de buen gusto reconocido. Por ello, sin dejar enfriar los ánimos, tres días después le contesta una de las más jugosas e ilustrativas cartas del epistolario; enumera cuantas razones se le alcanzan, aunque no dé su brazo a torcer —¡dejaría de ser Valera!—. Niega en redondo que sea cuestión de gusto individual: "No hay gusto individual que valga. Los versos son buenos o malos y la poesía es poesía o no lo es, con perfectísima independencia de todos los gustos o disgustos individuales" [18].

Mas sigue inclinado a creer que la prosa es "inmensamente superior a la poesía" en nuestra Edad Media. Y entre líneas, pero

---

[15] O. C., II, pp. 408 y ss.
[16] *Epistolario Valera-Menéndez Pelayo*, ed. citada, pp. 524-529.
[17] *Epistolario Valera-Menéndez Pelayo*, obra citada, p. 525.
[18] Idem, p. 528.

claramente para el lector familiarizado con Valera, se percibe mucha reserva, total incomprensión y muy poco, o ninguno, amor hacia la lírica primitiva.

RECAPITULACIÓN. VALOR
DE SU CRÍTICA DE LA
LITERATURA MEDIEVAL

Salvo los dos extensos ensayos, escritos para ser leídos en sendos discursos académicos, dedicados específicamente a estudiar la poesía popular, uno, y las *Cantigas,* el otro, los restantes trabajos de Valera sobre tema medieval están hechos "a propósito" de la aparición de algún libro o trabajo erudito. Es decir, que salvo en las dos ocasiones en que escribe para la Academia, no pretendió Valera analizar ni criticar directamente esta materia. En los siete trabajos restantes —algunos de ellos de considerable extensión— no se puede hablar de intención crítica *a priori;* a lo sumo podría hablarse de una crítica "derivada", es decir: tangencial. Don Juan expone su sentir frente a las ideas de los demás.

Hemos dicho más atrás que nuestro autor solamente criticaba lo que de algún modo le producía un cierto placer estético. Se indicó también el poco gusto que por lo medieval sintió. De esta falta de interés nace la dureza de sus juicios para con esta literatura "primitiva y ruda", según sus palabras. De esta especie de desprecio instintivo contra el que, justo es decirlo, intentó luchar (animado por su fraternal amigo don Marcelino Menéndez y Pelayo), sin conseguirlo, se derivan sus juicios negativos. Se aparta voluntariamente de cuanto no sea fruto de una civilización refinada y exquisita. Llega a llamar a nuestra poesía lírica primitiva "artificial, docta y estudiada" [19]. A su juicio, carece de todo valor literario intrínseco; de existir algún resto de poesía popular, está "muerta y enterrada

---

[19]   "La literatura en la Edad Media", O. C., II, p. 152.

en los libros; viva en boca del vulgo sólo hay poesía vulgar" [20].
A épocas bárbaras no pueden corresponder más que poesía y arte
bárbaros. Los versos de los cancioneros de Stúñiga, Baena, Don
Dionís y Resende no son para él más que "discreteos prosaicos"
donde tal vez "... el anticuario, el filósofo, el filólogo y el historiador hallen sin duda un tesoro inagotable de noticias y revela-
ciones; pero al hombre de buen gusto, que no pretende desentra-
ñar el pasado, le cansan y le hastían" [21]. Confiesa luego con franqueza desacostumbrada en Valera que "apenas pueden sufrirse las
poesías líricas de la Edad Media española", pues son "pedantescas
y frías" cuando no adolecen de "completa idiotez o de enfadosa
pedantería" [22]. Jamás estuvo el correctísimo don Juan, el "dulce
Valera" de don Marcelino Menéndez Pelayo, menos dulce y tan
poco correcto en sus juicios como cuando los hacía sobre este
campo de nuestras letras.

Echemos ahora una mirada hacia su crítica positiva: al *Poema
del Cid,* como se ha visto, comenzó negándole todo valor literario
para enmendarse no muy convincentemente en momentos en que
la crítica —incluida la de sus tradicionales amigos (don Marcelino
Menéndez Pelayo, especialmente)— se puso en contra suya [23].

A Berceo le concede únicamente valor arqueológico. Le molesta
al crítico el que todo un poeta descienda al nivel del pueblo para
hablarle "en fabla". Comparar los versos del cantor de Santa María
con los del Dante le parece a Valera "una blasfemia".

A *Las Cantigas,* su mejor trabajo crítico de los consagrados a
lo medieval, repetimos, tampoco las encomió como hubiera debido.
Halla más interesante el lado "épico de las Cantigas". Lo que hay

---

[20] "La poesía popular de Milá", O. C., II, p. 203.
[21] "Las cantigas", O. C., III, p. 1129.
[22] "Sobre la poesía popular de Milá", O. C., II, p. 210.
[23] Vid. O. C., II, p. 150 y *Epistolario Valera-Menéndez Pelayo,* obra
citada, p. 528.

de rudeza del idioma, lo que tiene de agreste pintura y bello colorido. Pero el delicado temblor poético se le escapó totalmente.

Muy poco antes de su muerte, cuando preparaba la edición antológica de los poetas del siglo XIX, vuelve a la carga al redactar la nota crítico-biográfica de Milá. Dice con naturalidad que, a su entender, "si se exprimen en la más moderna prensa hidráulica todos los serventesios, lais, tensiones y pastorelas de los antiguos trovadores, ha de salir poquísimo jugo de auténtica poesía" [24].

Resumen las líneas que anteceden la postura de toda su vida de no querer admitir la existencia de nuestra primitiva lírica popular como verdadera obra artística. Terco como nunca, sólo alcanza a ver lo que de poético tenían las vidas y aventuras de los autores de los versos. Sus andanzas por un mundo misteriosamente bello como el de la Edad Media, mundo al que Valera idealizaba cuando quería, sí que le resultaban poéticas. Pero sus obras no fueron más que tentativas meritorias, balbuceos poéticos incipientes.

Don Juan Valera, pues, no realizó en el campo de lo medieval una tarea crítica al modo como lo hicieron años más tarde un Menéndez Pidal, o el mismo don Marcelino Menéndez Pelayo, que con un amor extraordinario por todo lo primitivo rastrearon y hasta recrearon muchas de las composiciones que se creían perdidas. Mas no olvidemos que Valera, a pesar del título que suele llevar en los manuales de literatura de "eruditísimo", no fue, en el sentido propio de la palabra, un erudito. Era hombre de un caudal enorme de lecturas, de excelente memoria y, por tanto, de rara y valiosa erudición. Le faltaban el estudio y la meditación fructíferos. Tenía muy poca paciencia y no fue, como hemos dicho, el sabio que trabaja incansable para estudiar y hacer progresar, consciente de sus responsabilidades, la cultura patria. Fue el elegante prócer que, en los ratos libres en que su amada *high life* (para decirlo en inglés, como él gustaba) se lo permitía, gozó con la lectura y nos regaló con sus ocurrencias casi siempre valiosísimas para ayudar al lector.

---

[24] "Notas biográficas y críticas", O. C., II, p. 1300.

LAS LETRAS DE LOS SIGLOS DE ORO

La poesía auténtica, según Valera, comienza en nuestro país con Garcilaso. Solamente unas contadas excepciones anteriores al poeta de las églogas pueden recibir el título de obras de arte: "Algunos versos del Arcipreste, las *Coplas* de Jorge Manrique, el *Amadís* y la *Celestina*".

Mas no se piense que la parquedad en el número de ellos significa que don Juan les dedicó análisis detallados; la simpatía que siente hacia esas obras no pasa de ser —al igual que la antipatía que sintió por la poesía medieval— una especie de idea fija, un prejuicio que no pretendió explicarse ni explicarnos.

Del Arcipreste no sólo no encontramos alabanzas sino ni siquiera un simple análisis de sus versos. Las regocijadas páginas del *Libro de Buen Amor* no debieron hacer mucha gracia a Valera, no sólo por la rudeza de la lengua en que están escritas, sino también por esa falta de pudor de "no velar con pleguerías" lo que Juan Ruiz pinta con tan alegre desenvoltura. Era demasiado realismo para el gusto valerino.

De las *Coplas* de Jorge Manrique es bastante revelador el respetuoso silencio que guardó para con ellas. Y en esta obra sí que no tenía pretexto alguno para poner inconvenientes.

Con el *Amadís* es un poco más explícito; su admiración por dicha obra se nos antoja más directa, más fruto de la lectura. Es un libro de entretenimiento en el cual el lector encuentra siempre multitud de aventuras fantásticas y esa verosimilitud artística que Valera pedía a las obras de imaginación. Debió leer con detenimiento las aventuras del fiel enamorado de Oriana; su delicado gusto encontró el placer que deja traslucirse en comentarios y alusiones cuando tiene oportunidad, ya que no en artículos largos dedicados a analizarla.

Escribió dos artículos sobre este tema como consecuencia de la lectura del estudio que del *Amadís* y sus orígenes había hecho el doctor alemán Ludwig Braunfels. Pero no fue muy lejos en sus análisis. Discurren galanamente, escritos en un español pulido, verdaderamente valerino, y vemos cómo se interesa más en apoyar con su opinión propia la españolidad del primitivo *Amadís de Gaula* que en estudiar las bellezas que él encontraba en dicha obra. Sin querer que se nos tache de osados nos parece ver, en el silencio que guardó a este respecto, una prueba palpable de que a don Juan no le parecían tan acabadas las bellezas literarias del libro.

Le gustaba el *Amadís* porque era un ejemplo más de "novela libre", fantástica y que no se atenía a cánones ni leyes de ningún género. Tuvo siempre muy en cuenta las palabras de Cervantes en el escrutinio del cura y el barbero. No se molestó en contradecirlas, pero tampoco las apoyó con otras de su cosecha. Lo calificó —y es la única nota encomiástica que en los dos artículos encontramos— de "libro bellísimo" y, dispuesto a ensalzarlo, continúa haciendo una cálida alabanza del *Quijote,* saliéndose así por una inesperada tangente que le ahorra el elogio que no parece salirle de muy dentro del alma. El héroe manchego es mejor que Amadís "porque no es tan llorón como él, y no es menos valiente, discreto y leal enamorado" [1].

Con *La Celestina* le ocurre algo muy parecido. Aunque es muy posible que la admiración que sintiese por esta obra fuera superior a la que acabamos de mencionar. Pero tampoco nos dio los claros estudios que su agudeza crítica, su buen gusto y su saber le hubiesen permitido hacer. Conocía, como ya se indicó, los trabajos que sobre la tragicomedia famosa habían visto la luz en toda Europa. Los tuvo muy en cuenta cuando de ella habla y quizás por ello nos privó de juicios más originales y extensos. Debió pensar don Juan que el público lector español, su público, no tenía demasiado interés en conocer tan "beneméritas antiguallas". Y como nada original —sin un trabajo mucho más profundo del que él mismo era capaz— podría salir de su pluma para el otro público lector, el erudito, si más limitado también más exigente, optó por tocar otros temas menos comprometedores.

Un solo artículo de periódico, y no muy extenso, dedicó concretamente a la *Celestina* cuando apareció la edición de don Marcelino Menéndez Pelayo. Sabe don Juan el interés de dicha edición; le consta el valor que al libro —ya de por sí muy valioso— dan el prólogo y las notas de don Marcelino, y aprovecha la oportunidad para discurrir sobre la obra. Quiere alabarla sin cortapisas... y no lo logra. Pese a sus buenas intenciones, no sabe callarse si algo hay que no le satisface; no quiere ir "contra corriente" y acepta como buenos juicios que eran, en su opinión, muy discutibles. Pero se nota en el fondo de lo que escribe una especie de descontento íntimo que no concuerda con lo expresado. Nunca como ahora se verá más claro lo que don Juan nos había dicho muchos años antes:

"El diablillo crítico que me atormenta, y por el que estoy no sé si obseso o poseído, no consiente que diga yo, cuando escribo,

---

[1] "El Amadís de Gaula", O. C., II, p. 493.

aquello que quiero decir, sino aquello que él quiere que yo diga" [2].

Se propone alabar sin tasa, porque la obra lo merece y porque su prologuista y anotador gozaba de sus mejores simpatías. Mas las alabanzas, que no faltan, suenan a frialdades. No hay crítica "en contra" mas, entre líneas, por las digresiones de que don Juan se vale, percibe el lector atento los verdaderos sentimientos de Valera.

El hombre que en 1861, incidentalmente, había hablado de la "desenfrenada y obscena *Celestina*" [3] no olvida que, junto a las bellezas innegables de la tragicomedia, hay un realismo en los detalles que le parece grosero y no para ser descrito. Que incluso puestos, como están, en boca de criados y gente de baja condición, no dejan de ser atrevimiento de muy dudoso gusto. ¿Cómo puede alabar el exquisito don Juan Valera las procaces expresiones de Pármeno, Areusa o el fanfarrón Centurio...? ¿Son para olvidadas las escenas que ocurren en casa de la vieja, los excesos, la libertad con que el desconocido autor analiza las almas y las acciones de sus personajes? Aquel "pasmoso realismo y tan bien observada y expresada pintura de caracteres y afectos" no podía por menos de causar asombro al elegante don Juan [4]. Pero estas mismas realidades eran demasiado fuertes, estaban dibujadas demasiado a lo vivo para que captasen por entero la voluntad y el aplauso del refinado hombre de mundo.

Este realismo un tanto brutal y descarnado, estas escenas tan "naturalistas", para emplear una de sus expresiones, de las primitivas grandes obras de nuestra literatura son las que se yerguen frente a Valera como murallas almenadas que le impiden un acercamiento cordial. En la lírica fueron la rudeza de formas y la falta de elegancia y compostura —¡él decía de sencillez!—. En la naciente novelística, en la dramática, son los abundantes pasajes llenos de atrevimiento los que le desaniman.

[2] "Cartas americanas", O. C., III, p. 238.
[3] "Protección a la literatura dramática", O. C., II, p. 276.
[4] "Nueva edición de La Celestina", O. C., II, p. 1035.

LA PRIMITIVA LITE-
RATURA DRAMÁTICA

Nada encontramos tampoco que se refiera a la primitiva literatura dramática española, excepción hecha del artículo en que discutía con Cañete y de que ya dimos cuenta [5].

¿Es posible que nada significaran para Valera el teatro de Juan de la Encina, Torres Naharro y Gil Vicente? Suponemos que su insaciable curiosidad le llevó en más de una ocasión a la lectura de ellas, a "desempolvar" obras que sabía muy bien estaban en manos de los eruditos. Su silencio debemos interpretarlo como elocuente calificación de falta de interés por dichas obras. Que carecían de los más elementales valores literarios, según su criterio.

Otra causa que cooperó a que don Juan no se dedicara con más interés a escribir artículos críticos sobre todos estos temas, para nosotros hoy tan interesantes, debió ser el hecho de que Valera encontraba una tremenda falta de interés en el lector medio en el siglo pasado. No merecía la pena escribir largos ensayos críticos en un país en el que "no leen más que los que escriben" [6]. Ante todo había que ganar lectores, formarlos y ser, para ello, ameno, breve y divertido. Con demasiada frecuencia encuentra don Juan difícil el compaginar brevedad y diversión en escritos dedicados a estudiar obras de importancia que nadie, salvo la erudición, se tomaba la molestia de leer.

LA POESÍA LÍRICA

No se le ocultó la importancia de la poesía de Garcilaso. (Repitió constantemente que con él nació la verdadera poesía lírica es-

---

[5] "Sobre el discurso acerca del drama religioso español, antes y después de Lope de Vega", O. C., II, pp. 331-342.
[6] "Otras cartas", O. C., III, p. 616.

pañola de calidad.) Su buen gusto natural y su afición a lo clásico le habían inclinado desde muy temprano a familiarizarse con el Siglo de Oro.

Las nuevas tendencias del siglo xix no hacen sino empujarle —por reacción contra lo nuevo— más y más hacia los clásicos. La mayoría de las obras románticas le parecían una "melopea insoportable" que pretendía, sin conseguirlo, producir nuevas notas musicales. En cuanto a las innovaciones modernistas (o las de las nuevas escuelas francesas), le reafirman en sus ya citados prejuicios contra lo que no fuese "cultivo de las letras a la manera tradicional". Garcilaso, Herrera y Fray Luis eran sus preferidos. Las frecuentes citas y referencias en toda la obra de Valera así lo demuestran.

Pero esta predilección, este cariño que sintió por ellos no se tradujo en amorosos estudios. Nunca los analizó pensando en ilustrar a otros lectores menos afortunados que él; en mostrarles las bellezas que a él se le aparecerían tan claras.

Ningún arma hubiera sido más eficaz para combatir lo que él llamaba "la barbarie moderna y los excesos que pretendían crear algo nuevo" que unos comentarios inteligentes a las obras que tanto deleite le causaran. Sin embargo, nada de esto salió de su pluma. El temor, por un lado, de que, estragado el gusto de los escasos lectores por "la mala poesía al uso", no los estimaran, y, de otro, su constante deambular por la vida diplomática y su poca afición al trabajo de biblioteca, hicieron que tampoco nos dejara ningún estudio de esos autores a quienes consideraba como maestros de la lírica universal, esos autores a los que volvía con devoción y amor una y otra vez.

LA MÍSTICA

Aún son más de sentir estas lagunas en lo que se refiere a nuestros místicos, a quienes dedicó Valera "lo mejor de mis años de madurez". Estudiándolos no sólo con amor de *dilettante*, sino como estudioso que pretende sacar de ellos una personal filosofía.

Como muy sagazmente demostró Jean Krynen en su estudio *Juan Valera et la mystique espagnole* [7], buscó don Juan en la literatura mística respuestas ciertas a las preguntas que su alma de esteta, que su concepto personal del arte le planteaban. No nos interesan estas cuestiones en un trabajo de la índole del nuestro; nos atendremos exclusivamente a estudiar el posible influjo literario que de tales lecturas de los místicos pudo sacar nuestro autor y trataremos de ver si esta misma afición crítica que le dominaba le condujo a analizar obras tan interesantes.

Desgraciadamente, tras una rápida ojeada al temario de la crítica de Valera, vemos que prácticamente no existe una labor encaminada a valorar tales obras. Y en ningún otro terreno como en éste hemos de sentir esta pereza valerina, pues, conociendo el campo a fondo, valorando para sí la poesía de San Juan, la prosa inimitable de Santa Teresa, nos dejó sin unos estudios que le hubieran elevado a las cimas de la mejor crítica. Las pocas páginas que conservamos, que, aun siendo pocas, tienen cierto interés, no son más que la prueba de que su agudeza mental percibió claramente el valor superior de tales obras.

Llegó a estudiar a los místicos en su afán por buscar argumentos con los que defender a los krausistas contra la acusación de que mantenían un panteísmo místico. Fruto inmediato de estas lecturas fue su *Pepita Jiménez*. Cuando doña Emilia Pardo Bazán le acusa en *La cuestión palpitante* [8] de tener un estilo "harto atildado y primoroso" por mirar demasiado de cerca el estilo de nuestros místicos, aconsejándole la autora gallega que lea obras de nuestra picaresca, contesta Valera muy amostazado:

---

[7] *Bulletin Hispanique*, XLVI, 1944, pp. 35-72.
[8] Emilia Pardo Bazán, *La cuestión palpitante*, Madrid, 1891, pp. 263 y siguientes.

"Yo afirmo enteramente lo contrario; que nuestros autores picarescos pecan de afectados, y los místicos no, y que en nuestros libros de devoción hay que ir a buscar no el arcaísmo, sino el verdadero naturalismo; esto es, la sencillez, el candor, la total carencia de artificio de quien habla o escribe de buena fe, porque tienen algo que decir, salga como salga de sus labios o de su pluma" [9].

Que Valera, como alumno, aprendió bien su lección lo demuestra toda su producción novelística. Jamás autor alguno antes que Valera, en el siglo XIX, llegó a bucear en las almas de sus personajes —en la suya propia— con la valentía y la soltura con que él lo hizo. Sus novelas, calificadas como de verdaderos estudios psicológicos, demuestran que don Juan hablaba convencido de la veracidad de sus palabras. No recomendaba a los naturalistas la lectura de los místicos por elegante esnobismo en aquellos momentos en que estaban tan olvidados, sino con la plena conciencia de la utilidad de dicho estudio y lectura.

Toda su vida fue Valera un lector fervoroso de las obras de nuestros más grandes escritores místicos. Desgraciadamente, tales lecturas no le fecundaron para, so pretexto de comentarlas, elevarse como se elevó al margen de otros autores y obras de mucha menor importancia [10].

Solamente en dos ocasiones, en dos discursos académicos precisamente (lo que revela, como sospechábamos más arriba, que sólo trata de los temas místicos cuando considera que su auditorio, sus lectores, merece que se ocupe de tales temas, pues pueden escucharle y entender sus palabras), se ocupó de problemas de la literatura mística.

Ambos discursos son contestación a los de recepción en la Real Academia Española del Conde de Casa Valencia y de don Marce-

---

[9]   "Sobre el nuevo arte de escribir novelas", O. C., II, p. 646.
[10]   Sí influyeron tales lecturas, sin embargo, en el Valera novelista. Su *Pepita Jiménez* acusa estas influencias, según el propio autor confesó y lo que la crítica moderna ha opinado.

lino Menéndez Pelayo. En el primero —"Elogio de Santa Teresa"— solamente la parte final, poco más de dos páginas de lectura, es verdadera alabanza de la obra de la Santa. Y nos parecen elogios escritos un poco de prisa y corriendo, como para salir del paso —del compromiso— de la mejor manera posible. No hay una crítica auténtica, un análisis detenido de la obra que tan bien conocía.

El segundo es una muestra de lo que don Juan hubiera podido hacer de haber tenido más tiempo y una mayor afición al trabajo erudito. Trata de los escritores místicos en general; no se atreve a llamarlo ni siquiera discurso, sino que modestamente los llama "apuntes". Magníficos apuntes, en todo caso, que no hacen sino dejarnos con la miel en los labios, pues no cala en el tema con la hondura y la profundidad de que él era capaz [11].

Percibe agudamente la peculiaridad de nuestro misticismo con respecto al de otros países; nuestros místicos buscan a Dios, se unen con Él, le ponen en todo lo creado, sin caer por ello en un panteísmo egoteísta ni endiosar tampoco a la naturaleza. El alma de nuestros místicos no se aniquila al contacto divino. Sale de esa prueba "más hábil e idónea para la vida activa". Mística que tiene su fruto inmediato en la lucha por la predicación de la verdadera fe que llevan a cabo nuestros misioneros entre los pueblos bárbaros recién descubiertos.

El esfuerzo requerido para buscar a Dios en lo más intrincado de la mente humana conduce al alma a observar y analizar sus reflejos más ocultos, llegando a intimidades donde sólo los más pacientes y sutiles psicólogos podrían llegar, resultando así una especie de nueva psicología práctica, agudísima, "un estudio claro del yo, con todos sus afectos, facultades y propensiones".

Menciona luego los extravíos del amor falsamente místico para con la mujer, que no es sino "aberración y herejía del misticismo legítimo y ortodoxo".

---

[11] "Elogio de Santa Teresa", O. C., III, p. 1148 y "Del Misticismo en la Poesía Española", O. C., III, p. 1153.

Ve cómo en la poesía de Fray Luis hay mucho de objetivo para ser verdaderamente mística, aunque religiosa lo sea siempre. Pone esclarecedores ejemplos de tan bellos versos y analiza luego con brevedad la importancia que dentro de la poesía mística, y de nuestra literatura, tuvo San Juan de la Cruz.

EL QUIJOTE

En muy pocas ocasiones brilla con tanta fuerza la capacidad crítica de don Juan Valera, ni su elegancia y primor de estilo están más patentes en cuanto escribió, como cuando dedica sus pensamientos al tema de su predilección. El libro inmortal que él consideraba no sólo lo más excelente de nuestras letras, sino la cima de todas las literaturas: *El Quijote*.

Se diría que la gracia narrativa de Cervantes se comunica, como un milagro de simpatía, a la pluma de quien escribe. Que el razonador frío y cerebral de otros ensayos se transforma, al contacto del tema, en el más enamorado, dulce y tierno comentador que, dejando hablar a su corazón, nos explica una extraordinaria lección con encendidas frases de amor y entusiasmo verdaderos. El escéptico Valera nunca lo fue menos ni penetró un tema con más hondura y habilidad que en los ensayos dedicados a la inmortal novela.

Lector incansable de ella (confesaba en 1862 haberla leído "treinta o cuarenta veces") [12], cada vez que vuelve a ella lo hace con más devoción y amplitud de espíritu. Y creemos que fue consciente de la superior calidad de sus escritos consagrados al *Quijote*, pues dijo, hablando de uno de ellos, "que es en mi sentir lo menos malo que he escrito, aquello de que estoy más satisfecho" [13].

El *Quijote* fue para Valera "la novela", el espejo donde había que contemplarse, el ejemplo a seguir para todo escritor que se

---

[12] "Sobre la estafeta de Urganda", O. C., III, p. 288.
[13] *Epistolario Valera-Menéndez Pelayo*, obra citada, p. 21.

proponga hacer arte verdadero. Es, en su opinión, la más acabada de las perfecciones literarias. (Le reservó el lugar de excepción en el Parnaso literario y cuando algún crítico quiere poner a la misma altura a Shakespeare dice que "entonces habría que poner también a Tirso, Lope y Calderón, que igualan, si no sobrepasan, al genio inglés, pero sin llegar ninguno a la grandeza del manco genial") [14]. Es la novela que divierte y entusiasma al lector, a la vez que le eleva el alma por la contemplación de la belleza más pura. No porque haya en ella explicaciones morales, ni enseñanzas de otro tipo, que si las hay están allí como "por añadidura", pues Cervantes nada de eso se propuso al escribirla, sino porque el autor, al pintar las almas de sus personajes, supo poner en ellas lo mejor y más bello que tenía en la suya. Según Valera, Cervantes era un genio lego que se sorprendió a sí mismo escribiendo lo más extraordinario que el arte novelístico ha producido. Le dedicó tres ensayos largos, dos artículos cortos de menos importancia y multitud de referencias en otros artículos de los más variados temas.

El primer ensayo vio la luz en 1862. Trata de echar abajo las afirmaciones de Nicolás Díaz de Benjumea, según el cual el *Quijote* estaba lleno de una oculta filosofía que sólo se revela a los que, con mucha paciencia y tras profundos estudios, llegan a dar con el verdadero sentido de la obra de Cervantes. A Valera le parecen tales afirmaciones de una pueril ingenuidad. Toda la novela es de una claridad meridiana, según él. Son muy estimables las noticias curiosas que el investigador puede descubrir acerca de la vida y hechos de la sociedad que rodeaba a Cervantes; pero dedicar tiempo y fatigas a descubrir tesoros ocultos en libro tan claro le parece inútil; en los libros "buenos o malos, no hay más escrito que aquello que está escrito". Las ocultas filosofías que Benjumea creía descubrir no existieron sino en su imaginación, no en la de Cervantes,

---

[14] Véanse idénticas razones en el artículo "Sobre Shakespeare", O. C., II, pp. 371-375.

y añade Valera con un rasgo de humor: "no consentimos que la fama de Cervantes crezca a expensas de su modesto comentador" [15].

Cervantes —sigue Valera— no hizo sino copiar la realidad, hermoseándola con su fantasía y el ideal artístico de que estaba dotado. Ni siquiera sería lícito decir que Cervantes hizo alegorías cuando tomó rasgos propios, o de quienes le rodeaban, para inventar sus personajes. Es obra autobiográfica en lo que toda obra de creación tiene de autobiografía, mas no como el autor del folleto pretendía, "una alegoría cervantina". Negar el parecido que la creación tiene con la realidad sería tan infantil como afirmar que un cuadro de la Sagrada Familia no es tal sagrada familia sino las alegorías de tales y tales personas amigas del pintor que le sirvieron de modelos para inspirarse.

Benjumea hace depender el valor de una obra de arte del beneficio que presta a la humanidad y no de la belleza en sí. Ya sabemos lo que a este respecto piensa don Juan: que quienes tales verdades afirmaban mantenían también que un manual de agricultura cualquiera vale más que *Las Geórgicas,* y un mal tratadillo de botánica sería por lo mismo superior a *Las estaciones,* de Thomson.

Valiéndose de los argumentos de que el único fin del arte es la creación de la belleza, va demoliendo con humor y malicia las afirmaciones de su oponente. Ni siquiera la conocida afirmación de que Cervantes se propuso acabar con las novelas de caballería puede ser tomada al pie de la letra; tal fue el pretexto que la motivara, pero sólo el pretexto para crear una hermosa fábula, único y verdadero fin que movió la pluma de Cervantes.

Por otro lado, los grandes críticos que se habían ocupado de analizar el *Quijote* [16] no encontraron las ocultas filosofías de Benjumea, sino las superiores bellezas que saltan a la vista de quien lo lea.

---

[15]   Vid. O. C., II, p. 280.

[16]   Se refiere don Juan a Federico Schlegel, Gioberti, Pictet y Hegel, a quienes cita en varias ocasiones.

No niega Valera que tenga el *Quijote* su moral, pues los elevados sentimientos del autor se depositan naturalmente en su obra; pero tampoco era éste el fin de la obra. Benjumea confunde hermosura con utilidad. Con gracia verdaderamente valerina, esto es, de la mejor, termina don Juan su precioso ensayo animando a Benjumea para que estudie el *Quijote* cuanto quiera, sin que por ello tenga que achacar sus conclusiones personales al artista que la trazara y cuya grandeza brilla con luz propia.

El más largo ensayo que sobre este tema saliera de su pluma, el discurso leído ante la Real Academia el 25 de setiembre de 1864, es, sin duda, la más bella pieza de literatura crítica que don Juan escribió [17]. Ensayo en el que el amor y comprensión que sintió por la obra, el estudio emocionado y el ánimo de profundizar llevan a Valera a escribir, en su mejor estilo, páginas imborrables, en las que el lector ve brillar no sólo la agudeza crítica y el seguro discurrir de nuestro autor, sino una pasión, un entusiasmo que separan este trabajo de la manera ordinariamente cerebral y fría con que juzga don Juan, elevándole a la altura de los mejores ensayistas modernos que han escrito sobre tan inmortal libro.

Con el mismo tierno amor con que Valera "vio" a Cervantes escribiendo su mejor obra, mirando en torno y copiando a la humanidad amorosamente, con infinita y desacostumbrada ternura analiza aspectos interesantes que, sin llegar a ser descubrimientos novedosos o sensacionales, nos dan una exacta visión de su total comprensión de la obra y a la vez nos ayudan a entenderla mejor y amarla.

Ve las diferentes maneras en que, a lo largo del tiempo, se ha ido interpretando el *Quijote*. Cada época procuró sacar de esta obra el modelo de sus ideales viendo en ella las virtudes propias retratadas y magnificadas. Enumera las alabanzas que le dirigieron desde los

---

[17] "Sobre el *Quijote* y sobre las diferentes maneras de comentarlo y juzgarlo", O. C., III, pp. 1065-1086.

más opuestos rincones, a veces atribuyendo a Cervantes "méritos que ni tuvo ni quiso tener, ni soñó, en vida", sin entender muchos otros que en realidad tiene. Cómo el XVIII lo convierte en "terrible erudito, moralizador, purista escrupuloso, atildado hablista, un siervo de las reglas...". Otros lo llaman "ilustrador del género humano", psicólogo sutilísimo, refinado político y hasta médico consumado. Todo le parece a Valera exageradísimo y falto de veracidad.

Otros, como el crítico Clemencín [18], en su afán por ensalzarla, la analizarán con tal detalle que la convierten en menudas partículas, encontrando defectos como las impropiedades mitológicas [19], o gramaticales, que no hacen sino demostrar que Cervantes era un sencillo escritor humano, y, como tal, sujeto a error [20]. No escribió —ni se lo propuso— disertaciones académicas; dejó volar su pluma al compás de su fantasía genial. Estos y otros defectos que los críticos querían descubrir en la obra son, para Valera, objetos de finos argumentos. En cuanto a las acusaciones de que Cervantes remedó los libros de caballería, en lo que no fueran las acciones vulgares, como las de atar el caballo a un árbol, cabalgar o descabalgar, etc., le parecen a Valera totalmente faltas de verdad. Si hizo una parodia de los l.bros de caballería, fue *in genere,* no de una obra o más obras en concreto.

Cervantes parodió el género porque lo amaba, ya que sólo lo que se ama es digno de ser parodiado. Explicando lo cual, hace Valera, a nuestro juicio, la aportación más valiosa y personal para la interpretación del Quijote: todo poeta, en el momento de parodiar, eleva el objeto parodiado ante sus ojos "como un bello ideal que le enamora el alma y arrebata el entendimiento", aunque aquel

---

[18]   *El Ingenioso Hidalgo D. Quijote de la Mancha,* ed. Diego Clemencín, Madrid, 1833.

[19]   Idem, pp. XXVIII y ss.

[20]   "... no tenía ideas científicas del arte de escribir, ni había meditado mucho sobre el asunto". Clemencín, obra citada, p. XXIX.

bello ideal no responda a la realidad circundante por parecerle "ilógico o anacrónico" [21].

El español, continúa Valera, no tiende, como el francés, a la burla ligera, sino que se inclina a la parodia profunda, por lo mismo que estamos más inclinados al amor violento y al entusiasmo más fervoroso. Ningún otro pueblo asimiló más fuertemente que el español el espíritu caballeresco de la Edad Media. Y Cervantes no se burlará de él despiadadamente, sino que "parodió en su *Quijote* el espíritu caballeresco, pero confirmándolo antes que negándolo" [22].

Confirmación que tal vez nació en él poco a poco, a medida que iba escribiendo. Sigue después un estudio de lo que entiende él por literatura caballeresca; cómo de los ciclos épicos cosmopolitas nacen las rudas epopeyas meramente nacionales. Señala don Juan que los héroes españoles son más de carne y hueso, están más enraizados en la realidad que "la fantástica, libertina y afectada poesía caballeresca de otros países". Nuestros héroes son más auténticos, más reales y sin aquella vaguedad que tenían los de la *Table Ronde*. El Cid Campeador es una figura histórica ensalzada por la fantasía popular, pero sin perder por ello su individualidad. Y estos héroes de nuestra épica no serán los antecedentes de las figuras de los libros de caballería. Éstos mirarán a las aventuras importadas, tomadas a préstamo de los ciclos, ya agónicos, extranjeros. Nuestra fantasía no se acomodó copiando bajo otra forma, sino que se trazó como meta el superarlas. Sacó nuestra literatura multitud de héroes disparatados y quiméricos, entre los que descuellan Amadises y Palmerines. Contra tal género decadente va la descubierta sátira de Cervantes: "Surge entre un género que acaba y otro que comienza y de ambos es el más acabado y hermoso modelo" [23].

---

[21] "Maneras de comentar el *Quijote*", O. C., III, p. 1069.
[22] O. C., III, p. 1069.
[23] Idem, p. 1074.

Se cuidó muy bien Cervantes de ridiculizar las ideas caballerescas del honor, la lealtad, cantidad y fidelidad de sus amores. *Don Quijote,* al encarnarlas todas, es la figura más bella de toda la historia y hasta su locura tiene más de sublime que de ridícula.

No acepta tampoco don Juan la idea, bastante en boga entonces, de que don Quijote y Sancho encarnan lo ideal y lo real. El intuitivo sentido poético de Cervantes le hace pintar seres vivos, como Homero, como Shakespeare; seres vivos, figuras humanas, aunque reales, muy hermosas. No buscó la creación de prototipos.

Estudia Valera también las cualidades humanas de caballero y escudero; los acerca a nosotros poniendo en la tarea el mismo amor que Cervantes puso en la creación. Examina la grandeza de alma de Cervantes al estudiar su sátira, nunca amarga o misantrópica. ¡Con cuánta ternura nos lo muestra, sirviéndose don Juan de su mejor prosa!

La tan proclamada unidad de acción del *Quijote* no alcanza Valera a verla; apenas halla verdadera acción en esa serie de aventuras admirablemente enlazadas, pero sin progreso en la fábula que prepare y precipite el desenlace. La unidad reside en el pensamiento de los protagonistas, no en la acción [24].

---

24 "... La unidad del *Quijote* no está en la acción, está en el pensamiento, en Don Quijote y Sancho unidos por la locura", O. C., III, página 1077.

D. Américo Castro, en su admirable colección de ensayos titulada *Hacia Cervantes,* Taurus, Madrid, 1960, ratifica el pensar de Valera. Confróntese, por ejemplo, lo que éste dice respecto a la estructura del *Quijote* con el ensayo, del mismo título, de Castro. De él entresacamos lo siguiente: "Las aventuras son solicitadas y urdidas, menos por lo que haya en ellas de suceso divertido que por su virtud de poner en un brete a Don Quijote y a cuantos bullen a su lado... Cervantes ha ido acumulando aventuras, ocasiones de toda índole para, a través de ellas, continuar el proceso iniciado por los libros sobre Alonso Quijano; es decir, a fin de que sus personas y cosas den a luz sus latencias y se hagan irradiantes de posibilidades, poetizándose al encarnarse en la incitación advenida a ellas" (p. 276).

Quita importancia Valera a las alusiones que han creído descubrir algunos críticos a seres vivos del tiempo del autor. Claro que Cervantes se sirvió de la realidad, pero tomó los datos para completar las figuras que estaba trazando, no para satirizar a los vivos. También usó rasgos reales en los que no puso sátira alguna.

No encuentra las alusiones "liberales o antimonárquicas" que algunos ponían en boca de Cervantes. Antes al contrario: quien alaba tan candorosamente a Felipe III, resulta absurdo que satirice a Carlos V y Felipe II. Su pluma no fue servil, pero tampoco resentida.

Analiza la religiosidad de Cervantes, profunda y sincera a pesar de las burlas que se permite contra los clérigos, y nos demuestra Valera que tales burlas más proceden de la "general relajación en las costumbres y depravación en la moral" de la época. Dice que en cuanto parece haber parodia de la religión hay más intención de lograr la risa del lector que de burlarse de las cosas santas, y así debió entenderlo la Inquisición, pues las dejó pasar [25].

Percibe Valera como los dos polos del alma de Cervantes la ambición y el amor a la gloria, de una parte, y cierto menosprecio del mundo y cierta ternura mística, por otra. Polos que se mani-

---

Y en cuanto a la encarnación de lo ideal y lo real en las figuras de D. Quijote y Sancho, encarnación que Valera niega, véase lo que dice Castro:

"Olvidemos, por tanto, la inveterada rutina de llamar a D. Quijote 'idealista' y a Sancho 'realista', pues ambos tienen de lo uno y de lo otro..." (p. 283).

Para terminar con este punto: "No se oponen, por tanto, el idealismo y el materialismo sino la voluntad proyectiva de D. Quijote y la voluntad receptiva de Sancho". (A. Castro, obra citada, p. 290.)

[25] "Maneras de comentar el *Quijote*", O. C., III, pp. 1081 y 1082. Resulta muy interesante —para percatarse de la agudeza valerina— comparar cuanto dice Valera acerca de la religiosidad de Cervantes, con lo que opina el profesor A. Castro en el capítulo "Cervantes y la Inquisición" de su citada obra (pp. 185-193).

fiestan de una manera muy sutil en el diálogo del capítulo VIII de
la segunda parte, en el que caballero y escudero mantienen cada
uno su punto de vista, terminando por quedar el sentimiento religioso triunfante sobre las ambiciones de gloria y poderío de los
caballeros, sin desdeñar el que se compaginen las aventuras y el
ardor guerreros al servicio de la patria.

Mírese el *Quijote* por el lado que se mire, puede demostrarse
que Cervantes dista mucho de querer burlarse del espíritu caballeresco. No es su novela, como quería Montesquieu, "la reacción y
la mofa del espíritu nacional español". Todo lo contrario: según
él, es la síntesis del espíritu guerrero y religioso cargado de sano
realismo sin dejar de entusiasmarse con lo bello y lo grande.

En otras dos ocasiones vuelve don Juan a ocuparse, con cierto
detalle, del *Quijote*. La primera en 1898, con motivo de la publicación en Edimburgo [26] de una nueva edición a cargo del hispanista
británico James Fitzmaurice-Kelly; la segunda resultó ser la obra
póstuma de nuestro autor [27]. La muerte le sorprendió cuando dictaba un nuevo discurso que la Academia le había encargado para
el centenario del *Quijote*. Hizo así el destino que se despidiera don
Juan del cultivo de las letras trabajando en un tema que era muy
de su predilección. Ni el artículo, por su brevedad, ni el discurso,
por haber quedado inconcluso, añaden mucho a las observaciones
que había hecho anteriormente.

Lástima grande, volvemos a repetir, que la manera de ser de
Valera, su pereza y poca afición al trabajo de investigación crítica
verdadera nos haya privado de unos estudios fundamentales en tema
tan español como interesante. Su agudeza de ingenio y su simpatía
por la obra se compaginaban a maravilla para haberlo hecho. Podemos repetir las palabras de Clarín escritas a principios de siglo:

---

[26] O. C., II, p. 983.
[27] O C., III, p. 1246.

"Cosa rica sería... un libro de Valera dedicado al *Quijote* por dentro, y acaso es el español de hoy más a propósito para tal empeño ." [28].

LA NOVELA PICARESCA

Tres cualidades de *la novela picaresca* disgustaban a don Juan:

a) Su pretencioso didactismo.

b) Las descripciones "excesivamente realistas", para su gusto.

c) El retorcido estilo que, en busca de bellezas, se complica más y más llegando hasta la afectación, oponiéndose al natural fluir de la prosa que era el ideal de Valera.

Tres pretextos suficientes para que cierre sus ojos críticos a tal tema y nos deje ayunos de consejo, puesto que las raras notas que encontramos referentes a él son siempre de carácter negativo, sin esforzarse lo más mínimo para darnos a conocer el juicio que *El Lazarillo*, *Guzmán* o *Don Pablos* y sus andanzas por el mundo literario le merecían. Si tal le ocurría con la picaresca, se comprende fácilmente el poco amor que por Quevedo y Góngora sintió.

QUEVEDO

A Quevedo le estudió como pensador y filósofo, dedicándole cuatro largos ensayos, en donde se percibe el horror que a Valera le producía el conceptismo (no menor que el que sintió por el culteranismo). Considera a Quevedo "altísimo ingenio" pero "insufrible y enmarañado culterano" en ocasiones [29]. No le perdona tampoco al señor de la Torre de Juan Abad la capacidad satírica, puesto que "exacerbó nuestra inclinación a la sátira fundada en la

---

[28] Leopoldo Alas, *Siglo pasado*, Madrid, 1901, p. 69.

[29] "Correspondencia", O. C., III, p. 779.

caricatura, torciendo nuestros espíritus como se ponen convexas algunas partes de los espejos, a fin de que lo que en ellos se refleja aparezca más feo, deforme y dislocado que en la realidad y promueva a risa" [30]. Si bien admira la lírica de Quevedo, no se tradujo tal simpatía en algún análisis crítico que nos lo confirme.

GÓNGORA

Con el autor de las *Soledades* aún fue menos generoso, pues, aunque admite que fue extraordinario poeta en los romances y letrillas, lo llama autor de "desatinos y extravagancias" y encuentra cosas de "perverso gusto" en las *Soledades* y el *Polifemo* [31]. Juicios que nos evitan, por lo elocuentes, comentario alguno y nos vuelven a mostrar al hombre incapaz de vencer sus principios, esos prejuicios que le impiden ver con toda imparcialidad, agrandando así las lagunas de su crítica.

EL TEATRO

Tanto más es de lamentar la falta de trabajos salidos de su pluma sobre nuestro teatro de los Siglos de Oro, cuanto que fue un tema que le satisfizo siempre y al que consagró muchas horas de lectura. No encontramos más disculpa que la consabida pereza valerina y el temor de comprometerse a un trabajo en el que le constaba había que andarse con pies de plomo, pues era campo en el que practicaba lo mejor de la crítica europea.

Muy pocas son las notas originales y no siempre muy acertadas. Comparar a Lope de Vega con el océano y a Shakespeare con un lago nos parece fruto de ese españolismo orgulloso de que él

---

[30] "Nuevas cartas americanas", O. C., III, p. 451.
[31] O. C., II, p. 8 y O. C., III, p. 215.

mismo nos habló[32]. Considera a Lope como el más grande dramaturgo español, si bien prefiere a Tirso como artista superior, ya que,
sin tener el genio creador de Lope, sabe perfeccionar, pulir y her-
mosear lo que aquél había inventado primero[33]. Afirmación que demuestra su independencia de criterio frente a los reconocidos juicios
que admitían la superioridad dramática y el genio calderoniano
sobre todos nuestros autores, como querían los críticos alemanes.
No olvidemos que a Tirso le estudió sin respaldarse mucho en otras
obras que las del fraile mercedario, mientras que para Lope o Calderón tiene siempre presente una buena dosis de erudición; a Tirso
debió leerlo con su genio crítico en libertad y proclamar abiertamente sus conclusiones, aunque no vayan muy de acuerdo con las
de otros.

Mas los análisis que hace de las obras de Tirso no son, por
desgracia, tan extensos como para poder ser considerados magis-
trales.

Para juzgar a Lope de Vega se vale de los prólogos y notas que
a la edición de las obras completas estaba realizando don Marcelino Menéndez y Pelayo.

A Calderón, al que dedicó un largo artículo destinado al *Diccionario Enciclopédico* ya citado, le analiza siguiendo muy de cerca
la obra, también de su amigo don Marcelino, *Calderón y su teatro,*
lo que no impedirá que Valera exponga sus propias opiniones, a
veces en completo desacuerdo con las del autor de *Los Heterodoxos*[34].

No le parece muy justo el trato que para con Calderón ha tenido la crítica. Primero fue juzgado por defecto, más tarde por
exceso, por los críticos del XVIII y el XIX, respectivamente.

---

[32] "Sobre el drama religioso en España", O. C., II, p. 341.
[33] *Ibidem.*
[34] "Pedro Calderón de la Barca", O. C., II, pp. 767-780.

La Devoción de la Cruz es para don Juan una de las obras superiores de Calderón. Es a la que dedicó su más personal análisis, en el que, frente al sentir de don Marcelino, la encuentra natural de estilo y lenguaje, versificación perfecta y no echa de ver en ella los "tiquismiquis culteranos" de la época.

El drama "de honor" del teatro de Calderón no le parece a Valera ni más poético ni más dramático que el drama de celos de Shakespeare. Encuentra alambicada, demasiado poco natural esa preocupación exagerada por la honra, de los personajes calderonianos. Al marido podría decirse que se le da un comino del engaño de su mujer; sólo lo siente por su honra, la cual ha de ser reparada por un crimen mayor que el pecado, el asesinato a sangre fría, lo que le parece absurdo, aunque en la época del autor esto fuera lo natural.

En cuanto a las comedias de capa y espada, son más convencionales y más falsas que las de Tirso. Acusa a los galanes y damas de Calderón de estar todos ellos "vaciados en el mismo molde". Le cansan los "discreteos archicultos e impertinentes" de estas damas en sus diálogos de amor y celos. Ni tan chistoso como Lope ni tan buen constructor dramático como Tirso es Calderón a los ojos de don Juan.

Conociendo los gustos de Valera podemos concluir, tras la lectura de este artículo, que Calderón no le apasionaba como autor dramático. No se atrevió a ir contra la opinión general, nacional y extranjera, pues ello le iba a exigir un esfuerzo superior a sus fuerzas. Tomó el camino del medio: señaló los defectos de modo superficial, haciendo una crítica negativa que él mismo había condenado por ineficaz y parcial.

Para terminar con este punto, establezcamos la "calificación por méritos" que asignó Valera a nuestros dramaturgos clásicos: En primer lugar, y fuera de toda posible comparación, Lope de Vega. (Sin que olvidemos que personalmente don Juan prefirió a Tirso.) Le sigue "el fraile de la Merced", que "perfecciona y eleva las obras de aquél", que si eran geniales también eran imperfectas. Por último, Calderón, Alarcón, Moreto y Rojas, formando un sólido grupo [35].

GRACIÁN

Hay un autor con el que don Juan nos parece que fue a todas luces injusto. Un autor que era la "mezcla más insufrible de conceptismo y culteranismo", las dos enfermedades más graves de nuestras letras, según el cerrado —en esta ocasión— criterio valerino. Nos referimos al jesuita Baltasar Gracián. Le dedicó un breve artículo —tan breve como feroz— en una de sus cartas americanas, al publicarse una nueva edición de *El héroe* y *El discreto*. Conocía don Juan las alabanzas que de Gracián había hecho Schopenhauer, autor por el que no sintió nunca muchas simpatías, dadas las características de pesimismo y amargura que encontraba en él, tan opuestas a su personal filosofía de "encontrarlo todo bien en esta vida". Y, movido un tanto por el deseo de contradecir al filósofo nórdico cuanto llevado de su desamor por el culteranismo y el conceptismo, escribió contra Gracián uno de los ataques más duros que salieron de su pluma [36]. Recordemos cómo había tratado a Góngora y Quevedo, y digamos, no para justificar a Valera sino para dejar en claro su postura, que mantenía que la crítica podía ser "feroz y despiadada" solamente cuando el atacado había desaparecido muchos años o siglos antes. ¡Sólo a los muertos se les debe justicia total!, repite varias veces, como si justicia significara siempre castigo.

Hay muchas otras referencias de toda índole a lo largo de la obra crítica de Valera, que atañen a nuestros autores del Siglo de

---

[35] O. C., II, p. 780.
[36] "Cartas a la Nación", O. C., III, p. 581.

Oro. Como siempre van expuestas como ejemplos explicativos que confirman sus puntos de vista y son, además, demasiado breves en su mayoría, si bien las tenemos en cuenta para la valoración global del crítico, no son analizadas aquí por separado.

Capítulo VI

EL SIGLO XVIII

La postura de Valera con respecto a los autores del siglo XVIII español no resulta muy clara la primera vez que el lector se enfrenta con sus juicios. Pretende reconocer los defectos del siglo, por un lado, y se muestra empeñado en encontrar y hacer resaltar las virtudes, por el otro. Se diría que, más que nunca, con las letras del siglo de las luces se encuentra incómodamente preso entre sus prejuicios y la realidad de los hechos. Había negado obstinadamente que la literatura española hubiese pasado por etapas de marcadas influencias extranjeras. Épocas en las cuales nuestras letras habían perdido su casticismo y se tiñeron de los colores de los países de más allá del Pirineo.

Para don Juan —defensor de la personalidad radicalmente incontaminada e independiente de nuestra literatura— las influencias que llegaron, en ocasiones, a nuestro país fueron tan por completo asimiladas que produjeron nuevos frutos, más cercanos y similares a los que de siempre habíamos tenido, que "los del jardín ajeno" de donde procedían. Para decirlo con sus palabras: "Que en la literatura española no hubo nunca solución de continuidad". Que era incierto afirmar que el espíritu grandioso de nuestros Siglos de Oro no había tenido digna continuación a lo largo del XVIII.

Con objeto de probar tan arriesgada tesis se verá obligado, si no a elogiar por demás a escritores en quienes no puede por menos de reconocer defectos e influencias, sí al menos a disculpar con un discreto y sagaz silencio los nombres y obras que menos le satisfacen. Pero no tan discreto como para que no descubramos, en silencios tan elocuentes, el verdadero sentir de Valera.

Si no puede negar que la nueva dirección que imprimió al espíritu español el movimiento iniciado por Luzán venía de fuera, que era "anticastizo" en sus orígenes, afirma que "dejó vivo el espíritu de nuestro pueblo, el germen de su pensamiento y hasta las formas en que debía manifestarse". Los brotes de gusto francés encuentran "abundante caudal en la rica vena del ingenio propio", con lo que, lejos de ahogar las antiguas plantas de la civilización española, le sirvieron como de poda rejuvenecedora, privando al árbol de sus ramas inútiles [1].

Otra de las virtudes que achaca al llamado seudo-clasicismo francés fue "que nos sacó del aislamiento en que vivíamos", rompiendo aquella especie de cordón sanitario a que nos había sometido la suspicacia religiosa, temerosa de contagios dañinos. La vuelta a los escritores clásicos griegos y latinos, como en el Renacimiento, produjo las mejores traducciones en español [2].

Por encima de los remedos franceses, por encima incluso del tinte de las doctrinas enciclopedistas y revolucionarias que tan bien habían asimilado, se alzan las quintillas de la "Fiesta de toros en Madrid" y la "Oda a Pedro Romero" de Nicolás Fernández de Moratín.

---

[1] "Ventura de la Vega", O. C., II, pp. 577-594.
[2] Idem, p. 578.

Valera, llevado del afán de restar importancia a cuanto tomaron de Francia nuestros poetas neoclásicos, apunta como otra fuente la lírica italiana del mismo período. Sostiene que la escuela que había fundado Giuseppe Parini tuvo su eco entre los poetas españoles, como lo había tenido la poesía de principios del xvi; huellas felices de tal imitación pueden rastrearse en las composiciones de Gallego y Quintana, así como en las sátiras de Jovellanos y, por la forma, en muchos de los versos de don Leandro Fernández de Moratín [3].

EL TEATRO

En lo único que admite Valera copia servil de los franceses es en la tragedia neoclásica, que fue según él "un completo fracaso" [4].

En lo cómico, donde se conserva la mejor tradición clásica, brillan los nombres de dos autores que son dignos continuadores de nuestro mejor teatro; Moratín, hijo, "admirable por su aticismo, sobriedad y elegancia", había creado casi por entero "la verdadera comedia de costumbres española", y don Ramón de la Cruz, demócrata por instinto, que fustiga a la "caída y depravada nobleza" poniendo en el pueblo bajo, en medio de su grosera y graciosa ignorancia, las heroicas virtudes que mostrará en la lucha por la independencia.

Estos dos autores, Moratín y don Ramón de la Cruz, cada uno por su estilo y a pesar de todos sus defectos, representan mejor que los poetas líricos el grito castizo, una muestra del genio de la raza, según Valera, en el pretendido siglo afrancesado. Desgraciadamente, aunque demuestra que su agudeza supo columbrar la importancia exacta de ambas figuras, en especial la de Moratín, no escribió un detallado análisis de la obra que parecía conocer tan bien como

---

[3] O. C., II, p. 579.
[4] "El Duque de Rivas", O. C., II, p. 733.

nadie. (El artículo dedicado a don Ramón de la Cruz [5] —de circunstancias, escrito con motivo de la colocación de una placa en la
casa en que vivió el famoso sainetista— no es más que un extracto
declarado del libro de don Emilio Cotarelo *Don Ramón de la Cruz
y sus obras,* publicado en Madrid, 1900.)

LA LÍRICA

Tampoco dedicó especiales análisis a los poetas líricos del XVIII
que, según sus declaraciones en varios lugares, atraían su atención.
Consideraba a Quintana y Meléndez Valdés como dignos de figu-
rar entre nuestros más grandes líricos. Sólo dio algunas referencias
para apoyar la mencionada tesis de que nuestro neoclasicismo no
fue tan francés como querían demostrar.

La escuela salmantina del XVIII había sido el primer brote de
un renacer poético que mirando hacia lo nacional (Fray Diego González a Fray Luis de León, Cadalso a Villegas, Iglesias siguiendo
a Quevedo y Góngora) hizo posible la aparición de Juan Meléndez
Valdés.

Con Meléndez fue Valera un poco más generoso. Analizó con-
cisamente su obra y la influencia que tuvo sobre sus dos discípulos,
Quintana y Gallego. El exceso de almíbar en la sensibilidad de Meléndez es acaso la razón por la que el lector de hoy no se entusiasma con sus versos. Era un mal general en la época y, por tanto,
disculpable. Sus olorcillos campestres, sus delicados pastores y za-
galas tal vez nos resulten demasiado alquitarados —dice don Juan—
para nuestro gusto. El abuso de los diminutivos "cariñosos y meli-
fluos" que se perciben en la obra de Meléndez arranca notas un
tanto burlonas en la crítica que le dedica; pero más que defectos
verdaderos, más que manchas, son "verdaderos lunarcitos". Defecti-
llos que se compensan con la virtud principal de un estilo "que

---

5 "Ramón de la Cruz", O. C., II, p. 1013.

enlaza la espontánea y natural sencillez a la refinada delicadeza que jamás le abandona ni le deja caer en prosaísmo". Supo cantar el sano amor quizá "un tantico sensual y desenvuelto" con la ternura que nadie pondría después [6].

A Quintana, por quien Valera declaró siempre haber sentido el máximo grado de admiración, tampoco le dedicó sino brevísimo espacio en el análisis general que puso al frente del *Florilegio de poesías castellanas del siglo XIX* (Madrid, ed. Fe, 1900).

Defendiéndole contra Menéndez Pelayo (quien en su libro *Horacio en España* había atacado con dureza al cantor de la libertad y del progreso), lo declara "el primero de nuestros líricos, salvo Espronceda y Fray Luis", exageración evidente que podemos perdonarle por el cariño que sentía hacia aquél [7].

Valera no olvidó a otros dos poetas españoles que se vieron obligados a vivir fuera de España, llevados de un excesivo extranjerismo en las ideas de que estaban imbuidos: el Abate Marchena y José María Blanco White. Percibió con agudeza que ambos eran más interesantes por sus peripecias vitales que por su producción poética. Analiza la obra en español del autor hispano-británico (hijo de madre española y padre irlandés), la que califica de "elegante medianía", y dice que para llamarle gran poeta habría que recurrir al famoso soneto *Death and Night,* tan alabado por Coleridge. Marchena, más erudito que poeta, tiene, según Valera, estimables versos escritos antes de su ruptura con la Iglesia.

---

[6] "Juan Meléndez Valdés", O. C., II, pp. 1016 y ss.

[7] O. C., II, p. 389. Vuelve a repetir esta afirmación en el artículo "Horacio en España", O. C., II, p. 504.

EL ROMANTICISMO

CONTRADICCIONES VALERINAS

Algunas de las contradicciones que en los artículos de Valera pueden encontrarse han de ser achacadas, más que a miopía crítica, a su encend:do "españolismo". El calor, la pasión que pone al defender la literatura de su amada España le lleva a tomar posturas que más tarde le obligarán a contradecirse. Por ejemplo: hemos visto su terquedad, su obstinada negación a admitir el claro influjo francés en nuestras letras del XVIII. Le vimos hacer maravillas de silencios para no hablar de las comedias a la francesa de Moratín, hijo, de las adaptaciones y traducciones que del país vecino tomó para España. Habla del casticismo de los autores llamados "afrancesados". Pues bien: cuando dirige su lente hacia otros problemas, parece olvidar los sofismas que ha tenido que utilizar anteriormente, o, si no los inventó entonces, se verá obligado a crearlos ahora. Así, por ejemplo, cuando le vemos estudiando el romanticismo, su primera gran afirmación nos deja un tanto confusos:

"Entre nosotros [el Romanticismo] vino a libertar a los poetas del yugo ridículo de los preceptistas franceses y a separarlos de la imitación superficial y mal entend:da de los clásicos, y lo consiguió" [1].

"Yugo ridículo de los preceptistas franceses" que había negado toda su vida.

Negar que el Romanticismo era un movimiento literario cuyas raíces habían llegado a nuestro país desde Alemania, a través de Francia, le pareció demasiado a don Juan. Los hechos eran tan evidentes, la revolución literaria tan próxima a él, que sus afirmaciones hubieran sido fácilmente rebatidas por los mismos poetas que la comenzaron. No negó, porque sería negar lo evidente; pero puso todo su empeño en descubrir las cualidades originales que va adquiriendo el Romanticismo en nuestro país a med:da que va arraigando en él. Estudiando lo que hubo de genuinamente español y señalando lo extranjero más como defecto que como virtud. Otra vez su "españolismo" haciéndole falsear los datos; con su consabida sagacidad, ilumina las partes que sabe se asientan sobre la tradición más española, mientras deja voluntariamente en sombra los ángulos que le parecen extranjeros. Y cuando proyecta su luz sobre ellos lo hace con "la sana intención" de mostrar sus imperfecciones al lector. Guardó tal actitud singular en cuantos artículos se refieren a esta materia, y son varios y de no escasa importancia [2].

Ya en su juvenil artículo sobre el Romanticismo —escrito en 1856— había dicho Valera: "El romanticismo no ha de cons:derarse, hoy día, como secta militante, sino como cosa pasada y perteneciente a la historia" [3].

---

[1] "Del Romanticismo en España", O. C., II, p. 9.

[2] Quizá, de entre todos, el más importante sea el consagrado al Duque de Rivas, O. C., II, pp. 729-767.
Véanse también los estudios que puso al frente de su "Florilegio de poetas castellanos", O. C., II, pp. 1187 a 1381.

[3] O. C., II, p. 9.

SU   PERSONALÍSI-
MO   ROMANTICISMO

Si tenemos en cuenta estas palabras, entenderemos esa especie
de "enorme distancia" que parece poner Valera entre el momento
en que él escribe y la vuelta a España de los emigrados, y con ellos
la fiebre romántica. Contempló el romanticismo siempre desde fuera, como espectador. Lo más curioso es que recibe, aunque no lo ad-
mita nunca, muchas de las características de los héroes de sus
novelas. Antonio, don Faustino en especial, están aquejados de muchos de los males románticos. Morsamor, la misma Rafaela la generosa, que no es más que una rebelde a ese sino que la condena
a ser lo que ella no quiere, tienen la rebeldía romántica de que don
Juan se burla tan a menudo. No es éste el lugar adecuado para
analizar cuantos detalles románticos pueden espigarse entre las
creaciones de Valera, pero podemos afirmar que tuvo mucha más
influencia de lo que nos decía en su divertida autobiografía. Si es
cierto que "se curó pronto de la fiebre romántica" fue, a nuestro
juicio, solamente del "sarpullido romántico" de lo que se curó. Lo
externo, las burdas imitaciones que se traslucen en sus versos juveniles. Dejó pronto de hacer versos "a lo Espronceda" y "a lo
Byron". Mas lo que Valera continuó haciendo toda su vida —inconscientemente, claro— fue discurrir sobre muchos puntos con las
mismas características de que se burlaba en *Las inquietudes del
Doctor Faustino*.

Jean Krynen, el hispanista francés, en su estudio "L'esthétisme
de Juan Valera" también lo ve así: *Le tempérament artistique de
J. Valera, romantique d'inspiration, répugne à la complaisance romantique à l'égard de la nature et à l'effusion sentimentale* [4].

----

[4] J. Krynen, "L'esthétisme de J. Valera", en *Acta Salmanticensia*, II,
2, Salamanca, 1946, p. 10.

Don Juan, puesto a analizarse, se consideraba seguidor solamente de los clásicos. No sospecha lo que su personalidad tiene
—todo lo escondido que se quiera— de personaje romántico. Su
frialdad de razonador es cierto que no era romántica. De aquí el
que, cuando se analice, no perciba que, cuando se trata de obrar,
cuando hay algo más que el puro cerebro en movimiento, la frialdad y mesura de los clásicos desaparecen para dar paso al hombre
impetuoso y apasionado de los románticos.

La desgana, aquella melancolía que le domina otras veces en
cuanto la actividad mundana le permite un reposo, o cuando encuentra que sus deseos más íntimos están muy lejos de ser satis-
fechos; esa especie de malestar consigo mismo que veremos aflorar
tantas veces en sus escritos públicos o privados, ¿qué son sino
notas o posos románticos asimilados por él mucho más profundamente de lo que imaginaba?

Nada más lejos de nuestra intención que pretender pintar a don
Juan como figura romántica. Pretendemos señalar solamente que
ni su obra ni su persona quedan tan lejos de la época romántica
como él repitió en tantas ocasiones.

Contemplaba el espectáculo romántico como lo contempló todo:
con la frialdad de su claro razonar, que le mostraba, tal vez exageradamente, los pros y los contras de cada doctrina. No aceptó voluntariamente los dogmas que le mostraban, de donde provienen sus
negaciones. Pero muchas de aquellas experiencias, de aquellas modas literarias que él negaba, fueron moldeando, con los años, su
alma y allí quedaron para siempre. Combatirá aún con más fuego
y pasión el naturalismo y el realismo.

Ni romántico, ni realista, ni naturalista. Pretendió —mas sin
conseguirlo realmente— ser fiel a un clasicismo de espíritu que no
se doblegaba a lo que consideraba influjos pasajeros y mucho menos
cuando éstos llegaban de otros países.

Su afán por encontrar en nuestro romanticismo el mayor número posible de características nacionales le hizo ver con agudeza una

especie de preparación ideal, como de anuncio profético de lo que iba a ser el nuevo movimiento literario, preparación que empezó mucho antes de la vuelta a España de los emigrados. Señala la afición por los romances de don Agustín Durán, a quien llama el profeta del movimiento; el desarrollo de los estudios de los arabistas; y una especial mentalidad casi enfermiza en las gentes que preceden inmediatamente a la época romántica, un algo de soñador y tétrico y un pesimismo "ya lánguido ya desesperado que inducía a buscar la bienaventuranza en pasados tiempos fantásticos" [5].

La vuelta de los emigrados, en 1834, señala el comienzo de una nueva era política y literaria. Pero "nuevo", para Valera, no significa "extranjero". Venían los emigrados con lo mejor de sus ideas fermentadas al contacto con lo de fuera. Pero ideas españolas, antes que nada. Traen una literatura que se levanta en protesta contra el poder que pretende encerrar el pensamiento nacional y dirigir las ideas por un cauce determinado [6].

Según don Juan, los defectos principales del romanticismo son: el sentimentalismo exagerado, la misantropía y el fingido odio a la humanidad y a la civilización, males que procedían de Rousseau. El poeta tenía que ser "planta maldita" y dar "frutos de perdición", no pudiendo amar más que a la mujer ideal, la cual no se encuentra personificada en este bajo mundo. Pero el verdadero y más notable de los defectos románticos le parece "la verbosidad". Esa pompa y pretendida armoniosidad no logran encubrir lo vacío de sentido de muchas de sus obras. Abusaron de la utilización de frases y palabras como "esponjado tulipán", "ágil y pintado colorín", "negro capuz", "lúgubre son", "fúnebre ciprés", "flotante tul", "pliegues del viento y raudo torbellino", etc. [7].

---

[5] "Poesía lírica y épica del siglo XIX", O. C., II, pp. 1195-1196.
[6] O. C., III, p. 739.
[7] O. C., II, p. 12.

Tampoco le gustaba la hipocresía del romanticismo español. Fingían demostrar una fe que estaban muy lejos de poseer. Como era de esperar, tales defectos los achaca Valera a las influencias extranjeras.

Analiza brevemente, pero con bastante objetividad, la labor de los emigrados "mayores y menores".

MAURY Y MARTÍ-
NEZ DE LA ROSA

A Juan María Maury, el poeta malagueño, le encuentra notas comunes con otro malagueño ilustre, don Serafín Estébanez Calderón, en cuanto ambos "cincelan", pulen y esmaltan el idioma. Ve lo que de clásico y de romántico hay en la producción de Maury, ensalzando sobre todo el singular poema "Esvero y Almedora", compuesto sobre el asunto del célebre *Paso honroso* de Suero de Quiñones; la obra de Maury, a pesar de lo enmarañado de su argumento y de su poca popularidad, es libro digno de estudio por sus primores y excelencias poéticas.

Don Francisco Martínez de la Rosa "no traspasa los más altos grados de la medianía". No disimula Valera demasiado la poca simpatía que le inspira la obra del conocido político. Como don Juan no gusta de la crítica adversa, se abstiene de castigar con dureza, aun cuando deja bien claro que no le estima en mucho como poeta.

Poco entusiasmo debió sentir hacia la obra de José Joaquín de Mora; la juzga, si no con maliciosa bondad como la del anterior, con elocuente frialdad.

EL DUQUE DE RIVAS

Reservó las alabanzas mejores, así como el más largo y acabado ensayo de los que dedicó a nuestros románticos, al Duque de Ri-

vas [8]. No sólo por ser el Duque, para Valera, el mejor ejemplo de
"poeta-señor" que el siglo XIX español podía mostrar al mundo;
no sólo por el recuerdo y la amistad de sus años de juventud
en Nápoles (alegres días de juvenil y despreocupada holgazanería
poética en grado sumo), sino también por sincera admiración hacia
la obra poética de aquél. Claro que, conviene que recordemos, la
obra de Rivas se ajusta, en su mayor parte, al ideal poético de don
Juan. Porque puede decirse, ante el aire clásico de muchas de sus
composiciones, que el Duque es el menos romántico de nuestros
románticos, cuidándose muy bien Valera de ensalzar especialmente
las obras menos "teñidas de los defectos románticos". Encarnaba
también el Duque el ejemplo español de poeta que había recibido
savia y alimento vivificador del extranjero, sin dejar por ello de tener
enraizadas sus plantas en lo más castizo de nuestras letras. Ensalzando al Duque, a la vez que obra en justicia, puesto que es la
obra que más estima, daba don Juan con habilidad el último toque
a sus principales teorías sobre la importancia del casticismo en
todas las manifestaciones literarias de valor.

El Duque no significa (contra lo que opinaba en su trabajo
"Le Duc de Rivas", publicado en la *Revue des Deux Mondes* [9], el
erudito francés Charles de Mazade) un renacimiento de nuestra
poesía, sino que se encontró a sí mismo "en una época de floreci-
miento literario y poético todo lo español y todo lo original y castizo que era posible entonces".

Bajo el ejemplo y la emulación de Gallego, Arriaza y Quintana, se forma en la mejor poesía clásica española durante sus años
de estancia en Cádiz; en aquellas lecturas habría que buscar la raíz
de su clasicismo. Naturalmente, es esta poesía de los primeros tiempos la que más ensalza don Juan. Niega, además, que el poeta in-

---

[8] "El Duque de Rivas", O. C., II, pp. 729-767.
[9] Charles de Mazade, "Le Duc de Rivas", en *Revue des Deux Mondes*, 1846, 13, pp. 327 y s.

glés John Frere, en la isla de Malta, iniciara al Duque en las lecturas y el mundo de nuestros clásicos, como mantuvo Cueto en su obra *Bosquejo de la poesía*. Pudo aconsejarle en alguna ocasión sobre otros puntos poéticos, pero, cuando los avatares políticos condujeron al Duque a la isla del Mediterráneo, ya iba —en opinión del crítico— cargado con las mejores virtudes poéticas nacionales. Allí, como los demás emigrados en otros puntos, no haría "sino madurar sus anteriores conocimientos". Muy poco debió a las letras inglesas, salvo algún reflejo del falso Ossian, ni nada tampoco a los alemanes. Sus mejores poesías ("Al Faro de Malta" y "A las estrellas") son las "más clásicas, las más horacianas y las más académicas". Baja mucho en calidad en sus composiciones políticas, a las que califica Valera de "declamaciones falsamente apasionadas" [10].

Entre los "poemas épicos" del Duque establece un orden de bellezas: el primer lugar lo ocupa "El moro expósito", seguido por los "Romances históricos", los poemas "El paso honroso", "Florinda" y las leyendas "La azucena milagrosa", "El aniversario" y "Maldonado".

El excesivo encomio que Valera hizo del *Paso honroso,* en contra de la opinión de la mayoría de la crítica, sospechamos que se debe a que la obra fue escrita en 1812, en plena juventud del Duque. Tal dato era un argumento más en favor de la tesis valerina.

Analiza con detención estas y otras obras del Duque, en especial los romances, iluminando con agudos comentarios y verdadero amor tan extenso ensayo.

Termina estudiando en detalle los dramas del Duque. Alaba como el mejor el *Don Álvaro* y lo defiende de la acusación que le habían hecho de estar inspirado en una obra de Mérimée —la novela *Les âmes du purgatoire*—, siendo la realidad, según Valera, todo lo contrario, puesto que el Duque había escrito y dado su obra al escritor galo (traducida previamente al francés por Antonio

---

[10] "El Duque de Rivas", O. C., II, pp. 742 y ss.

Alcalá Galiano) con objeto de que aquél la hiciera poner en escena en el teatro de la Porte Saint-Martin. El manuscrito estuvo en poder de Mérimée mucho tiempo y parece ser que se perdió, y cuando, vuelto el Duque a España, la reclamó y no se la devolvieron, hubo de retraducirla al español, o escribirla de nuevo. La coincidencia con la novela de Mérimée, por otro lado, es mínima, y ambos autores valían suficientemente como para no "plagiarse".

ESPRONCEDA

Menos espacio que al Duque, aunque no menor comprensión, estudio y admiración, dedicó don Juan a Espronceda, autor, en su opinión, "el más romántico de España" [11].

En uno de los primeros artículos (de 1854) analizó con aguda visión el movimiento romántico y a las figuras que consideraba capitales: El Duque de Rivas, Zorrilla y Espronceda. Y ya entonces percibimos la especial admiración que siente por el cantor de Teresa. Admiración que tiene más valor si consideramos que Espronceda, como poeta romántico, es casi la suma total de las virtudes contrarias a las que Valera consideraba que debían adornar a todo gran poeta. Precisamente aplaude en él la pasión, el gran corazón que "se convierte en versos maravillosos" [12].

Supo amar y expresar el amor como nadie, porque "sólo explica bien el amor el que sabe sentirle e inspirarle". ¡Qué diferencia entre la raíz verdadera de don Félix de Montemar y el tremendismo fanfarrón del *Tenorio*, de Zorrilla! La prodigiosa imaginación,

---

11 "Del Romanticismo en España y de Espronceda", O. C., II, páginas 7 a 19. Véase también el artículo del "Florilegio", O. C., II, pp. 1318-1322.
12 "Del Romanticismo en España y de Espronceda", O. C., II, páginas 14 y siguiente.

la profunda melancolía del "cuento del estudiante", son difícil-
mente superadas en cualquier otra producción romántica.

No niega Valera las influencias que ejercieron otros poetas sobre Espronceda: Lord Byron (a quien en ocasiones, la carta de
doña Elvira por ejemplo, casi traduce, aunque "primorosamente y
más llena de sentimiento que la del poeta inglés"); Béranger, cuya
"Canción del cosaco" inspiró la del mismo título a nuestro poeta,
y Goethe, cuyo *Fausto* toma Espronceda como fuente de inspiración para su *Diablo Mundo*. Mas por encima de estas imitaciones
está la castiza y pura condición, el ser original y grande del poeta
español. Incluso admitiendo la inferioridad del estudio, de una
cultura profunda cual la que adornaba a los creadores del *Fausto*
y *Childe Harold,* podemos los españoles calificar de genio a Espronceda tan legítimamente como califican a los otros dos en Alemania e Inglaterra. Aunque los supere —en algunos trozos geniales de elegancia de la mejor y en fuerza emotiva— en determinados
pasajes, Espronceda es más desordenado y desigual que Byron, y
sus obras carecen de los espléndidos planes a que se atienen las
del alemán.

Sin que la pasión ciegue al crítico, valoró justa y claramente la
obra poética de Espronceda sin el acostumbrado frío razonar de los
temas que no le apasionaban.

ZORRILLA

No menor cariño sintió Valera por Zorrilla, el "más nacional
de nuestros románticos", sin que por ello le dedicara más espacio
que a Espronceda. Al igual que a aquél, siempre que tiene ocasión
le llama "altísimo poeta", lo que no impide que, al analizar sus
obras, señale los defectos que se le aparecen como sobresalientes.
Defectos que le perdona gustosamente don Juan en gracia a "su
irreflexiva fantasía, fácil y rara elocuencia y su rica y poderosa
imaginación".

En el artículo de juventud, dedicado al padre del Tenorio, se encuentran enumerados muchos más defectos que los que pueden verse en otros escritos más tardíos sobre el mismo tema; seguro que con los años fue Valera admirando más las buenas cualidades de la poesía de Zorrilla y disimulando —ya que no las oculta— lo que consideraba faltas. Admiraba en él sobre todo lo que había de trovador con ansia de agradar, la sencillez y el candor con que dice las cosas y no con la obligada "pose" que Valera afeaba en Baudelaire y en Hugo. Le perdona incluso lo que de alambicado y tenebroso ponía a veces en su obra.

No olvidó tampoco a otros poetas de menor importancia, como Nicomedes Pastor Díaz, que "trajo a Zorrilla a escena" y se "retiró después modestamente", Mariano Roca de Togores, Marqués de Molíns, el Duque de Frías y Miguel de los Santos Álvarez, quien, pese a lo desordenado y extravagante de su escasa obra, demostró en ella ingenio y buen gusto.

Para completar cuanto llevamos dicho respecto a la personal actitud de Valera frente al romanticismo, citaremos unas palabras que nos parece resumen con claridad la que se nos antoja postura de pueril patriotismo:

"Lo que tuvo el romanticismo de manía, de moda y remedo vino a España de Francia; pero lo esencial no vino de parte ninguna, como no vienen de Francia los frutos del otoño, ni las flores en la primavera, por más que coincidan en ambos países" [13].

Valera no prestó ninguna atención a la novela romántica salvo las ocasiones en que deja ver indirectamente su poca estima por las producciones de Fernández y González, a quien consideraba capaz de escribir mejor de lo que en realidad escribió.

---

[13] "El Duque de Rivas", O. C., II, p. 741.

EL TEATRO

No se molestó tampoco en analizar la tragedia romántica, a la que dedica sin embargo tibias alabanzas, pero siempre como escapando del compromiso de tener que estudiarla.

Podemos afirmar que el único autor dramático de la época (si se exceptúa el Duque de Rivas) al que Valera dedicó algún estudio, fue el menos afectado por el nuevo credo político, el más clásico: don Ventura de la Vega. El que había pasado a través de toda la fiebre romántica sin contagiarse, conservando su clasicismo más puro, con muy escasas tentativas románticas, las que abandonó inmediatamente para burlarse no poco de ellas.

Alaba especialmente la tragedia *La muerte de César*, a la que analiza comparándola con las del mismo tema de Shakespeare, Voltaire y Alfieri. A todos gana el español en la maestría con que observa las reglas del arte, en el primor y atildamiento del estilo y el orden con que huye de las extravagancias y monstruosidades. Pero en arte, continúa don Juan, no es esto todo, ni siquiera lo más importante. Alfieri supera al español en la profunda pasión que da origen a su inspiración, en el entusiasmo que echa de menos en el español y que "arde y palpita" en las páginas de aquél. En cuanto a Shakespeare, si más correcto y esmerado el español en la forma, no le alcanza en la consistencia y relieve que aquél dio a sus personajes. Lo que menos satisfizo a Valera de la obra de don Ventura fue el propósito pedagógico que movía la pluma del autor, al pretender servirse de la escena para dar una lección que no sentía.

A Ventura de la Vega le falta ese amor, esa compenetración con el personaje que se percibe en Shakespeare. Donde se aparta del autor inglés es menos bueno, donde "le imita o se inspira en él, quizá le sobrepuja"; y lo aclara estudiando una escena "inspirada" en otra similar de Shakespeare, comparando las frases en español y su fuente original en inglés.

La muerte de César le parece una obra sobresaliente, sólo comparable con la *Virginia* de Tamayo. Es incluso superior al *Pelayo* de Quintana e infinitamente mejor que el *Edipo* de Martínez de la Rosa y que las tragedias clásicas del siglo XVIII [14].

Aunque *El hombre de mundo,* comedia del mismo autor que la tragedia, gustase menos a don Juan, no dejó de reconocer en ella virtudes y méritos que la hacen ser como el germen de la moderna "alta comedia", género que don Jacinto Benavente perfeccionará y hará tan popular [15].

Mucho menos espacio dedicó a Bretón de los Herreros. Conoció y estimó en mucho la obra del costumbrista, lo que no impide que en uno de sus artículos, en las páginas de *El cócora* (año 1860), le propine un torniscón más que regular si se tiene en cuenta que don Juan no era partidario de la crítica violenta. Su pluma se volvió de una acidez desacostumbrada analizando la comedia *Elvira y Leandro,* y, enojado tal vez por considerar al costumbrista con mayores posibilidades de las que hacía gala en la comedia, o porque contribuía con su más que mediana pieza a incrementar el número de las de "baja calidad" con que se adornaba nuestro teatro de la época, lo cierto es que le censuró con una rigidez desacostumbrada. Don Juan, perdida la paciencia y los "buenos modales", fustigó a Bretón de los Herreros con una de las críticas más duras de las que salieron de su pluma. Censuras que levantaron una serie de réplicas y ataques al crítico en todos los periódicos y una carta del propio autor, a las que contestó don Juan en el número siguiente de su periódico ratificándose en su juicio, dando explicaciones a las explicaciones y pidiendo a Bretón que "pues es un gran autor, escriba como tal" [16].

---

14   O. C., II, pp. 355-361.

15   Véase también el estudio titulado "Ventura de la Vega", O. C., II, páginas 577-594.

16   "Revista de Teatros", O. C., II, pp. 184-185.

En su "Florilegio" [17], muchos años después, hace una crítica mucho menos apasionada y alaba el talento de don Manuel en su justo punto.

Muy raramente cita don Juan al maestro de la crítica satírica Mariano José de Larra, cuya popularidad contempló en todo su apogeo. Tal vez sea una explicación a este silencio la poca afición de nuestro autor por la sátira, género al que tenía verdadero horror, mas es lo cierto que las pocas líneas que le consagra dejan ver que nunca le tuvo en mucha estima [18].

---

[17] "Florilegio. Notas biográficas y críticas", O. C., II, pp. 1278-1283.
[18] O. C., II, p. 1303.

SEGUNDA MITAD DEL SIGLO XIX

"CUQUERÍA VALERINA"

A medida que el lector de la crítica de Valera avanza siguiendo un cierto orden cronológico en las obras analizadas, hasta llegar a las de sus contemporáneos, percibimos una especie de dificultad —a veces verdadera imposibilidad— para llegar a la valoración real que de la obra nos hace el crítico. En otras palabras: que no es fácil saber siempre con exactitud lo que don Juan quiere decir, pues tales son los repliegues, los circunloquios y los mil y un rodeos de que se vale para exponernos sus juicios sin herir susceptibilidades.

Tal postura dio lugar a que sus críticos llegaran a la conclusión de que, despojado del estilo y la gracia que en todos sus escritos puso Valera, no quedaba nada.

Jamás llegó Valera a las asperezas de Clarín o de Revilla, es cierto, pero tampoco es verdad que sea tan "bonachón", tan "dulce" como sus modales y la incomprensión de muchos lectores han hecho creer. Diríamos que es preciso un saber leer lo que escribió, un estar acostumbrado a los "juegos de magia" de su prosa y de su ingenio para captar en su totalidad los juicios casi siempre honestos y acertados, salvo cuando el error, en forma de teoría personal, le domina. En este caso, las pleguerías no son lo suficientemente densas como para que haya lugar a dudas.

Don Juan se nos aparece mucho más benévolo de lo que en realidad fue, porque temió la severidad excesiva. Teme hacer daño, "hacer sangre" en las carnes del autor y la obra criticados. Para "administrar" su crítica se valió siempre del "cloroformo" de que humorísticamente hablaba Ramón Pérez de Ayala. Este cloroformo de sus buenas maneras, la sutilísima ironía, a veces ocultan el juicio que en otros críticos menos temerosos aparece en la superficie de cuanto escriben.

Para encontrar la opinión sincera, desnuda de concesiones, hay que recurrir a sus cartas a los amigos. En ellas le oiremos hablar con una franqueza que asombra, teñida de un humorismo más pronunciado que en sus críticas publicadas.

No sólo son elocuentes los silencios valerinos. También son elocuentes, para quien logra prescindir de las "pleguerías" y veladuras, las alabanzas reticentes con que llenó muchos de sus escritos. Sírvanos de ejemplo uno dedicado a ensalzar un libro de versos. Uno de los muchos prólogos que su bondadosa condición y sus muchas amistades le obligaron a escribir, incapaz de negarse a quien se lo solicitaba.

Se trata del librito *Poesías hasta cierto punto*, de un señor Mesía cuyo nombre no ha pasado a la posteridad de los grandes poetas. Don Juan sabe que el "poeta hasta cierto punto" espera de él las obligadas alabanzas. Y en lugar de negarse a escribirlas, como hubiera hecho cualquier crítico menos benévolo, o de castigar severamente, prefiere recurrir a una ironía más desenfadada que de ordinario y escribe un artículo lleno de humor, en el que, sin negar que el libro carece de toda poesía, entretiene al lector durante un buen rato a la vez que satisface la vanidad del "artista". "¿Qué mal hay en ello...?", nos parece escuchar de sus sonrientes labios [1].

---

[1] "Poesías hasta cierto punto", O. C., II, pp. 361 y s.

Idéntica postura —rebajando tal vez las notas irónicas y, lo que es peor, las humorísticas— veremos que adopta en otras ocasiones.

LÓPEZ DE AYALA

Jamás participó Valera de la opinión de Hartzenbusch que calificaba a López de Ayala como un "Calderón redivivo". Como tampoco hizo caso de la opinión general que proclamaba a don Adelardo como el mejor dramaturgo con que España contaba. Sin embargo, en la única crítica que hizo a una de sus comedias (*El tanto por ciento*) no deja sino entrever "muy por lo profundo" que López de Ayala no era, ni con mucho, el genio que la gente creía. Que no hacía más que escribir medianas obritas de ambición clásica [2].

Discurre largamente alrededor (y nunca mejor empleada la palabra) de esta obra, pero con tanta cautela que al lector entusiasta de Ayala le deja la impresión que el crítico gustó de la obra, y al lector poco partidario del dramaturgo, la de que el crítico es de su misma opinión. El lector desapasionado, el que busca la opinión clara del crítico, concluirá que aquél no quiere decidir. De tal modo son complicadamente evasivas las razones de Valera cuando no se atreve a "atacar de frente", para decirlo con sus propias palabras.

El lector de hoy, más afortunado que los de su época, cuenta con la correspondencia privada del crítico, que forma la pieza auxiliar imprescindible para completar y calibrar sus juicios. Al contrario de lo que ocurre en sus artículos, encontramos en las cartas las conclusiones despojadas del "cloroformo" y las buenas maneras; las verdades más duras sin los velos con que iban envueltas allí. Juicios críticos que, en su brevedad, suelen ser de gran eficacia humorística y una franqueza que a veces raya en el descaro.

---

2 "El tanto por ciento", O. C., II, pp. 227-232.

Nadie podría imaginar luego de leer el artículo de que hablamos, tan comedido, tan lleno de delicadezas, que de la misma pluma salieran frases como ésta: "...las cosas de Ayala, que fuera de España y de los que admiraron sus ojos y sus bigotes no se pueden aguantar..." [3], en carta a don Marcelino; o las que dirigió a su amigo Narciso Campillo:

"Ayala seguirá muchos años aún pasando por un genio, aunque nadie lea ni aguante ya lo que ha escrito, y todas las ñoñerías cursilonas de los pequeños poemas y de no pocas doloras serán consideradas como maravillosas, concisas y hondas sentencias filosóficas, y como la poesía más elevada, docente y propia del ilustrado siglo XIX" [4].

TAMAYO Y BAUS

Es de lamentar, repetimos, la conducta de don Juan, puesto que sus juicios más agudos y esclarecedores, su visión crítica más sagaz y sincera, la reservó para comunicarla a un grupo muy reducido de amigos íntimos, mientras sirve al gran público una crítica inoperante, a veces, a fuerza de ser aséptica. También es de lamentar la crítica positiva que, por pereza, dejó de hacer. Por ejemplo, la del dramaturgo Tamayo y Baus.

Era este autor, en opinión de Valera, el mejor escritor teatral de la época, incomparablemente superior a todos los demás, incluido el favorito de todos —críticos y público—, don José Echegaray. A pesar de que el teatro de Tamayo le gustaba, y de que era este autor uno de sus mejores amigos (como lo demuestran las cartas publicadas por Ramón Esquer Torres) y de reconocerle públicamente como el mejor, no se tomó nunca la molestia de analizar con

---

[3] *Epistolario Valera-Menéndez Pelayo*, ed. cit., p. 179.

[4] Vid. "Carta a Narciso Campillo", en *Revista de la Biblioteca, Archivo y Museo del Ayuntamiento de Madrid*, T. III, p. 439.

atención los dramas de aquél. Solamente en un artículo de cierta
extensión y de la época de juventud de don Juan (escrito con ocasión del estreno de *La bola de nieve,* obra que fue bastante censu-
rada por los enemigos de Tamayo), defiende el crítico las buenas
calidades de la obra, analiza su argumento y declara, contra la opinión de los demás, que estaban ante "un gran poeta".

En otra ocasión, revisando un libro de crítica de Boris de Tannenberg, volverá a juzgar la obra de Tamayo, muerto ya éste, y la
encuentra "eminentemente española por la pureza del lenguaje, por
la fuerza del estilo y el carácter de su autor". Confiesa que "cuantas menos tesis hay, mejores son los dramas de Tamayo" [5].

Había proclamado en varias ocasiones a la tragedia *Virginia* como
la mejor entre las españolas; en el artículo que citamos, declara a
Locura de Amor y *Un drama nuevo* los mejores dramas, ya que en
ellos trató el autor de representar "la realidad purificada" (que era
el ideal poético de don Juan, como se recordará) mostrando la hermosura y sublimidad patética y trágica que produce la lucha de la
pasión vehemente con los sentimientos más nobles.

ECHEGARAY

Si, como ya vimos, a don Juan no le satisfizo el teatro romántico —salvada en cierto grado la tragedia—, entenderemos perfectamente su reacción contra el drama neorromántico de don José
Echegaray, el dramaturgo "del honor super-calderoniano", como ha
sido llamado por algún crítico. Aunque el ilustre premio Nobel de
nuestra literatura ocupe toda una época en la historia de nuestras
letras, satisfaciendo los gustos de una sociedad, no contó nunca
con el aplauso del crítico. Huyó siempre de tener que analizar la
obra del autor de *El Gran Galeoto.* Y en las dos únicas ocasiones

---

5   "La España literaria", O. C., II, pp. 1127-1137.

en que se vio obligado a escribir para el público acerca de él, le vemos hacer maravillas evasivas, recurrir a toda su capacidad de "escapismo" y de circunloquios que le evitan el tener que decir claramente que el teatro del matemático le parece muy flojo, cuando no malísimo.

Maravillosa disculpa fue la magnífica actuación de doña María Guerrero en la representación del mediocre drama de don José *La duda,* el único que Valera tuvo que criticar. Encomiando las dotes de gran actriz, alabando su talento interpretativo, sobre el que hábilmente hace recaer el peso del éxito del drama, dando una de cal y otra de arena, pero sin demasiadas concesiones al autor, llena don Juan las obligadas cuartillas de una crítica con pretensiones de amable, sin lograrlo [6].

Y menos pretexto encuentra cuando el organizador del homenaje a Echegaray —el año 1904 le había sido concedido el premio Nobel— solicita de él unas cuartillas para la publicación. Vuelta a la cuerda floja del equilibrio imposible y a las tangentes más inesperadas; llega casi a confesar en este artículo que Echegaray y su teatro le parecían "el fruto de una rica inventiva e imaginación desaforada" pero de mala calidad [7].

Tenemos que volver a su correspondencia privada para encontrar —en la brevedad de unos pocos renglones— el juicio verdadero. A Tamayo le habla del estilo "de cocinera redicha", de los errores gramaticales y el mal gusto que halla en las obras de Echegaray [8]. Y a don Marcelino, con motivo del drama *El loco Dios,* le dice: "Presumo que ha de ser un cúmulo de vaciedades y disparates de muy perverso gusto. Bien quisiera yo admirar a Echegaray como autor dramático..., pero la admiración y el entusiasmo no dependen de la voluntad, por fina y briosa que sea" [9].

---

[6] "La duda", O. C., II, pp. 969-974.
[7] "Homenaje a Echegaray", O. C., II, p. 1179.
[8] *Correspondencia de D. Juan Valera,* obra citada, p. 205.
[9] *Epistolario Valera-Menéndez Pelayo,* obra citada, p. 55.

BÉCQUER

De toda la poesía del siglo XIX español la que más alta estima alcanza en la admiración de Valera es la desnuda y pura lírica de Gustavo Adolfo Bécquer. Siempre que tiene que referirse al poeta de las *Rimas* lo considera como el mejor, el más alto lírico del siglo. Desgraciadamente, esta que parece sincerísima admiración no le movió a vencer su perezosa inercia y escribir un estudio en el que se justificase su admiración demostrando que la obra del sevillano era de la calidad de que el crítico nos hablaba. Hubiera sido la primera gran voz que se hubiese levantado, con derecho propio para hacerlo como nadie, para ilustrar a aquel público que aplaudía hasta destrozarse las manos los poemas de Núñez de Arce, Campoamor y demás poetas que no son sino satélites comparados con el poderoso astro poético del XIX.

Aunque no acaba de gustarle el tono lastimero de las quejas becquerianas, se las perdona con gusto por ser "las más bellas, las más sobrias, limpias y melodiosas" que jamás la poesía romántica española había producido. Que percibió la distancia abismal existente entre las rimas de Bécquer y las medianías de Campoamor y los demás poetas triunfantes, no hay la menor duda, puesto que en todo momento y en diferentes artículos de vario tema reserva siempre los mejores adjetivos para aquél. Mas no le consagró un solo ensayo de cierta extensión. Solamente las obligadas páginas en el *Florilegio,* en las que, sin ahondar demasiado, enumera las buenas cualidades de la poesía de Bécquer [10].

Lo defiende contra las acusaciones de "imitador de Heine" que alguna parte de la crítica (entre los que se encontraba don Marcelino Menéndez Pelayo, que había escrito un ensayo sobre la obra del poeta alemán) le había achacado. No niega don Juan que nues-

---

[10]   O. C., II, p. 1235 y ss.

tro poeta hubiera leído atentamente a Heine, incluso el que se perciba cierta influencia ideológica de éste sobre aquél. Pero mantiene que son dos poesías totalmente distintas. Si acaso, la semejanza estriba en que ambos poetas gustan de las estrofas de pocos versos, afición que el español pudo tomar del alemán. Pero nada del humor "cínico y desvergonzado" de Heine puede rastrearse en el fondo delicado y dulce de Bécquer.

También defiende a Bécquer de la acusación de que "usaba demasiadas comparaciones" en sus versos. Le parece a Valera pueril que un poeta no pueda usar cuantas imágenes crea convenientes, siempre que el resultado final sea la obtención de "un lenguaje poético natural y sin afectación".

CAMPOAMOR

Tampoco tuvo el suficiente valor como para declarar abiertamente su verdadero sentir acerca de la poesía de don Ramón de Campoamor. Nos parece que el daño que en este caso hace Valera fue doble, puesto que ni supo corregir al poeta de sus "desmanes", ni enseñó al público lector lo que había de flores artificiales en aquel invernadero de plantas de gusto muy dudoso.

Valera, frente a una miopía general que consideraba al autor de las "doloras" como el poeta más sublime que en España se había dado; frente a la opinión del que le parecía el mejor crítico con que contaban nuestras letras, Clarín, que se había declarado defensor de Campoamor en varias ocasiones, y frente a la amistad que le unía con el mismo Campoamor, no se sintió con fuerzas suficientes como para, en aras de una crítica desinteresada y honesta, declarar cuánto de falso e inartístico descubriera entre los versos del "genio oficial" del último tercio del siglo XIX, aunque ello hubiera significado el tener que defender su criterio frente a todos. Y el más favorecido hubiera sido el poeta, pues sin duda que, ante las palabras de don Juan, habría podido detenerse a estudiar su propia obra para "limar" las asperezas de calidad inferior que la afeaban y que le menguan hoy considerable valor. No tuvo el consejo de Valera y probablemente nadie tampoco se atrevió a decirle algo parecido a lo que éste pensaba de su obra.

Solamente romperá su prudente diplomacia al hablar con sus mejores amigos. En su correspondencia con Menéndez Pelayo y Tamayo y Baus hallamos las censuras más acres, las acusaciones más duras que Campoamor haya podido merecer nunca. Mas estas acusaciones valieron de poco, puesto que el autor no pudo sospechar que el gran crítico pensaba tan mal de su obra; ni el público pudo mejorar su gusto leyendo una explicación bien hecha acerca del poco valor artístico de algunas de las composiciones que ellos consideraban como "de oro puro", sin ver lo que había de falsos dorados. Porque si don Juan fue capaz de descubrirlos con gran perspicacia, no quiso mostrarlos a aquel público para el que "la crítica honrada debía ser la ayuda, la luz y la guía". Por otra parte, aquellos a quienes Valera se atrevió a comunicar su verdadero sentir eran los menos necesitados de consejo y guía, puesto que veían muy bien por sus propios ojos.

La "prudentísima cuquería" anulando —o por lo menos frenando— unas dotes de crítico excepcionales. Prefiere la cómoda senda de la alabanza más o menos irónica. Los palmetazos que dio al poeta en 1856, al criticar las *Obras poéticas,* iban tan empapados en cloroformo que proporcionaron seguramente no un castigo, sino más bien un dulce sueño. Tanto, que tomando estas palabras valerinas por alabanzas de buena fe, las colocó al frente de su segunda edición, hecha en París por Baudry, como un gran honor que el excelente crítico le hubiera hecho. Detalle que nos parece el colmo de la "astucia" diplomática de don Juan, pues, leído hoy el artículo, no deja de traslucirse en él una ironía más que regular en todo lo que afirma. Si el propio autor de los versos tomó las palabras del crítico por alabanzas, huelga decir lo que entendió el público medio.

El tono de encomiástica burla, disfrazado de amistoso cariño, es tan suave que, tras una lectura superficial, no se ve con certeza el verdadero sentir del crítico. Solamente una vez parece querer descubrirnos el velo de la amabilidad para que veamos lo que no se atreve a decir. En su resumen final, hablando de las "doloras", dice: "Falta saber si este género es bueno o malo. Pero algo ha de dejar el crítico por decidir, para que el público lo decida" [11].

Inesperada conclusión que le evita dar a conocer su opinión sincera acerca de la obra juzgada, propósito que se deja ver en todo el artículo, por otro lado.

Veamos algunos de sus juicios privados sobre Campoamor: a Menéndez Pelayo le dice en 1882 que ha leído un pequeño poema "que muerde de cursi, de falso sentimentalismo y de prosaísmo ridículo en la expresión, que quiere ser sencilla y es afectada" [12]; hablando de la Poética: "Será la proclamación y legalización de la barbarie" [13]; las "humoradas" le parecen "frialdades vulgarísimas y ultrapedestres. Es vergonzoso que semejante colección de simplezas se aplauda" [14]. Y enojado porque Clarín había alabado los versos titulados "Los amores de una santa": "... me parecen peores que la más rastrera y desmayada prosa, y me aturde que en tal mezcla de vulgaridad, prosaísmo y sensiblería vea la obra de un egregio genio poético nadie que esté en su juicio..." [15], etc.

Pero donde la extrañeza del lector de estas "expresivas muestras", que hemos escogido entre otras muchas, llega al máximo es en la siguiente afirmación:

"Campoamor, si hubiera crítica en España, hubiera hecho cosas estimables, porque no carece de ingenio; tiene muchísimo; pero la

---

11 Vid. O. C., II, p. 56.
12 *Epistolario Valera-Menéndez Pelayo*, obra citada, pp. 124, 156, 250, 268 y 286, respectivamente.
13 *Ibidem.*
14 *Ibidem.*
15 *Ibidem.*

adulación ignorante le ha depravado; ha hecho su ignorancia más atrevida y no escribe sino barbaridades y ñoñerías" [16].

Valera parece haber olvidado completamente que él mismo, antes que nadie, formaba parte de aquella "inexistente crítica" a la cual apostrofaba. Que también él había adulado, con sus pleguerías y sutilezas, al poeta lo mismo que los otros con sus encomios de buena fe. Y la falta de don Juan se nos antoja mucho más imperdonable si se considera que él vio claramente donde los otros no pudieron separar el metal puro de la ganga, las florecitas de trapo y colorete artificial, de las bellas y delicadas rosas naturales. Con su "prudente silencio" contribuyó al cultivo de las "malas hierbas" que casi ahogaron los macizos de las flores naturales. Peca por cómoda e inoperante cobardía.

NÚÑEZ DE ARCE

Aunque con Núñez de Arce guarda don Juan una postura semejante, puede decirse que el resultado, en conjunto, es menos injusto. Si es cierto que sus alabanzas —según confesión propia, excesivas— no dejan de confundir al poeta, no lo es menos que se perciben mejor los defectos señalados por el crítico en la obra del vate de Valladolid.

Tenemos que tener muy presente el cambio de gusto que nos separa de aquella época para darnos cuenta del acierto de Valera al juzgar ya entonces con severidad lo que la mayoría de los críticos (incluidos en algunos casos Clarín y Menéndez Pelayo) aplaudieron con todas sus fuerzas. Si, habida cuenta de la distancia que nos separa, se puede presentar hoy como válida buena parte de la crítica que Valera dedicó a Núñez de Arce, es prueba palpable de que su criterio analítico iba más acorde con los criterios del porvenir que con los de su propio tiempo.

---

[16] *Ibidem.*

Pero enfrentarse de plano con los gustos y criterios de la época hubiera significado una lucha sin cuartel, en la que muy probablemente iban a lucirse malos modales, gritos e improperios de los que tanto asustaban a don Juan. Prefirió alabar con salvedades, sonreir irónicamente cuando escribe su crítica larga al libro *Gritos del combate* [17], sin osar decir a las claras los muchos defectos que le encontraba, mas sin ocultarlos del todo tampoco. Llegando a una especie de malabarismo inigualable en el discurso de elogio que la Academia le encargó a la muerte del poeta.

Con los amigos, como siempre, fue mucho más sincero. Escribe sin las sutilezas de los artículos, aunque se note menos dureza que en el caso de don Ramón de Campoamor. Repite sus acusaciones menos veces que contra aquél. En carta desde Lisboa, de 1883, con motivo del discurso de contestación al de ingreso en la Academia, que hizo don Marcelino Menéndez Pelayo, le dice Valera a su amigo que le parecen excesivos los elogios que le dedica. Aclarando: "Harto sabe Vd. como yo, que las poesías políticas de Núñez de Arce, sin excepción, son artículos de fondo de periódico, declamatorios y huecos, con metro y rima ... Son malos artículos de fondo, muy huecos y vacíos ... Son filfa y hasta el título es risible por lo pretencioso sin fundamento" [18].

No ocultó sus apuros don Juan a los amigos cuando, en 1903, la Academia le encargó el discurso de elogio por la muerte del poeta. Otra vez la espada de la opinión general —que había que respetar— oprimiéndole contra la pared de su perspicacia y agudeza crítica. No tiene valor para desafiar a la primera ni para traicionar a la segunda. Y así escribe a don Antonio de Zayas, su amigo: "He andado apuradísimo escribiéndolo... No sé si he logrado salir de él hábilmente. Era menester elogiar mucho a don Gaspar y dejar entrever, no obstante, que en todo lo que toca a sus dudas y a sus

---

[17] O. C., II, pp. 446-455.
[18] *Epistolario Valera-Menéndez Pelayo*, ed. cit., p. 178.

filosofías, hay algo de nebuloso y vago, como le acontece al que oye campanas y no sabe dónde" [19].

ROSALÍA, CORONA-
DO Y AVELLANEDA

Quizá el mayor defecto de la crítica de Valera —y lo repetimos aunque se nos tache de reiterativos— es su política de diplomático. La crítica honrada exige al que la ejerce saltar por encima de amistad y conveniencias sociales. Exponerse, en pro de la verdad, a tener que olvidarse de los lazos amistosos, para señalar los defectos que se encuentren en la obra. Don Juan manejó muy discretamente los silencios, respecto a las obras de baja calidad. Pero no pudo estar callado siempre; sus lazos sociales le obligaban a escribir el prólogo de obrillas que dejaban mucho que desear, y a las que no hubiese dedicado, de otra manera, ni una sola línea. Gastó desgraciadamente muchas páginas —demasiadas horas de lo que pudo haber sido preciosa labor crítica— en poner ante sus ojos lindezas más o menos mediocres, brotadas de plumas de ilustres desconocidos, mientras dejaba por hacer análisis completos de autores que los estaban reclamando con urgencia. Y no habría nada que reprochar (puesto que por lo general todos estos articulitos de que hablamos están escritos en una prosa de la mejor clase y llenos del más fino ingenio valerino) si, junto a estas "cositas", nos encontráramos con otros dedicados a revisar, por ejemplo, la poesía de Rosalía de Castro, autora a quien Valera ignoró; que le pasó inadvertida ante los ojos; una de nuestras más finas poetisas, mencionada solamente en dos ocasiones en toda la obra de don Juan. La primera, entre una lista de nombres hoy perfectamente desconocidos, lo que prueba el poco valor que don Juan le concedía, y la otra, señalando la ausencia de su nombre en una antología de

_____
[19]   *Correspondencia de D. Juan Valera*, obra citada, p. 285.

versos gallegos de la que dio noticia. (No incluyó ni un solo verso de la tierna lírica gallega ni dio noticia alguna de su vida y obra en el *Florilegio*. ¿Querría Valera contrarrestar así la omisión de que se lamentaba...?)

Tampoco pueden tacharse estos artículos de ser demasiado elogiosos, ya que, leídos como toda la crítica de Valera requiere ser leída, se perciben claramente las burlonas ironías de don Juan, que, consciente de la endeblez poética del librito analizado, no se recata de manifestar su sentir, si bien disimulándolo convenientemente entre amabilidad y finas sonrisas, atacando de lado, como era su política.

Ni los versos del primer marqués de Castel Rodrigo, ni el libro *Laureles* de don Ángel del Arco, ni *Jirones* de Ramón A. Urbano, ni las poesías del duque de Almenara Alta —¡por muy duque que fuera!—, ni las del segundo duque de Rivas, ni las elegantes y "bilingües" producciones de la señora marquesa de Bolaños (por no citar más que unos pocos nombres que la bondad de don Juan apadrinara) han quedado para la posteridad literaria como cosa digna de atención; ¡y lo que es más grave es que don Juan lo sabía perfectamente!

De las tres grandes poetisas del siglo (Gertrudis Gómez de Avellaneda, Carolina Coronado y Rosalía de Castro) ya hemos visto cómo pasó ante sus cerrados ojos la cantora de Santiago de Compostela. Con la obra de Carolina Coronado, aunque confesó tenerle gran admiración, tampoco va muy allá a la hora de juzgarla. Obligadas alabanzas en el *Florilegio* y ligeras reflexiones sobre el misticismo que encuentra en algunas de las poesías juveniles.

A Gertrudis Gómez de Avellaneda fue a la única que don Juan consagró un detenido estudio [20].

---

[20] Véanse los artículos: "Sobre el drama *Baltasar*", O. C., II, pp. 111-117; "Poesías líricas de Gertrudis Gómez de Avellaneda", O. C., II, páginas 375-386, y *Florilegio*, "G. Gómez de Avellaneda", O. C., II, páginas 1357-60.

Analiza muy hábilmente la obra lírica de la poetisa en un largo artículo y se ratifica en sus alabanzas treinta años más tarde, al repasar su labor para el *Florilegio*, en donde resume lo que allí había dicho. No encontramos absurdas hipérboles como él temiera, sino la que nos parece una justa estimación de la poesía de la Avellaneda. La declara inferior como novelista a Cecilia Böhl de Faber y la compara como poetisa a Victoria Colonna, por encontrarle muchos rasgos comunes con ella.

No deja de notar Valera la falta de "facilidad descriptiva", lo que empobrece en cierto modo la producción, así como la de sentido patriótico y de verdadera profundidad religiosa, pues está muy lejos de llegar al misticismo [21].

FERNÁN CABALLERO

La postura que Valera adoptó con las novelas de Fernán Caballero venía determinada, de un lado, por el concepto personal que del género tenía nuestro autor; y de otro, por el prurito de "españolismo" que determinaba un cambio en el espíritu de su crítica, de ordinario muy tolerante, para hacerse de una intransigencia rayana en la injusticia cuando tenía que analizar cuanto venía —o sospechaba que venía, como era el caso de *La gaviota*— del extranjero.

El que la novelista se propusiera "moralizar" en sus novelas causaba tal enojo e irritación a Valera que las virtudes que por otros estilos encontraba en la obra no eran suficientes para hacerle olvidar lo que él consideraba "manía de sermoneo".

No dejó de percibir lo que de evolución de la materia romántica hacia el costumbrismo de la novela regionalista tenía la más famosa novela de Fernán Caballero, *La gaviota*. Y así lo declara en breve nota dedicada a ésta y a *Un verano en Bornos*, en *Revista de Ma-*

---

[21]   O. C., II, pp. 382-383.

drid, 31 de julio de 1856 [22], si bien le hallaba el inconveniente de querer "moralizar y catequizar", cosas que "amén de aburrir a los frívolos lectores, fastidiaban a los lectores serios e instruidos".

A su juicio, Fernán Caballero no es escritor castizo. Ni por su lengua ni por la manera de expresar cuanto ve. Son ojos de extranjero más que de español los que contemplan la región andaluza y la vida de sus gentes. Se fija especialmente en lo pintoresco. Los antecedentes de la escritora no se hallan en nuestra literatura castiza, sino en la novelística romántica europea, en especial en las novelas *Paul et Virginie*, de Bernardin de Saint-Pierre, y *André*, de George Sand.

Años más tarde, ante las que consideraba excesivas alabanzas dadas en la *Revista de Edimburgo* a Fernán Caballero, volverá a reiterar lo que él consideraba defectos de la autora. Pero más con la intención de contradecir al articulista escocés (que afirmaba con gran escándalo de Valera que nuestras letras no habían producido nada de interés tan grande después del Teatro del Siglo de Oro hasta la aparición de Fernán Caballero) que con la de atacar a la novelista [23].

ALARCÓN

Muy a gala tuvo siempre don Juan el haber servido como de presentador oficial, en su primera salida al campo de las letras, del poeta andaluz y novelista don Pedro Antonio de Alarcón. La amistad profunda que les unió de por vida fue sincerísima. Y las alabanzas que le dedica don Juan en el prólogo de aquel libro primero de versos, como cuantas le dedicará después, no lo fueron menos. Alarcón, por muchas razones, pero especialmente por su idealismo literario, su manera de ver y sentir el arte, al igual que por sus

---

[22] O. C., II, pp. 85-86.
[23] "Sobre las obras de Fernán Caballero", O. C., II, pp. 232 y s.

cualidades humanas —gracejo y desenvoltura— congeniaba perfectamente con Valera.

En los versos de Alarcón celebra don Juan, sobre todo, el humor y el desenfado, la espontaneidad y ternura con que están escritos. El humor burlón y sin amargas ironías que surge especialmente en las parodias de versos célebres, lo que no impide que admire también la "robusta y correcta versificación y su lenguaje castizo, elegante y propio". Pero aún estimaba en más el crítico las cualidades de "narrador en prosa" de que estaba adornado su amigo. Lo considera el restaurador de la novela de costumbres. Lo que había pretendido Fernán Caballero sin conseguirlo plenamente, la universalización de lo popular español, lo consiguió Alarcón porque "es español por los cuatro costados" [24]. No se percibe su entronque —si lo hay— extranjero. Realistas y naturalistas se dejan llevar por las influencias de los novelistas ingleses, franceses y rusos. Alarcón, en cambio, echaba sus raíces en lo más original de nuestro pueblo. *El sombrero de tres picos* no es otra cosa que la "purificación idealista de un aire popular del más irreflexivo e insolente desenfado" que todavía se cantaba, acompañándose a la guitarra, en las tabernas de Andalucía.

De entre todas las novelas alarconianas no es la más popular, con todo, la que goza de las preferencias de don Juan, sino *El niño de la bola,* según declaró en varias ocasiones. Desgraciadamente, no contamos con estudio alguno que nos explique y justifique las preferencias del crítico.

PEREDA

Muy poco fruto debieron surtir los consejos de don Marcelino Menéndez Pelayo, repetidos en muchas de sus cartas, para que don Juan se animara a leer las novelas de don José María de Pereda.

---

[24] Véase O. C., II, p. 1369.

A las cariñosas sugerencias del amigo responde Valera con un silencio glacial. No participó nunca del entusiasmo de Menéndez Pelayo por Pereda. En general, la novela regionalista (al igual que el cuento, pues a Trueba lo trató con manifiesta injusticia, ignorándolo en varias ocasiones) le interesó muy raramente. Dicha novela le pareció siempre "demasiado tendenciosa" [25]. Si a esto se une el poquísimo interés que hacia la descripción de paisajes sintiera siempre Valera, se explica, en cierto modo, la incomprensión. Consideró a Pereda como un buen amigo y lo pone (junto a Galdós y a doña Emilia Pardo Bazán) al frente de nuestros novelistas mejores. Pero de ahí a interesarse verdaderamente por su obra media un abismo. Abismo de silencio que no rompió jamás.

GALDÓS

Tarde y no sin pocos recelos llegó don Juan a la lectura de las obras de Galdós. En julio de 1878 escribe a don Marcelino: "Se anuncia una nueva novela de Galdós. ¿Quiere Ud. creer que nada he leído de este fecundo y celebrado novelista? Usted, que lo lee todo, habrá leído sus novelas. ¿Qué le parecen?" [26].

Conviene recordar que por aquellas fechas don Benito Pérez Galdós había publicado ya seis novelas (entre las cuales estaban *Doña Perfecta, Gloria* y *Marianela*) y las dos primeras series casi completas de sus *Episodios*. Que su popularidad era grandísima [27]. Nos parece muy revelador el que un hombre como Valera, tan inclinado siempre a la curiosidad literaria que le empujó a buscar los nombres nuevos en todas partes, llegue con tan relativo retraso a la

---

[25] Llegó incluso a negarla, en un artículo para *El Correo de España* de Buenos Aires cuando Pereda leyó su discurso de ingreso en la Real Academia. Véase O. C., III, pp. 496-498.

[26] *Epistolario Valera-M. Pelayo,* ed. cit., p. 32.

[27] J. Casalduero, *Vida y obra de Galdós,* ed. Gredos, 1951, p. 22.

obra de nuestro mayor novelista del siglo xix. ¿Cuál pudo ser la causa..?

De ninguna manera un descuido involuntario. Conocía muy bien Valera lo que se publicaba en España y fuera de ella, por pequeño que fuera el valor de lo publicado. No pudo pasarle inadvertido tan fecundo y celebrado novelista. En otra carta a don Marcelino encontramos ya una explicación a este retraso: "el temor de no encontrarlo de su gusto". Prefiere no saber cómo son dichas obras —cerrar los ojos ante una realidad que todos alaban— antes que tener que confesar que no le agradan. Una vez más, el lastre de sus prejuicios en contra de su agudeza crítica. Temía que muchos de los amigos del novelista fueran a tomar a mal las palabras que dijera "en caso de que no le gustaran dichas obras" y escogió el camino más cómodo: no leerle para no tener que decir nada de él. ¿No serían celos disfrazados de temores? ¿Por qué iban a ser sus juicios forzosamente contrarios...? ¿Por qué iban a ser tomadas sus palabras como envidiosos ataques de un novelista a otro?, y otras muchas preguntas que se nos vienen a las mientes.

Tras muchas dudas leyó, por fin, *La familia de León Roch.* Y he aquí que no le decepciona. Antes al contrario: "Me ha parecido inmensamente mejor de lo que yo había figurado" [28].

No encuentra a Galdós "tan cursi como lo imaginaba" (¡nos gustaría saber por qué esperaba Valera que el autor de los *Episodios* fuera un cursi!). Aunque nota que imita a Dickens y otros autores, lo hace como se debe y no "copiando desmayadamente".

Encuentra también que los personajes de la novela de Galdós son hijos espirituales de *El comendador Mendoza,* aunque los suyos, los de Valera, menos preocupados de probar una tesis que los galdosianos, se emplean más en sus asuntos y son más humanos y reales que éstos.

---

[28]   *Epistolario Valera-M. Pelayo,* obra citada, p. 57.

Se explica Valera la popularidad de Galdós por aquel "espíritu de partido" que a él le faltaba y que es cualidad "que da calor y brío a cuanto don Benito escribe".

Los defectos principales que encuentra en la obra galdosiana son: el no conocer bien la sociedad elegante que describe, algunas desarmonías en los diálogos (que nacen del prurito que tiene por parecer natural), en los que halla palabras bajas y feas de puro familiares, algunos galicismos y deslices gramaticales (como el uso del dativo de plural del pronombre personal masculino en lugar del acusativo) y otras menudencias [29].

Salvo el brevísimo comentario que dedicó a *Misericordia* en una de sus "Cartas americanas", nada escribió don Juan para criticar la novela de don Benito. La encontró buena... pero no de su gusto. El género de novela galdosiana aburría tanto a Valera como las de Pereda, o como los "sermones" de Fernán Caballero. En el caso del escritor canario no se atrevió, como con el autor de *La gaviota*, a hacer pública su opinión. Siempre que a Galdós ha de referirse, le concede la primacía entre nuestros novelistas; pero ni una sola vez demostró que conocía a fondo su obra. Tal vez por esta falta, y como para contrarrestarla, pidió a Menéndez Pelayo que fuera elegido académico el gran novelista.

PARDO BAZÁN

Muy diferente es la actitud del crítico hacia doña Emilia Pardo Bazán. Reconoció el valor de la escritora gallega y jamás le escatimó alabanzas, sin que por ello cayera nunca en la más pequeña exageración. Lo que molestaba a Valera fue lo que él llamaba "el prurito de aclimatar extrañas corrientes, en los cauces propios de nuestras letras", que manifestaba doña Emilia.

---

[29] Véase *Epistolario de Valera-M. Pelayo*, obra citada, pp. 57 y s.

La defensora del realismo contra el crítico y paladín del idealismo. Mas si prescindimos de las diferencias, las disputas y hasta de los enfados transitorios que en la obra crítica de una y otro se dejan ver, don Juan admiró sinceramente el talento de novelista de la condesa de Pardo Bazán, así como su facilidad y buen estilo de narradora.

Como vemos por las cartas del epistolario, no opinaba igual don Marcelino Menéndez y Pelayo. En sus críticas privadas llega hasta el insulto menos fino. Es curioso ver cómo Valera, a los improperios de aquél, opone un mesurado tono de respeto hacia la escritora. Respeto que no nacía esta vez de su habilidad diplomática, pues sabemos que en sus cartas privadas, en especial las dirigidas a don Marcelino, no se recataba de decir cuanto se le venía a la pluma.

Contestó a la autora de la *Cuestión palpitante* con su *Nuevo arte de escribir novelas* [30] porque consideraba absurdas las teorías que aquella escritora mantenía. Mas no iba —lo repite machaconamente— contra "la excelente escritora". Lo mismo cuando doña Emilia defiende a los escritores rusos. Contestó don Juan con un largo artículo [31], pero hemos de reconocer que, en tal disputa, la razón estaba de parte de la condesa, pues los débiles argumentos que Valera oponía habían nacido antes de conocer y juzgar debidamente las novelas de que hablaba. Como tantas otras veces, utiliza argumentos preconcebidos y, por lo tanto, de muy poca consistencia.

No sabemos hasta dónde llegaba el conocimiento y admiración verdaderos que la escritora decía sentir por los grandes escritores rusos; cabe admitir, como sugiere don Juan, que esta admiración le llegara a doña Emilia "vía Francia"; pero sí sabemos —porque don Juan lo confesó— que él no las había leído; que los primeros contactos con tal literatura los tuvo en alemán, es decir, en traducciones.

---

30 O. C., II, pp. 622-710.
31 O. C., II, pp. 715 y s.

Nos parece que el amor propio de Valera le hizo tomar una postura errónea para justificarse a sí mismo. Había estado en Rusia cerca de dos años y nada de aquella literatura, ni entonces ni más tarde, había llamado su atención. Doña Emilia resultaba la "descubridora" de obras de suma importancia que él había ignorado por completo. Y una prueba de "miopía" de tal envergadura hería el orgullo del crítico. Para no sentirse vejado, la solución más fácil le pareció que era restar importancia a las novelas que la condesa alababa y él no había siquiera entrevisto. De aquí la poca fuerza de sus argumentos; pretender enfrentar la obra de Puchkin, Lermontov, Gogol, Turgueniev, Dostoyewsky y Tolstoy a los nombres portugueses, españoles y americanos que don Juan cita resulta de todo punto infantil.

En otra discusión mantenida con doña Emilia, lució Valera con mejor fortuna el gracejo que le caracterizaba. Fue en la que podría titularse "Las mujeres y las Academias" [32], donde burlonamente expone don Juan los motivos por los cuales una dama de bien no podría llegar a ser "individua de número".

No fue muy generoso en lo que se refiere al número de críticas dedicadas a la fecunda novelista. Analizó con cierto detalle solamente *Morriña* [33] de entre las novelas largas y *El tesoro de Gastón* y *La Chucha* [34] entre las novelas cortas y los cuentos. Y valoró siempre muy favorablemente la producción de la escritora. Se percató muy bien de que el naturalismo de que doña Emilia hacía gala no era más que un realismo extremado y que no fue naturalista más que en teoría.

EL PADRE COLOMA

Al escandaloso éxito que arrancó la novela del Padre Coloma *Pequeñeces* contestó don Juan con un folleto anónimo (titulado *Pe-*

---

[32] O. C., II, pp. 863-875.
[33] O. C., II, pp. 801-804.
[34] O. C., III, pp. 541-2 y 559, respectivamente.

queñeces, Currita Albornoz al P. Luis Coloma, Madrid, 1891), que produjo no menor escándalo que la citada novela [35].

Crítica y público habían recibido la novela con entusiasmo desacostumbrado y, hasta el anónimo folleto de Valera, nadie había discutido los valores de aquella sátira del ambiente moderno que era *Pequeñeces.* Don Juan se atrevió a hacerlo amparado en el anónimo, aunque el mundo de las letras reconoció inmediatamente a la personalidad que se escondía tras él. No era difícil averiguarlo, incluso por los detalles personales que contiene la carta. Repite párrafos completos que figuran en otros escritos suyos, además de que el estilo de Valera es inconfundible.

En un divertido tono de burla amable, hace una crítica de la novela, en la cual enumera las virtudes y defectos principales; caló bien en los méritos y defectos de la obra y, como nota curiosa, diremos que en dicho escrito se documenta por primera vez la palabra "esperpento" [36]; la cual, según J. Corominas, fue más tarde recogida por Pastor Molina como madrileñismo, y por Segovia como americanismo, haciendo su entrada en el diccionario de la Academia en 1899 [37].

EL PENSAMIENTO

Resulta curioso que una figura como la de don Juan, tan preocupado por el pensamiento y la filosofía de su época, no preste atención a las figuras más significativas del pensamiento de la segunda mitad del siglo XIX. Sabemos la atracción que sintió por el krausismo y su introductor en España, don Julián Sanz del Río, y del temprano abandono o separación de unas teorías que no acabaron

---

[35]   O. C., III, pp. 848-863.

[36]   "...Me presenta usted ya tan ajada y marchita que parezco un esperpento". "Pequeñeces", O. C., II, p. 862.

[37]   J. Corominas, *Diccionario Crítico Etimológico de la Lengua Castellana,* ed. Gredos, Madrid, 1954, p. 389.

de convencerle. Las escasas críticas que se refieren a estos temas son más bien censuras al "poco castizo estilo" erizado de fórmulas que usaban los krausistas.

Ni la figura de Sanz del Río ni la de su discípulo, F. Giner de los Ríos, ocuparon su atención. Tampoco la obra de don Manuel Bartolomé Cossío, y nada nos dice de Joaquín Costa, pensador que coincidía en muchas ideas con el grupo mencionado.

Donoso Cortés no agradaba a don Juan ni por las ideas que defendía ni por el estilo de sus escritos. Dedicó una serie de artículos a contradecir el famoso *Ensayo sobre el catolicismo, el liberalismo y el socialismo.* Lo que él llamaba "las estrecheces de ideas de los neocatólicos" le enojaban y, más que crítica literaria del libro, hizo una refutación filosófica de él [38].

Con Castelar fue don Juan muy severo; si a Donoso le criticó las ideas, a éste le censurará también —y con dureza— el estilo y forma en que las vertía. Las pleguerías valerinas al escribir las críticas a Castelar no encubren tanto los ataques: "Con el pretexto de lisonjear el mal gusto reinante, llena sus escritos y discursos de adornos superfluos"; lo llega a llamar "Zorrilla de la elocuencia", y no le gustan los "lirismos archifloridos y archipomposos". Y es aún más duro en sus cartas a los amigos, en las que pueden verse frases como ésta: "... saca a relucir el pésimo gusto, los falsos floripondios y las huecas composiciones de nuestro Demóstenes" [39].

---

[38] O. C., II, pp. 1383-1399.
[39] Véanse los artículos "Refutación a Castelar", O. C., III, p. 636, *Epistolario Valera-M. Pelayo,* obra citada, p. 333, y *Correspondencia de don Juan Valera,* obra citada, p. 260.

Capítulo IX

LA CRÍTICA

Podría decirse que don Marcelino Menéndez Pelayo fue uno de los grandes descubrimientos de don Juan Valera crítico. Lo mismo que a Rubén, vaticinó muy certeramente don Juan, desde los primeros escritos que del joven estudioso cayeron en sus manos, lo que aquél iba a ser más tarde. La gloria que a nuestras letras iba a proporcionar por su sabiduría y capacidad de trabajo.

A nadie trató con más amor, justicia y sagacidad en sus consejos y advertencias —cuando las creía necesarias— que al joven don Marcelino. A nadie predicó el trabajo como a su joven amigo en los comienzos de su amistad, que iba a durar más de treinta años; él, que se pasaba semanas enteras sin tomar la pluma, ¡con qué cariño anima a su estudioso amigo a traducir —por ejemplo— la trilogía de Esquilo que planearon hacer en colaboración, y que don Marcelino llevaría a cabo, pues el vivir de don Juan no era el del reposado y fructífero estudio de aquél!

Afortunadamente, contamos con el voluminoso epistolario que recoge gran parte de la correspondencia cruzada entre ambos amigos, a lo largo de esos treinta años de amistad y devoción mutua.

Nada mejor que dichas cartas para percibir esa corriente de inteligencia y comprensión que se estableció entre ambos escritores cuando don Marcelino contaba poco más de veinte años. (Don Juan tenía sesenta y dos cuando recibió en su casa de Madrid la visita del joven recién salido de la Universidad, que se presentaba a él con una tarjeta de recomendación del catedrático de literatura y crítico, amigo de ambos, don Gumersindo Laverde.) Nada más elocuente para ver las mutuas ayudas que se prestan —pues en muchos casos los consejos son recíprocos— y la inteligente actitud de ambos en las cuestiones en que no están de acuerdo.

Tan opuestos en muchos rasgos de su personalidad como semejantes en otros, su afición a las letras, y especialmente a las clásicas, estrechará su amistad por encima de los altibajos y diferencias a que suelen estar expuestos, por lo general, hombres de su talla y responsabilidades.

El influjo es mutuo y, pese a que don Marcelino con su modestia ejemplar se consideró siempre discípulo de don Juan y su fiel admirador admitiendo su "especial tutela", también los puntos de vista del "joven sabio" (como gustaba Valera de llamarlo cariñosamente) harán meditar y hasta modificar criterios, en ocasiones, al autor de *Pepita Jiménez*.

Menéndez Pelayo no cesó —siempre con cariñosas disculpas— de estimular a don Juan para que escribiera más, y éste llegó a confesarle: "necesito sus estímulos para seguir escribiendo" [1].

Dijimos antes que, desde muy temprano, se percató Valera del enorme valer de don Marcelino. Recién salido de la Universidad y antes siquiera de concurrir a las oposiciones que le dieron la cátedra de Literatura en Madrid, ya admiraba nuestro crítico el "raro saber" y el "mejor talento crítico" que dejaban ver aquellas primicias de investigación, obra de aquel modesto "estudiantón" de aspecto provinciano que confesaba, a su vez, ser un entusiasta fervoro-

---

[1] *Epistolario Valera-M. Pelayo*, obra citada, p. 323.

so de la prosa de Valera. Probablemente tuvo mucha importancia, desde el punto de vista puramente humano, la influencia que Valera pudo dejar sentir en su amigo, en lo que pudiéramos llamar "detalles de índole social".

Desde el más antiguo artículo —dedicado a criticar el libro *Horacio en España*—, fechado en 1878, se ven clarísimamente las alabanzas y aun lo poco que de reprochable descubre en él. Habla de los "prejuicios de escuela" que siempre separarán a los dos escritores y que no fueron sino el criterio libre y racionalista que profesaba él, frente al "catolicismo a machamartillo" de don Marcelino. Era éste un "neo" menos intransigente que los seguidores de Donoso. Su postura de intransigente intolerancia —como dice su biógrafo Pedro Laín Entralgo— [2] tenía que chocar radicalmente con la cómoda actitud de librepensador que siempre mantuvo Valera. A pesar de tanta diferencia ideológica, en literatura están de acuerdo en casi todo.

Analizó muy agudamente don Juan la importante obra de Menéndez Pelayo *Los Heterodoxos* en tres largos estudios, en los que apunta las virtudes y los defectos que se le alcanzan. La mayoría de las afirmaciones del crítico siguen teniendo validez hoy en día, lo que demuestra su agudeza.

Fue uno de los primeros en proponer el nombre del joven profesor para la Academia y tuvo el placer de ser su padrino y, por tanto, contestar al discurso de su amigo. En él vuelve a analizar la obra y a alabarla debidamente. Sin exageraciones inútiles, pero con gran amor; lo considera gran crítico, excelente poeta y le profetiza en nuestro parnaso un alto puesto. Privada, como públicamente, Valera demostró siempre un especial cariño por el gran polígrafo; hasta el descuidado aspecto externo del sabio fue objeto más de una vez de las cariñosas reprimendas valerinas. Aquella "poca afi-

---

[2] P. Laín Entralgo, *Menéndez Pelayo*, Instituto de Estudios Políticos, Madrid, 1944, p. 176.

ción a la limpieza" provocaba graciosísimas lamentaciones del *dandy* refinado que fue siempre don Juan [3].

OTROS CRÍTICOS

Hemos dicho que Valera consideró siempre a don Marcelino como el único crítico de auténtico valor con que contaba el país. Y dedicado aquél a la labor de investigación y crítica profunda, la crítica cotidiana estaba en manos de "unos cuantos ignorantes" que "desollaban vivo al enemigo" y ponían sobre sus cabezas, por las nubes, a los amigos, así fuesen tan pedestres autorcillos como ellos criticuelos. De entre aquella turbamulta de autorcillos satírico-críticos —son palabras de Valera— descollaban Clarín y doña Emilia Pardo Bazán.

Nunca se extendió don Juan en el examen de la crítica de su tiempo, y éste es otro argumento que demuestra el poquísimo valor que le concedía. Solamente espigando textos que se le caen de la pluma al tratar de otros temas, o por referencias que hallamos en sus cartas, podemos saber la opinión que le merecían aquellos críticos a los que en conjunto, sin que osara mencionar nombres, calificaba con tan desfavorables adjetivos.

De la erudición crítica de la primera mitad del siglo XIX poco o nada dijo. A Larra como crítico ni lo entendió, ni aplaudió sus sátiras. Moderados encomios a Nicomedes Pastor Díaz, el marqués de Pidal —si bien se ocupaba de una materia, la poesía medieval, que a Valera le producía muy poco entusiasmo, como ya se dijo—, Milá y Fontanals y Amador de los Ríos, así como los hermanos Fernández Guerra. Pero son unas alabanzas tan tibias, para hombre tan magnánimo, que están denunciando la plena convicción del crítico de que la labor de aquellos investigadores no era tan importante como generalmente se creía. Negó la existencia de la crítica durante

---

[3] *Correspondencia de Don Juan Valera*, obra citada, p. 228.

toda la segunda mitad del siglo; existían —según don Juan— solamente en el país unos pocos hombres con mejores intenciones que formación y talento.

Don Manuel Cañete era "modelo de cortesía y de moderación para con los criticados". Si consideramos la gran amistad que les unió, las comedidas alabanzas que Valera escribe a la muerte del amigo, podemos deducir la importancia real que le concedía en cuanto crítico.

Negó todo valor y utilidad a la crítica de Antonio de Valbuena (seudónimo que utilizó el crítico Miguel de Escalada). Su sátira mordaz le desagradaba pues, con tal de hacer reir al lector, se ensañaba sin piedad alguna —y, lo que era mucho peor, sin razón— con los infelices autores que caían bajo su férula. Lo llama en varias ocasiones "crítico desaforado" e "imitador de Clarín", aunque sin su talento. Esta era la clase de crítica que don Juan detestaba más. "La escuela del mal humor de Clarín" llegó a llamarla. Imitaban al autor de *La Regenta* sin tener en cuenta que lo que hacía gracia y efecto no era la ferocidad en sí, descarnada y brutal, sino el chiste inteligente en que el crítico ovetense sabía envolverlas.

A don Gumersindo Laverde —a quien prologó un tomo de trabajos críticos— lo trató siempre con mucho cariño y respetuosa benevolencia, así como a Federico Balart.

REVILLA

Menos benévolo fue con don Manuel de la Revilla. El optimista temperamento de Valera no podía casar con el pesimismo y la amarga desesperación que Revilla vertía en sus escritos. Por otra parte, muy sensible don Juan a las críticas adversas, no consiguió olvidar tan fácilmente los torniscones que aquél le propinara cuando publicó *Pasarse de listo*. Ni las poco justificadas faltas que encuentra en la labor de don Juan al trazar, en sus *Bocetos literarios,* su retrato [4]. Por si todo ello fuera poco, se comprende con facilidad la distancia existente entre ambos críticos al estudiar los "Principios a que debe obedecer la crítica literaria", de Revilla [5]. Aunque se proclame partidario del arte por el arte, sus principios estéticos tienen poco o nada en común con los de Valera. No admite capacidad creativa en el crítico perfecto (lo que debió escocer a don Juan), así como tampoco capacidad crítica en el creador. El mejor ejemplo de crítico —para Revilla— era Larra. Y ya sabemos lo que pensaba don Juan del extraordinario satírico. *Et sic de caeteris.*

Cuando murió, en plena juventud, el crítico ex-krausista, escribe don Juan a su amigo el poeta Campillo en términos que no dejan ver admiración, ni mucho menos alabanzas. Lo llama "deplorabilísimo y desmayado coplero". Veinte años después, en la antología de poetas líricos, dulcificó algo los términos.

Al historiador de la literatura del siglo XIX, el Padre F. Blanco García, no le escatimó alabanzas, al tiempo que le señaló los lunares que en su obra se le aparecían.

CLARÍN

Conocía muy bien don Juan la sagacidad crítica de Clarín para determinadas materias, a la vez que no se le ocultaba la incapacidad material que tenía para apreciar en su justa medida y exacto valor la poesía lírica. Después de Menéndez Pelayo era Clarín, para don Juan, el hombre que, si no se dejaba llevar por la más amarga sátira, a la que fue tan aficionado, podía ejercer el oficio ideal de crítico en España con mayor dignidad y el mejor talento.

Pero, según el criterio de Valera, era Clarín demasiado apasionado, demasiado violento desgraciadamente en sus análisis, para que

---

[4] Manuel de la Revilla, "Bocetos literarios: Don Juan Valera", en *Revista Contemporánea*, 15-XII-1877.

[5] Manuel de la Revilla, *Obras*, Sainz, Madrid, 1883.

los resultados fuesen eficaces. Muy raras veces aprobó don Juan aquella especie de crítica "policíaca" que Leopoldo Alas confesaba practicar. Teniendo en cuenta la diplomacia de carácter de Valera, podemos explicarnos el que a duras penas le contradiga en su correspondencia privada. Lo que no impide que esté en completo desacuerdo con él en muchas ocasiones.

Por otra parte, Clarín fue el crítico más entusiasta con que contó Valera. Él y don Marcelino fueron sus mayores admiradores —sinceros admiradores, mejor dicho, pues muchos se llamaban así sin pasar de un "querer vivir a bien con el autor de *Pepita*"—. No podía, por tanto, contestar con improperios a las amabilísimas frases que le dedicaba Clarín en todas las críticas. Pero entre líneas —en lo que escribe don Juan para el público—, como abiertamente cuando escribe a los amigos, se deja ver claramente que estaba muy lejos de aprobar la severidad terrible de su amigo.

Nos parece bastante revelador el siguiente texto sacado de una de sus *Nuevas cartas americanas*: "Alguien podría observar y suponer que yo elogio mucho a Clarín porque él también me elogia. Lo único que en este punto acierto a decir en mi defensa es que, si yo no gustase de las obras de Clarín, no las elogiaría aunque él me elogiase; procuraría hablar de ellas lo menos posible" [6].

Esto decía en 1896. Ya había publicado Clarín sus más famosas novelas y buena parte de sus folletos críticos. Muy poco de esta labor había sido criticada por don Juan hasta esa fecha y nada analizó después. La conclusión a que se llega, si tenemos en cuenta las palabras finales del texto valerino, no deja lugar a dudas.

Estima al crítico, se duele de su virulencia... y procura con habilidad soslayar la crítica a la mejor obra de Clarín, la novelesca. Al hacer un brevísimo análisis de *Su único hijo* en *Nuevas cartas americanas* nos dice que "es muy inferior a la primera novela" —*La Regenta*— de la que nunca había hecho crítica alguna.

---

6 O. C., III, p. 462.

Callando, había evitado la áspera tarea de confesar que le parecía demasiado desagradable, demasiado "naturalista", la obra del crítico amigo. Clarín pintaba la verdad, pero era la clase de verdad —la desagradable— que a don Juan enfadaba como materia artística.

Las líneas que siguen nos parecen la expresión más sincera del juicio que, como crítico, merecía Clarín a los ojos de Valera: "Un crítico duro, cruel, injusto a veces y sobrado descontentadizo; pero (estoy seguro de que no me engaña la gratitud), de agudísimo ingenio, de erudición varia y sana y de singular chiste y discreción en cuanto escribe, cuando la pasión de secta no le ciega" [7].

También consideraba don Juan a doña Emilia Pardo Bazán con dotes y conocimientos más que suficientes para llevar a cabo una crítica eficaz y sana. Pero, como a Clarín, la encuentra demasiado apasionada, demasiado defensora de una escuela única en arte.

---

[7] Vid. "Poesías de Menéndez Pelayo", en O. C., II, p. 612.

Capítulo X

AUTORES NUEVOS

Con el precursor del modernismo en España (y más tarde seguidor de Rubén), el poeta malagueño Salvador Rueda, se mostró siempre don Juan cariñosamente benévolo. No por eso dejó de censurar en su obra lo que, con expresión equívoca para el lector de hoy, calificaba de "excesos naturalistas". Valera se negó obstinada e injustamente a conceder categoría de movimientos literarios a cuantos "ismos" habían hecho aparición después del naturalismo. Parnasianos, simbolistas, decadentistas y modernistas eran, según él, una especie de corruptela o planta enferma que había brotado del "tronco podrido del naturalismo". No encontraba en ellos el menor valor, si dejamos a un lado la excepcional obra del poeta nicaragüense, a quien descubrió y ponderó antes que lo hiciera nadie. Una vez más su obstinada terquedad, y sus prejuicios, le impiden ver con claridad y percibir los primeros vagidos de lo que iba a ser el modernismo y con él el nacimiento de la auténtica poesía contemporánea, todavía floreciente en bellísimas composiciones, en nuestros días.

Lo mismo en el que le pareció "escandaloso" *Himno a la carne* que en la novela *El gusano de luz* descubría Valera las excelentes virtudes del personalísimo estilo de Salvador Rueda; la riqueza de imaginación, la maestría en el manejo del lenguaje, la facilidad pasmosa para versificar —en el libro de versos publicado en 1897— eran valores que le hacían "uno de los más estimables poetas españoles de nuestros días"[1].

RUBÉN DARÍO

La mayor —y la mejor— muestra de agudeza crítica, sensibilidad poética y seguridad en el juicio, así como en el vaticinio, nos la dio Valera al analizar, muy poco después de su aparición, el librito de un poeta hispanoamericano totalmente desconocido antes en el mundo de las letras. El joven nicaragüense Rubén Darío, de veintiún años, había escrito y publicado un librito titulado *Azul*, que se apresuró a mandar al crítico. (Aunque había escrito varias cosas antes, este libro fue su primera publicación. El mismo año de 1888 vio la luz *Primeras notas,* pero el crítico tuvo ante sí solamente el volumen titulado *Azul* para juzgarlo.)

Bastaron a don Juan la prosa y los poemas que llenan las no muy numerosas páginas del libro para adivinar, proclamar y profetizar un rotundo y seguro éxito al originalísimo poeta que tras ellas se escondía. Le descubrió y presentó al público español e hispanoamericano antes que lo hiciera ningún otro crítico[2]. Y esta vez las palabras de don Juan no iban envueltas en "pleguerías", ni obligaron al lector a buscar entre líneas. Don Juan es claro, como clara es la idea que tiene del extraordinario valer que el poeta lleva en sí. No vacila en afirmar, desde el primer artículo, que Rubén será gloria de las letras hispanoamericanas.

---

[1] O. C., II, pp. 588-589.
[2] "Carta a Rubén Darío", en "Nuevas cartas americanas", O. C., III, páginas 291 y ss.

Las dos largas y bellas cartas dirigidas al autor, y en su elogio, no dejan lugar a dudas. Percibe el crítico el profundo conocimiento que el poeta tiene de los más grandes poetas franceses del xix y la influencia que sobre el novel ejercen. Por una vez, esta influencia será benéfica a los ojos de Valera. Porque el poeta sudamericano no ha copiado sandiamente, sino que ha sabido asimilar, digerir lo que de bueno ha estudiado:

"Y usted no imita a ninguno; ni es usted romántico, ni naturalista, ni neurótico, ni decadente, ni simbólico, ni parnasiano. Usted lo ha revuelto todo, lo ha puesto a cocer en el alambique de su cerebro y ha sacado de ello *una rara quintaesencia*" [3].

Esta rara quintaesencia, que subrayamos, será ni más ni menos que el modernismo.

Lo que en Salvador Rueda había tachado de excesos naturalistas se percibe en esta obra de Rubén más clara, noble y bellamente expresado. Es una auténtica nueva manera de hacer poesía y el crítico lo ha descubierto y aplaude gozosamente con todas sus fuerzas. Cuanto hay de clásico, como cuanto hay de moderno.

En especial, en los cuentos rubenianos es donde don Juan halla más que aplaudir. Esos cuentos fantásticos, libres como él mismo los quería, de princesas y ninfas, de mundos de ensueños y quimeras bellísimas que, aunque no mucho, algo tienen que ver con su "Pájaro verde" y otros cuentos valerinos.

La absoluta sinceridad de las palabras del crítico, el entusiasmo que sintió por Rubén Darío, se corrobora en su correspondencia privada. A Menéndez Pelayo le dice estar convencido del "poderosísimo y original ingenio de Rubén"; además del mestizo de español e indio encuentra en el joven poeta "el extracto, la refinada tintura de todo lo nuevo de la poesía europea, perfectamente asimilada con personalidad, acierto y buen gusto". No hay "afectación ni esfuerzo,

---

[3] *Ibidem.*

ni remedos; todo en Rubén es natural y espontáneo, aunque primoroso y como cincelado"[4].

En otras dos ocasiones volverá don Juan a criticar obras de Rubén Darío[5]. Aunque en ambas manifiesta su admiración por el poeta hispano-indio, nos parece ver en dichos artículos —no muy largos en extensión— una sutilísima —estuvimos tentados de escribir "valerinísima"— serie de razones que completan y, hasta cierto punto, modifican un tanto aquellas cartas famosas, el más resonante éxito crítico de Valera, como dijimos.

No son ya los reparos, claramente expuestos ahora. (En realidad, justo es decirlo, los había mencionado en su crítica a *Azul.*) Estos dos artículos dejan traslucir una actitud de prudente cautela que no tenían las cartas primeras. Sospechamos que tal cautela proviene de que don Juan, asustado un tanto de lo que había dicho años antes, cuando el resto de la crítica no había leído ni alabado tan espontáneamente como él lo hizo el primer libro de Rubén, ahora, ocho años más tarde, juzga oportuno replegar un tanto sus velas. Sin llegar a lo que algún malintencionado pudiera tomar por una vergonzante "marcha atrás" en su postura crítica, trata con sumo cuidado de poner los puntos sobre las íes.

En otras palabras: que, temeroso de que sus benévolos juicios del principio puedan ser mal interpretados, quiere señalar ahora, con toda claridad, lo que a él le parecían defectos en la poesía rubeniana. Repetimos que no es que quisiera desdecirse. Es simplemente prudencia (o cuquería) valerina.

Rubén, y se cuida Valera muy bien de subrayarlo, le sigue pareciendo un gran poeta; el primero de Hispanoamérica y uno de los mayores en lengua española de todos los tiempos. Mas el entusiasmo que el de Nicaragua siente por ciertos autores no es totalmente compartido por el crítico, como se ve en el artículo consa-

---

4 *Epistolario Valera-Menéndez Pelayo*, obra citada, pp. 447-448.
5 O. C., III, pp. 480-483 y 517-518, respectivamente.

grado a *Los raros*. En cuanto a *Prosas profanas*, comprendemos, por las razones de exquisitez y buen gusto ya apuntadas, el asombro de don Juan ante tan manifiesta, aunque hermosísima, sensualidad. (Recuérdese cuanto se dijo a propósito del libro de Salvador Rueda, criticado también crudamente por don Juan.)

Pide al poeta más hondura de sentimiento, menos cantos de amor carnal y, en definitiva, menos monotonía.

Desgraciadamente, la muerte impidió a Valera contemplar, como nosotros lo vemos hoy al estudiar la obra de Rubén, el cambio de signo que él pidiera a la poesía de aquél. En *Cantos de vida y esperanza* veremos a un Rubén menos juvenil, tan gran poeta como siempre, por no decir superior, lleno aún de vitalidad y fuerza, pero en el que el espíritu predomina sobre la carne. Lo sensual, sin dejar de existir —¡dejaría de ser Rubén!—, se adelgaza bellísimamente para dar paso a una serena luz de total hermosura poética y espiritual. Los difíciles años del vivir rubeniano lograron, justamente, aquella perfección que, por razones puramente estéticas, le pedía el crítico.

Muy comedidas fueron, en cambio, las alabanzas que a la obra de don Armando Palacio Valdés consagró nuestro crítico. Comedidas y escasas en número. Quizá fuera éste el motivo por el que Valera más tarde fue tan poco bien tratado por aquél.

LA GENERACIÓN DEL NOVENTAYOCHO

La conducta de silencio y prudencia que siempre practicó, guardando una cautelosa reserva ante toda obra que no le producía un inmediato entusiasmo, se fue acentuando con el paso de los años. No dejó de conocer cuantas de interés aparecían en España. Sabido es el impulso, o por mejor decir, el nuevo giro que la literatura toma en los años últimos del siglo pasado. Los que iban a formar la generación del noventayocho habían publicado muchas de sus más célebres obras en vida de don Juan Valera.

Y, sin embargo, salvados unos pocos artículos superficiales, el crítico se limitó a darse por enterado del valer de los nuevos escritores, sin entrar en análisis de fondo. (Debemos tener en cuenta, por otra parte, que en tales momentos la vista de Valera iba apagándose con rapidez. Que si su mente estaba más clara que en plena juventud, como él mismo repitió, sus ojos no le servían de mucho. Que tuvo que hacerse leer durante los diez últimos años de su vida, así como dictar sus artículos, lo que debió mermar enormemente su actividad.)

Mas, con todo, sospechamos que no fue sólo el impedimento físico (ya que conoció las obras principales, y a sus autores, pues muchos de ellos acudieron a sus famosas tertulias de la Cuesta de Santo Domingo) la única causa de su prudente silencio final. Sino que unido a la incapacidad iba, como siempre, el recelo; el temor a enojar, por una parte, a sus lectores (muchos de ellos en Suramérica) y, por otra, a los autores de los libros mencionados, con los que no siempre estaba de acuerdo. Varias veces había expresado este temor: "Es difícil, cuando se habla de autores contemporáneos, dejar contentos a los que son censurados, por blanda y delicada que sea la censura" [6].

Se disculpa muchas veces de no poder "cumplir tan ardua tarea por sentirse ya sin fuerzas y por carecer de autoridad suficiente" [7]. Deben tomarse sus palabras con toda reserva. No es que desconfíe, como dice, de sus posibilidades críticas. Teme las reacciones y la agresividad de los jóvenes. No quiere comprometerse, ya que le falta la energía juvenil requerida para sostener sus criterios en las discusiones.

---

[6] "Lit. Española en el siglo XIX", O. C., II, p. 897.
[7] "Laureles", O. C., II, p. 1099.

Tampoco convence plenamente, si bien hay en ella más de verdad que en las disculpas anteriores, otra de sus razones: "... por desengaño razonable y justo veo yo tales faltas en mi propia labor, que no me atrevo a censurar la de aquellos a quien la gran mayoría de mis compatriotas otorga aplausos y laureles" [8].

Analicemos, siquiera sea en esquema, la crítica hecha por Valera en los últimos años del siglo pasado y primeros del actual.

No es crítica profunda. Son artículos en su mayoría muy breves. A Pío Baroja —a su novela *Aventuras, inventos y mistificaciones de Silvestre Paradox*— le dedicó un corto pero interesante examen [9], en el que encontramos alabanzas y frases de aliento, animándole a que "continúe escribiendo para gloria de la novelística española". También conoció Valera *Camino de perfección,* leída primero por el autor en la tertulia literaria que el crítico mantenía en su casa de la cuesta de Santo Domingo [10], y *La busca,* de ninguna de las cuales quiso hacer crítica, aun cuando sabemos gustó de ellas. Conociendo, no obstante, el horror que por las notas descarnadas sentía Valera, el poco gusto que le producían las amarguras descritas en las obras barojianas, comprendemos su silencio. Aprobaba la pura creación artística de Baroja; vio en él un novelista completo y de gran porvenir, mas no apreciaba los temas que le servían para hacer arte. Reconoce las espléndidas dotes de escritor que tenía Baroja y lamenta la afición que manifiesta por pintar el lado triste de la vida. Además de la estructura personalísima de la

---

8   *Ibidem.*

9   O. C., II, pp. 1082-1084.

10   Pío Baroja, *Desde la última vuelta del camino,* Biblioteca Nueva, Madrid, 1945, p. 270 y ss. Cuenta Baroja cómo asistía a las famosas tertulias valerinas y su lectura de unos capítulos de *Camino de perfección.* Refiere la agudeza de Valera pues, pese al cuidado que pusiera Baroja en saltarse los párrafos que se referían a un personaje que era una contrafigura del propio Valera, éste, muy astutamente, conoció las intenciones del joven novelista y así se lo dijo días más tarde, entre sonrisas amistosas y comprensivas.

prosa, su fuerza expresiva y su belleza, alaba Valera el singularísimo humor del escritor vasco.

Solamente analizó un cuento —el titulado *Satanás*— de don Ramón del Valle Inclán [11]. Las alabanzas vuelven a brotar de su pluma con entusiasmo sincero. Encuentra el estilo "poderosamente atractivo", amén de mucha riqueza de color, capacidad para grabar en la memoria del lector los caracteres de los personajes todos, etc.

Resulta muy curioso, y no poco significativo, por otra parte, que, habiendo conocido don Juan las *Sonatas*, rehúse dedicarles un estudio detenido. En el fondo eran estas novelas —como muy agudamente señaló Ortega y Gasset [12]— "la novela libre de trabas con que soñara siempre Valera". Y, sin embargo, no las criticó. No debía encontrarse ya con fuerzas para analizar e interpretar obra tan interesante con la amplitud que el tema requería.

Palabras no menos elogiosas tuvo para *El alma castellana* del joven José Martínez Ruiz, que aún no había adoptado su popular seudónimo (pero tampoco escribió nada a la aparición de *La voluntad,* muy poco después). Aunque le afea el pesimismo general de la obra —como se veía también en las de los otros escritores que conocemos hoy como los del noventayocho— y le tacha de "demasiado derrotista", no puede por menos de ensalzar la magnífica calidad, la belleza inigualable de la prosa de Azorín [13].

---

[11] O. C., III, pp. 559-560. El periódico *El Liberal* había organizado un concurso de cuentos al cual presentó Valle Inclán el suyo. Componían el tribunal don Juan Valera, don José Echegaray y don Isidoro Fernández Flórez. Parece ser que Valera se inclinó a conceder el primer premio a *Satanás,* mas no así sus compañeros de jurado. No por razones de estética —pues que lo consideraban de gran calidad artística—, sino porque consideraban el tema un tanto escandaloso. Don Juan, no obstante, lo aplaudió vivamente y le concedió el honor de una crítica muy entusiasta, que debió calmar un tanto la furia de don Ramón.

[12] J. Ortega y Gasset, *Obras Completas,* Madrid, 1946, vol. I, p. 19.

[13] "Nuevas cartas americanas", O. C., III, pp. 576-577.

Conoció Valera los primeros escritos de Unamuno —a quien llamó en una ocasión "originalísimo escritor, filósofo y docto humanista"—, pero tampoco hizo crítica alguna a dichos escritos. (Se habían conocido personalmente años antes, en las oposiciones que dieron a Unamuno su cátedra en la Universidad de Salamanca, y en las cuales era don Juan miembro del tribunal.)

Tampoco pasó desapercibido al fino espíritu valerino el valor de los trabajos del "joven y docto filólogo don Ramón Menéndez Pidal", que comenzaba entonces a dar los primeros frutos de sus investigaciones sobre la poesía medieval. Ni los estudios "críticos e históricos de don Francisco Rodríguez Marín", y sus cualidades de poeta y escritor.

A don Jacinto Benavente —a su comedia *Gente conocida*— dedicó don Juan un corto pero encomiástico fragmento en una de sus últimas cartas americanas, al igual que a la obra de don Eduardo Marquina [14].

También vemos citados en sus artículos a los hermanos Álvarez Quintero, a Vicente Blasco Ibáñez y a don Gregorio Martínez Sierra.

Tenemos, pues, que nuestro crítico no abandonó en ningún momento, hasta el fin de sus días, el terreno amado de la crítica. Si bien no se atrevió (como lo hubiera hecho años antes, si la floración magnífica de escritores de fines de siglo se hubiera producido cuando todavía contaba don Juan con toda su energía física); si bien no se atrevió, repetimos, a enfrascarse en discusiones críticas para las que se encontraba sin vista y con escasas fuerzas, no por ello dejó de percibir el rumbo especial que, a partir de 1890, toman las letras españolas. Lástima grande que don Juan nos privara de sus opiniones acerca de la obra de aquellos escritores jóvenes, sobre los que, de algún modo, influyó la suya en mayor grado del que ellos mismos quisieron reconocer. (Solamente Azorín y en sus artículos de los últimos diez o quince años le reconoció "exquisito y admirado maestro".)

---

[14] *Idem*, pp. 466 y 561-562, respectivamente.

Capítulo XI

TEMAS DE LA LITERATURA UNIVERSAL
Y RECAPITULACIÓN

No queremos terminar este estudio del crítico literario sin referirnos —siquiera sea de manera esquemática— a su labor como aficionado y estudioso de las literaturas de otros países. Nos limitamos aquí a trazar lo que puede ser el guión de un trabajo a realizar en el futuro, para el que los límites del presente no nos dejan espacio.

Don Juan Valera fue quizá el primer crítico español que se preocupó de la literatura hispanoamericana. Menéndez Pelayo —y Unamuno luego— le secundaría más tarde con el estudio amoroso de la poesía de aquellos países. Mas Valera fue el primero que dio periódicamente noticia de cuanto se publicaba de interés en las nacientes repúblicas de la América hispana.

En sus artículos, analizó no sólo la labor de los escritores más importantes, sino las de otros mucho más modestos que, atraídos por la bondadosa actitud y el renombre del crítico, le enviaban sus obras pidiéndole consejo y su más sincera opinión. Para todos tuvo palabras de aliento. Quizá mucha de esta crítica, a la hora de valorarla, no pueda ser tenida en cuenta por su excesiva bondad de juicio. Mas debe tenerse muy presente que el mayor interés de don Juan al escribirla estribaba no en hacer un mero juicio crítico, sino en el más generoso de acercar a los lectores y escritores de ambos lados del Atlántico. Dio a conocer así a muchos nombres de escritores suramericanos totalmente desconocidos antes en España.

Entre los mejores análisis pueden contarse los que dedicó a don Ricardo Palma, a quien consideró como clásico de nuestra lengua, y los que consagró al ecuatoriano Juan Montalvo (al que consideró el mejor estilista de América del Sur) y que, juntamente con las cartas a Rubén Darío, nos parecen la mejor crítica de Valera sobre los escritores de aquellos países.

Durante sus estancias en Portugal, tuvo don Juan la oportunidad de hacer amistad con los poetas y escritores más famosos de aquel país y de conocer sus obras. Gozó de la amistad de Guerra Junqueiro, Latino Coelho, Oliveira Martins, Antero de Quental, etc. De todos ellos nos dejó muy interesantes noticias en artículos y cartas, así como de su devoción por el poema de Camoens.

Contra la literatura francesa se estrellaron los mayores prejuicios de nuestro autor. De un lado, por la "petulante postura" hacia todo lo español "que le parecía encontrar" en los escritores franceses. Y de otro, por la "cómoda y servil imitación" que encontraba en muchos de nuestros escritores. La lente de su más que nunca exacerbado españolismo le deformaba cuanto de aquel país sometía a su análisis. Ni tuvo razón al negar las bellezas de la lírica medieval española ni pudo juzgar unos trabajos que apenas conocía o conocía muy mal. Y no se hable de los escritores modernos de aquel país; baste señalar que sus favoritos fueron Gautier y Mérimée. Menospreció a los naturalistas, sin exceptuar a Zola, y abominaba a Rousseau. Renan le parecía indecente por su *Abbesse de Jouarre,* y Baudelaire, detestable. A Victor Hugo, a quien en el fondo consideraba gran poeta, le encontraba multitud de faltas.

Con la literatura en lengua inglesa —aunque no le consagrase análisis de importancia— fue algo menos injusto. Lo que no impide que considerase a Shakespeare inferior a Lope, Tirso y Calderón. Apreciaba a Byron, Shelley y Walter Scott especialmente y fueron no pocas las composiciones que tradujo al español, de poetas norteamericanos. Entre los mejores, según su criterio, estaban Longfellow, Edgar Allan Poe, Russell Lowell y Walt Whitman. De la literatura italiana, como de la alemana, fue siempre ferviente admirador. Uno de los mejores estudios suyos fue el largo ensayo sobre Leopardi. Y son también dignos de consideración los que consagró al *Fausto* de Goethe.

RECAPITULACIÓN

Dado el poco interés que la investigación ha manifestado hasta el presente por la crítica de Valera, teníamos la impresión, antes de habernos decidido a comenzar nuestro trabajo, de que el autor de novelas, el fino estilista y el elegante hombre de mundo habían hecho olvidar (o por lo menos lo habían relegado a un segundo plano) todo el mérito de sus trabajos críticos. Sin pretender llegar a descubrimientos sensacionales, escogimos la tarea de estudiar este aspecto menos conocido —o, lo que es peor, mal conocido— de quien siempre nos pareció uno de los espíritus más finos, no sólo de las letras hispánicas, sino de la Europa del siglo xix.

Nos acercamos a él, primero, tratando de comprenderle, de analizar sus trabajos sin pasión, con objetividad, intentando aclarar las dudas que se nos habían planteado, en la esperanza de que tal labor pudiese ser de alguna utilidad.

El camino que llevamos recorrido hasta aquí nos permite trazar ahora un resumen esquemático de lo que ha ido apareciendo ante nosotros.

Comenzamos por estudiar la figura del hombre, tratando de observar la proyección que pudiera tener en sus obras el azaroso vivir del diplomático, su formación y su carácter. Proyección que se nos antojaba como de importancia, si se tiene en cuenta que sus juicios fueron siempre dulcificados por aquella elegancia física y espiritual que le distinguió.

Valera no volverá a desprenderse de aquella formación clásica —el estudio de autores griegos y latinos— de sus primeros años. ("Nosotros somos clasicotes hasta los tuétanos", le dijo en una ocasión a don Marcelino.) Formación clásica que nos conducirá a una de las paradojas valerinas: lo mismo que le hizo dueño de un estilo purísimo del mejor sabor, le incapacitó para apreciar cuanto se saliera de los cánones de su cerrado clasicismo, ya se tratase de las sencillas y puras composiciones medievales, ya de las mejores novelas picarescas, o cuantas novedades —y no fueron pocas— se dieron en las letras de la segunda mitad del siglo pasado.

Tampoco pudo desprenderse (y esto se sale, por el momento, de los límites del presente trabajo) de las imágenes del paisaje andaluz que, como placas fotográficas, se habían grabado en su retina durante los primeros tiempos de su vida. Don Juan recordaría siempre aquel paisaje, embelleciéndolo más y más.

Aquel no afirmar ni negar nada, su escepticismo para muchos, se debió principalmente a que el espíritu desengañado de sus padres le había conformado el suyo; quizá con demasiada fuerza en los años de niñez y adolescencia. Igual que su "cuquería" en política.

Mas no se han de buscar las raíces de cuanto de negativo pueda verse en su figura, en las influencias que sobre él ejercieron aquéllos. No olvidemos cuánto de bueno —lo mejor de cuanto ella misma poseía— debe Valera a la figura de su madre. E incluso su padre, menos instruido que la marquesa de la Paniega, le daba consejos prácticos "para asentar más los pies sobre el suelo".

Y si el oficio de diplomático le apartó temporalmente de las letras, fue esa actividad la que primero le había conducido al lado de una de las figuras más elegantes de nuestro romanticismo: el Duque de Rivas y su corte poética de Nápoles, lo que no dejó de tener su importancia.

Si es cierto que los viajes le impidieron una labor más constante para el cultivo de nuestras letras, no lo es menos que aquellos frecuentes cambios le proporcionaban campo propicio para cosechar las primeras flores valerinas, el estilo y la gracia de sus cartas desde Rusia. (Don Juan Valera, de haber sido profesor provinciano, como Clarín, hubiera sido muy diferente de lo que fue. Su tarea de crítico se habría resentido —hasta la bilis colérica se echa de ver en las de Leopoldo Alas—, resentimiento que jamás aparece en las críticas valerinas.)

El elegante mundo de la diplomacia contribuyó a perfilar acabadamente el carácter ya en sí de esteta delicado y exquisito. De allí su falta de interés por todo lo que considera carente de belleza, su horror por el tremendismo, por lo feo.

También los amores y amoríos valerinos, tan mencionados y estudiados, tienen reflejo en su obra. Aunque más importante en la de pura creación que en la crítica, naturalmente. El conocimiento del alma femenina facilitaba, a su agudísimo ingenio, material para proporcionarnos esos paseos, de la mano de sus personajes, a lo largo de tantas páginas de sus novelas. Novelas de amores, las llamaba Montesinos. De mujeres enamoradas, diríamos nosotros.

E incluso el desengaño, o por mejor decir: la desilusión sufrida con la mujer de quien tanto esperaba, le hizo ser más comprensivo, más sabiamente humano al tratar de personajes femeninos en obras ajenas.

Buscando las raíces de la estética valerina, nos adentramos en su obra sin tener muy en cuenta lo que siempre se le había echado en cara, a nuestro juicio muy ligeramente: su bondad.

Que nació de una elegancia espiritual, de su tolerancia filosófica, de su alegría vital y sus finos modales, reflejándose en todo lo que hizo. También, y esto sí que nos parece importante, porque don Juan desconfiaba mucho de la eficacia de una crítica más dura.

Antes que segar cruelmente, aconseja que se abonen nuestros hambrientos campos, regándolos con amor y comprensión. No quie-

re criticar la obra de los tontos y se inclina por la defensa de la
de los discretos. Alabando cuando lo cree necesario, y aunque se
prodigó un tantico en las alabanzas —como ya señalamos—, no puede negarse que ayudó a muchos a mejorarse en el cultivo de las
bellas letras. Frente a la dureza de juicio de Revilla y Clarín, la
amable bondad de don Juan.

Se dedica a la crítica literaria para mejorar el estado de nuestras letras, no para ser verdugo de ellas. No señala sólo defectos,
sino que indica caminos a seguir, animando con sus frases toleran-
tes a los que las necesitan.

Su crítica, mejor que de una obra, podríamos decir que lo es
"a propósito de una obra". Lo que la hace un tanto peculiar a los
ojos de un público acostumbrado al latigazo y al comentario mor-
diente. La suya se sale de los cauces de la tradicional. Ateniéndose
siempre a una estética flexible, bien asimilada, elegante, como la
personalidad de su autor, pero no improvisada o hecha con los re-
tazos de otras mal digeridas, como solían hacer los critiquillos de
tres al cuarto.

No se le oculta la dificultad de aplicar rígidamente un "decálogo estético riguroso" para obras de la endeblez de las que caían
en sus manos las más de las veces. Con criterio más estricto que
el suyo, hubieran pasado muy pocas el examen.

El crítico, para don Juan, es un artista que, en lugar de crear,
juzga y estudia lo que hacen los demás. Por lo que su obra vale
tanto —y justifica al autor— como la de un novelista, dramaturgo
o poeta lírico, siempre que sea buena.

Valera como crítico, y como artista, fue paladín del más puro
idealismo. Su estética brota de las fuentes más clásicas; aunque no
dejó de conocer las más modernas estéticas, raramente se apartará
de las ideas aprendidas en los primeros años de estudiante de filosofía.

Su idealismo le llevó a cometer uno de los más graves pecados.
el no admitir más que a regañadientes que, fuera de las formas clá-

sicas, podía existir belleza pura. Cierra los ojos voluntariamente y con una terquedad asombrosa a toda otra sugestión.

El único fin del arte, para don Juan, es la creación de la belleza. Todo arte que ofenda gravemente a la moral no es arte.

En cuanto al concepto que de los géneros literarios tiene Valera, puede decirse con Clarín, "¡Todo son cosas de Valera!". Para él todo es poesía, todo es arte de la palabra y, como tal, libre de trabas.

Rompe cuando le conviene los vallados que separan a uno u otro género por considerarlos cosas de artificio. Predica con el ejemplo, haciendo sus "cuentos-novela" o sus "novelas-cuento", sin otra diferencia que la puramente formal.

Los fracasados intentos dramáticos de don Juan no hacen sino demostrarnos que, al igual que con la novela y los demás géneros, no se atuvo a los moldes tradicionales. Si su teatro a veces tiene aciertos, si resiste bien una lectura —porque está ingeniosamente escrito y en una lengua casticísima—, no es auténtico teatro.

Como ensayista, puede ser considerado don Juan antecedente clarísimo de la moderna literatura de ensayo; tanto por los temas de que se ocupó como por la especial manera de tratarlos, precede a los componentes de la generación del noventayocho. Justamente en el campo del ensayo es donde Valera se sintió más libre. Allí aquellas "cosas de Valera" chocaban menos, parecían menos nuevas.

Respecto de la literatura peninsular de la Edad Media, en especial la lírica primitiva, manifestó siempre don Juan una incomprensión radical que le impidió el acercamiento amoroso que toda poesía requiere para ser estudiada, entendida y admirada. Defendiendo su postura, ideó argumentos no muy convincentes a los que se aferró hasta el fin de sus días.

Brilló mucho más alto como crítico de las mejores obras de nuestras letras posteriores. Su más tierno amor, como tema de análisis, *El Quijote,* al que consagró tres importantes trabajos.

Quizá el mayor reproche que pueda hacérsele a don Juan Valera como crítico literario es que no dedicase más tiempo a su tarea. Amor, comprensión y estudio le sobraban para haber llevado a cabo una labor comparable, sin ningún género de dudas, a las de las más altas figuras de la crítica universal.

Mejor que hablar de los defectos de la crítica valerina, podría hablarse de las grandes "lagunas" que tal labor nos deja ver; de los huecos que nos hubiera gustado ver rellenos con sus comentarios sabios y oportunos a obras que lo merecieron. A veces, eran lagunas voluntarias que no se tomó el trabajo de "llenar", a causa del trabajo de biblioteca requerido. Otras veces, lo impedía el constante viajar por los países que más le atraían o el ver a gentes que requerían su deliciosa personalidad. No olvidemos que don Juan pasó por este mundo como asistiendo al más "maravilloso espectáculo", y disfrutando de él cuanto fuera posible. La vida fue para él —incluso en los momentos menos agradables, que también los tuvo— una fiesta deliciosa.

Antes que escritor, antes que crítico, trató simplemente de ser hombre. Y, a poder ser, hombre feliz. Salvo unos cuantos momentos difíciles, salió adelante con su empeño.

Disfrutó 81 años de una existencia llena de aquella alegría pagana que había descubierto en sus amados clásicos.

De regalo, nos dejó una labor de creación excelente. Y una tarea crítica de la mejor calidad, por su finura, su agudeza, su ingeniosa sagacidad y, sobre todo, por sus acertadísimos juicios. Sólo puede ser equiparada —sin perder por ello en la comparación— a la que realizaron otras dos grandes figuras de la crítica española y entrañables amigos suyos, don Marcelino Menéndez y Pelayo y Leopoldo Alas, Clarín.

Quizá la mejor alabanza que podamos hacer de tan interesante labor crítica sea decir que, pasados más de cien años desde la publicación de muchos de los artículos de Juan Valera, no han perdido actualidad. No han envejecido sus ideas. Aún siguen deleitando e instruyendo al lector que, de la mano de tan noble figura, se pasea encantado a través de las mejores páginas de nuestras letras, iluminadas bellamente por la clara luz del mejor espíritu valerino.

Leeds, setiembre de 1964.

TERCERA PARTE

BIBLIOGRAFÍA

Intentamos recoger en nuestra lista bibliográfica todos los trabajos consagrados a don Juan Valera de cuya existencia tenemos noticia hasta la fecha.

No nos han sido accesibles en su totalidad —de aquí el que alguna de las fichas vaya incompleta— y antes que silenciar su existencia hemos preferido mencionarlos acompañados de un asterisco.

Abbot, Alice Katherine: *A Study of the Women Characters in the Novels of Juan Valera*, Illinois, 1927.

Alcalá Galiano, A.: Prólogo a *Ensayos poéticos*, de Juan Valera, Granada, Edit. Benavides, 1844.

Aldama, Leonardo de: "Valera, la heterodoxia y la Hispanidad", en *Revista de la Universidad de Buenos Aires*, N. 12, año 1953.

Altamira, R.: "Genio y Figura", en *Revista crítica de Historia y Literatura*, mayo y junio de 1897.

Anónimo: "Valera", en *El Imparcial*, Madrid, 15 de abril 1905.

— "Littérature espagnole. Critique. Un diplomate romancier: Juan Valera", en *Revue Britannique*, 8 de agosto 1882.

— *Diccionario de la Literatura española*, Madrid, Revista de Occidente, 1964.

Anzoátegui, Ignacio B.: "Don Juan Valera, novelista andaluz", en *Cuadernos Hispanoamericanos*, XXXI, 1957, n. 88, pp. 94-102.

Araujo Costa, A.: "Giovanni Valera critico", en *Rivista Colombo*, Roma, II, 1927.

— "El cincuentenario de don Juan Valera", en *ABC*, 17 de abril 1955.

— "Valerismo", en *ABC*, 28 de octubre 1954.

Arias Abad, Francisco: *Las mujeres de don Juan Valera*, Andújar, 1935.

Arrarás, Joaquín: "Valera y el Quijote", en *ABC*, Sevilla, 24 de mayo 1947.

Arriaga, Joaquín de: "España y el clasicismo de don Juan Valera", en *Arriba*, Madrid, 9 de enero 1944.

Artigas, M., y Sáinz-Rodríguez, Pedro: *Epistolario de Valera y Menéndez Pelayo*, Madrid, Espasa Calpe, 1946.

Artigas, M. y Sáinz-Rodríguez, Pedro: *Epistolario de Valera y Menéndez Alcalá-Galiano*, A.: Prólogo a *Ensayos poéticos*, de Juan Valera, Granada, Azaña, Manuel: "Valera en Rusia", en *Nosotros*, Buenos Aires, LII, año 1926.

— *Pepita Jiménez*, prólogo y notas para la edición de "La lectura", Madrid, 1927.

— "La novela de Pepita Jiménez", en *Cuadernos literarios*, Madrid, 1928.

— *Valera en Italia. Amores, política, literatura*, Madrid, edit. Páez, 1929.

— "Asclepigenia y la experiencia amorosa de don Juan Valera", en *Plumas y palabras*, Madrid, Ciap, 1930.

— *Pepita Jiménez*. Edición, prólogo y notas para "Clásicos Castellanos", n. 80, Madrid, 1935.

— "Valera", en *La invención del Quijote y otros ensayos*, Madrid, Espasa Calpe, 1934.

Azorín: "Sobre Valera", en *Blanco y Negro*, 2 de noviembre 1907.

— "La estatua de Valera", en *ABC*, 2 de noviembre 1907.

— "Don Juan Valera", en *Los valores literarios*, Madrid, 1913, pp. 171-176.

— *El paisaje de España visto por los españoles*, Madrid, 1917.

— "Don Juan Valera", en *ABC*, 22 de noviembre 1946.

— "La sensibilidad en Valera", en *ABC*, 18 de febrero 1947.

— "Valeriana", en *ABC*, 10 de enero 1947.

— "Valera en Granada", en *ABC*, 12 de febrero 1947.

— "Valera y sus amigos", en *ABC*, 19 de marzo 1947.

— "Prólogo", en *Canciones del suburbio*, de Pío Baroja, Madrid, 1944.

— "Valera", en *De Valera a Miró*, Madrid, 1959, pp. 19-51.

Baig Baños, A.: "Cinco andaluces en Madrid", en *Revista de la Biblioteca, Archivo y Museo Municipal*, vol. V, Madrid, 1928.

Balseiro, J. A.: *Novelistas españoles modernos*, New York, 1946.

Baquero Goyanes, M.: "Juan Valera y la generación de 1868", en *Arbor*, XXXIV, 1956.

Barberán, Cecilio: "Los amigos de don Juan Valera", en *ABC*, 9 de diciembre 1933.

Barja, César: *Libros y autores modernos*, New York, 1924.

— *Literatura española*. Edición revisada y ampliada de la obra anterior, Los Angeles, 1933.

Baroja, Pío: *Desde la última vuelta del camino*, Madrid, 1945.

— "Las horas solitarias", en *Obras Completas*, vol. V, Madrid, Biblioteca Nueva, 1948.

— *Juventud, egolatría,* Madrid, 1917.

Bello, Luis: "La casa de Pepita Jiménez", en *La Esfera,* Cabra, 6 de diciembre 1924.

Bender, J.: "La correspondencia de D. Juan Valera", en *La Lectura,* XII, Madrid, 1913.

Benítez, R. A.: "Don Juan Valera", en *Revista de Educación,* La Plata, 1955.

Benítez Claros, R.: "Valera y el español", en *Anales del Instituto de Lingüística,* Mendoza, V, 1952.

Blanco García, F.: *La literatura española en el siglo XIX,* Madrid, Sáenz de Jubera, 1909.

Blennerhasset, L.: "Der moderne spanische Roman: Fernán Caballero, Valera, Coloma", en *Deutsche Rundschau,* 1895.

Bonilla y San Martín, A.: *Este es un decir antiguo que compuso Aphante Ucalego y se intitula "J. V.",* Barcelona, 1905.

Boussagnol, Gabriel: *Ángel de Saavedra, Duc de Rivas. Sa vie, son oeuvre poétique,* Toulouse, 1926.

Bravo Villasante, C.: "Idealismo y ejemplaridad de Valera", en *Revista de Literatura,* 1952, pp. 339-362.

— "Don Juan Valera en el Alamillo", en *Semana,* 22 de abril 1958.

— *Biografía de don Juan Valera,* Barcelona, edit. Aedos, 1959.

Brenan, Gerald: *The Literature of the Spanish People,* Cambridge University Press, 1951.

Brunetière, F.: "La casuistique dans le roman", en *Revue des Deux Mondes,* París, 15 de noviembre 1881.

Busuioceanu, A.: "Una historia romántica: Don Juan Valera y Lucía Palladi", en *Revue des Études Roumaines,* 1953.

— "El grande y no secreto amor de don Juan Valera: Lucía la muerta", en *Correo Literario,* marzo 1953.

Caballero Pozo, L.: "Valera y el embrujo andaluz", en *Revista de la Universidad de Buenos Aires,* 1953, pp. 135-200 y 403-460.

Camacho Padilla, J.: "Valera en el centenario de Goethe", en *Boletín de la Academia de Ciencias, Bellas Letras y Nobles Artes de Córdoba,* 1932.

Candela Ortells, V.: "El centenario del nacimiento de don Juan Valera", en *El mercantil valenciano,* 18 de octubre 1924.

Cano, José Luis: "Un amor de don Juan Valera", en *Quaderni Ibero-Americani,* Torino, diciembre 1954, pp. 487-489.

— "Valera siempre actual", en *Ínsula,* octubre 1959.

— "Don Juan Valera en el Brasil", en *Cuadernos Americanos*, XXII, Méjico, 1963, pp. 279-284.

Cánovas del Castillo, A.: "Prólogo a las novelas de don Juan Valera", en *Colección de Escritores Castellanos*, Madrid, 1888.

— "Prólogo" a *Las ilusiones del Doctor Faustino*, Madrid, 1901.

Cañamaque, F.: *Los oradores de 1869*, Madrid, 1879.

Cardona, María de: "El gran amor de juventud de don Juan Valera", en *Tajo*, 17 de mayo 1941.

— "Don Juan Valera", en *Tajo*, 23 de agosto 1941.

— "Don Juan Valera. Cartas inéditas y anecdotario", en *Tajo*, 30 de agosto 1941.

Carilla, Emilio: "Una novela de don Juan Valera", en *Cuadernos Hispano-Americanos*, n. 89, Madrid, 1957, pp. 178-191.

Casa Valencia, Conde de: *Necrología del Excmo. Señor don Juan Valera*, Madrid, 1905.

— *Necrológica en honor de don Juan Valera*, Madrid, 1907.

Castro, Cristóbal de: "Valera, la distinción y la gratuidad", en *La Esfera*, 1 de octubre 1927.

— "Valera periodista", en *ABC*, 8 de agosto 1952.

Cejador y Frauca, Julio: *Historia de la Lengua y Literatura Castellana*, Madrid, 1918.

Cervães e Rodriguez, F.: *A travez da Hespanha Literaria*, Porto, 1901.

Chiareno, Osvaldo: *Lettere di Juan Valera a Angelo de Gubernatis*, Génova, 1962.

Christianson, A. C.: *The Women Characters of Juan Valera*, Arizona University, Doctoral Dissertation, 1937.

Clarín: "Valera", en *Nueva campaña*, Madrid, 1897.

— "Entre bobos anda el juego", en *Ensayos y Revistas*, Madrid, 1892.

— *Solos de Clarín* (figuran los artículos "Un prólogo de Valera", "El comendador Mendoza", "Tentativas dramáticas" y "Doña Luz"), Madrid, 1891.

— "Revista literaria" (Crítica a *Juanita la larga*), en *Las Novedades*, New York, 1896.

— "Revista literaria" (Crítica a *Genio y Figura*), en *Los lunes del Imparcial*, 5 de abril 1897.

— "Revista literaria" (Crítica a *A vuela pluma*), en *Los lunes del Imparcial*, 19 de julio 1897.

— "Revista literaria" (Crítica a *Morsamor*), en *Los lunes del Imparcial*, 7 de agosto 1899.

— "Revista literaria" (Crítica a *Dafnis y Cloe*), en *Los lunes del Imparcial*, 26 de marzo 1900.

Clavería, Carlos: "En torno a una frase en 'caló' de don Juan Valera", en *Hispanic Review*, T. XVI, 1948, pp. 97-119.

Coello, Carlos: "Doña Luz y las novelas de Valera", en *La Ilustración Española y Americana*, XXIX, 8 de agosto 1879.

Condesa de Yebes: "Tres cartas inéditas", en *Boletín de la R. A. de la Historia*, CXLVIII, 1961, pp. 249-254.

Conejo, Ángel: "De las andanzas sentimentales de Valera", en *La estafeta literaria*, enero 1946.

Correa Calderón, E.: *El centenario de doña Emilia Pardo Bazán*, Madrid, 1952.

Cossío, José M.: *Rasgos políticos para una semblanza de don Juan Valera*, Madrid, 1947.

*Coster, Cyrus C. de: *The Theory and Practice of the Novels of Juan Valera: A Study in Technique*, Doctoral Dissertation, Chicago University, 1951.

— "Valera en Washington", en *Arbor*, Madrid, n. 98, febrero 1954, páginas 215-223.

— "Valera y Portugal", en *Arbor*, Madrid, n. 123, marzo 1956, pp. 398-410.

— *Correspondencia de don Juan Valera (1859-1905)*, edición, prólogo y notas por C. C. de Coster, Valencia, edit. Castalia, 1956.

— "Valera: Critic of American Literature", en *Hispania*, XLIII, 3, páginas 364-367.

— "Valera and Andalusia", en *Hispanic Review*, 1961, pp. 200-216.

— "Un fragmento inédito de una versión más antigua de la novela de Valera *Morsamor*", en *Boletín de la Real Academia de Ciencias, Bellas Letras y Nobles Artes de Córdoba*, 1956, pp. 138-142.

Covaleda, Antonio: "Juan Valera espectador y protagonista en la muerte de un siglo", en *La Estafeta Literaria*, 5 de mayo 1936.

Cruz Rueda, B.: "Un don Juan siempre es discutido", en *La Estafeta Literaria*, 15 de junio 1944.

Cuervo, Rufino José: *El castellano en América*, ed. El Ateneo, Buenos Aires, 1947.

Cusachs, C. V.: *Pepita Jiménez*, edición crítica para Norteamérica, New York, 1910.

Darío, Rubén: *España contemporánea*, París, Garnier, 1907.

Dato Iradier, E.: *Discurso leído ante la Academia de Ciencias Morales y Políticas*, Madrid, 1910.

Demidowick, John P.: "El Conde de las Navas y los contertulios de don Juan Valera", en *Revista de literatura*, 1957, pp. 154-165.
— "Una carta de don Juan Valera y el chascarrillo andaluz", en *Revista de literatura*, 1958, pp. 231-236.

Díez Echarri, E, y Roca Franquesa, J. M.: *Historia de la Literatura Española e Hispanoamericana*, Madrid, Aguilar, 1960.

Diego, Gerardo: "Barajas contra Luis Vives", en *ABC*, 5 de febrero 1947.
— "Vives derrotado", en *ABC*, 14 de febrero 1947.

Domínguez Bordona, J.: "Centenario del autor de Pepita Jiménez. Cartas inéditas", en *Revista de la Biblioteca, Archivo y Museo Municipal*, Madrid, T. II, 1925, pp. 83-108 y 237-252; T. III, 1926, pp. 430-462.

Donato, E.: "Don Juan Valera, ese casi desconocido", en *Boletín de la Real Academia de Ciencias, Bellas Letras y Nobles Artes de Córdoba*, 1961, pp. 135-137.

D'Ors, Eugenio: "Palique", en *ABC*, 14 de diciembre 1923.
— "Mímesis, o de las artes de imitación", en *Arriba*, 2 de julio 1944.
— "Il superamento", en *Arriba*, 4 de julio 1944.
— "Lo caduco", en *Arriba*, 23 de mayo 1946.
— "Nacional y castizo", en *Nuevo glosario*, O. C., Vol. I, Madrid, 1947.
— "Juan Valera", en *Nuevo glosario*, O. C., I, Madrid, 1947.
— "Valera el artista", en *Nuevo glosario*, O. C., I, Madrid, 1947.

Dos Fuentes, Marqués de: "Don Juan Valera. Un aspecto de su vida", en *Boletín de la Real Academia de Ciencias, Bellas Letras y Nobles Artes de Córdoba*, 1951, pp. 63-69.

Ellis, Havelock: *The Soul of Spain*, London, 1929. (Publicado también en *La España moderna*, abril de 1909.)

Enríquez Barrios, M.: "Florilegio", en *Boletín de la Real Academia de Ciencias, Bellas Letras y Nobles Artes de Córdoba*, 1956, pp. 136-137.

Entrambasaguas, J.: "Juan Valera", en *Las mejores novelas contemporáneas*, Barcelona, ed. Planeta, 1957.

Eoff, Sherman: "Juan Valera's Interest in the Orient", en *Hispanic Review*, Vol. VI, 1938.

Espinosa, Agustín: "Juan Valera", en *Almanaque literario*, Madrid, 1935.

Esquer Torres, Ramón: "Para un epistolario Valera-Tamayo y Baus", en *Boletín de la Real Academia Española*, enero-abril 1959, pp. 89-163.

Estrella Gutiérrez, F.: *Pepita Jiménez* (edición, prólogo y notas), Buenos Aires, Katelusz, 1958.

Falcão Espalter, M.: "El epistolario de Valera y Menéndez Pelayo", en *Criterio*, Buenos Aires, 1938.

Fernández Luján, J.: *Valera, Pardo Bazán y Pereda*, Barcelona, 1889.

Figueiredo, Fidelino de: "A lusophilia de don João Valera", en *Revista de História*, Lisboa, 1926.

Figueroa, Agustín de: "El primer amor de Valera", en *ABC*, 1 de julio 1948.

Fishtine, Edith: *Don Juan Valera. The Critic*, Bryn Mawr, 1933.

Fitzmaurice-Kelly, J.: *A New History of Spanish Literature*, Oxford University Press, 1926.

Ford, J. D. M.: *Main Currents of Spanish Literature*, London, Constable & Co., 1921.

Francés, J.: "Don Juan Valera", en *La novela semanal*, 31 de enero 1925.

Francisco, A. de: "La proyección internacional del pensamiento de J. V.", en *Revista de Estudios Políticos*, 125, setiembre-octubre 1962.

Francos Rodríguez, J.: "Valera y el periodismo". Conferencia leída en la Real Academia Española de la Lengua el 9 de diciembre de 1924.

Fray Candil (seudónimo de Emilio Bobadilla): *Grafómanos de América*, 2 volúmenes, Madrid, 1902.

Gallego Morell, A.: "Un teléfono en la literatura de Valera", en *La Estafeta Literaria*, n. 192, p. 10.

— "Las poesías de Valera", en *Poesía española*, n. 89, Madrid, 1960, páginas 29-32.

— "Valera y Alarcón se asoman al Vesubio", en *Índice*, n. 163, Madrid, 1960.

Gálvez, Rafael: *Don Juan Valera y Menéndez Pelayo*, Cabra, Imprenta Cordón, 1957.

García de Castro, R. G.: *Los intelectuales y la Iglesia*, Madrid, 1934.

Garciasol, Ramón de: "América, preocupación de don Juan Valera", en *Estudios Americanos*, Sevilla, XVII, 1959, pp. 217-234.

— "El escritor don Juan Valera", en *Cuadernos Hispanoamericanos*, 1948, n. 3, pp. 541-554.

Gil y Carrasco, Enrique: *Crítica literaria*, Madrid, 1893.

*Giménez Caballero, E.: *El índice de Valera* (discurso leído ante la exposición del libro portugués).

— "Conmemoración de don Juan Valera", en *Revista de Occidente*, T. VI, octubre 1924.

Giner de los Ríos, H.: "El vocabulario de *Juanita la larga*", en *El resumen*, febrero de 1890. Reproducido en *La España moderna*, febrero 1896.

Gómez Alfaro, Antonio: "A los cien años de la primera obra de Valera: Versos", en *Arriba*, 13 de abril 1958.

Gómez Carrillo, E.: *Cuentos escogidos de autores castellanos contemporáneos*, París, Garnier, 1894.

Gómez de Baquero, E.: "Juanita la larga", en *La España moderna*, mayo 1896.

— "Morsamor", en *La España moderna*, diciembre 1899.

— "La última novela de Valera. ¿Nuevo Persiles?", en *La España moderna*, setiembre 1899.

— "El ocultismo en Morsamor y en otros libros del Señor Valera", en *La España moderna*, setiembre 1899.

— "Florilegio de poesías castellanas del siglo XIX, formado por don Juan Valera", en *La España moderna*, agosto de 1902.

— "Dos muertos ilustres: Balart, Valera", en *La España moderna*, mayo 1905.

— *El renacimiento de la novela en el siglo XIX*, Madrid, 1924.

— "Don Juan Valera humanista", en *O Instituto*, Coimbra, LXXII, 1925.

— "El humanismo en Valera", en *La Vanguardia*, Barcelona, 11, 18 y 25 de febrero 1925.

— "Valera humanista", en *De Gallardo a Unamuno*, Madrid, 1926, páginas 75-100.

Gómez Reshipo, L.: *Las cartas americanas de Valera*, Bogotá, 1888.

Gomis, Juan Bautista: "Sentido católico de Juan Valera", en *Verdad y vida*, enero-marzo 1944.

González, Ceferino: *Historia de la filosofía*, Madrid, 1886.

González Blanco, Andrés: *Historia de la novela en España desde el Romanticismo a nuestros días*, Madrid, 1909.

González López, Luis: *Las mujeres de don Juan Valera*, Madrid, Aguilar, 1934.

— "La gracia, amigo", en *Boletín de la Real Academia de Ciencias, Bellas Letras y Nobles Artes de Córdoba*, XXVII, 1956, pp. 294-296.

González Román, Gonzalo: "Don Juan Valera, sus andanzas diplomáticas y su personalidad humana vistas a través de ellas", en *Boletín de la Real Academia... de Córdoba*, XXVII, 1956, pp. 157-186.

Gullón, Ricardo: "Valera leído por Montesinos", en *Ínsula*, n. 130, 15 de setiembre 1957.

Hart, W.: *Pepita Jiménez*, introducción y estudio a la edición alemana, Berlín, 1882.

*Herrero Mayor, A.: "Don Juan Valera", en *Revista de educación*, La Plata, vol. 1.

Icaza, F. A. de: "Crítica española y literatura hispanoamericana", en *Guía del lector*, I, 1924.

— *Examen de críticos*, Madrid, 1894.

Iruña, Fermín de: "Don Juan Valera autor de zarzuela: Una letra en busca de música", en *Semana*, 8 y 29 de noviembre 1942.

Jiménez, Alberto: *Valera y la generación del 68*, The Dolphin Book, Oxford, 1956.

Jiménez Serrano, J.: "Prólogo" a *Ensayos poéticos*, de Juan Valera, Granada, Benavides, 1844.

Juderías, Julián: "Don Juan Valera; apuntes para su biografía", en *La lectura*, 1913 y 1914, vols. XIII-XIV.

— "La bondad, la tolerancia y el optimismo en las obras de don Juan Valera", en *La Ilustración española y americana*, 1914, números 31, 32 y 33.

— "Don Juan Valera y don Gumersindo Laverde. Fragmentos de una correspondencia inédita", en *La lectura*, 1917, pp. 15-27 y 165-178.

Juretschke, Hans: *España ante Francia*, Editora Nacional, Madrid, 1940.

Krynen, Jean: "Juan Valera et la mystique espagnole", en *Bulletin Hispanique*, 1944, XLVI.

— "L'esthétisme de J. Valera", en *Acta Salmanticensia*, 1946.

Lacoste, Maurice: *Juanita la larga*. Edition presentée par..., Paris, 1959.

Lancashire, G. S.: "Juan Valera", en *The Manchester Quarterly*, July, 1917.

Laverde, Gumersindo: "Cartas al Sr. D. J. Valera sobre asuntos americanos", en *La España moderna*, 1890 y 1891.

Lida de Malkiel, María R.: "El Parsondes de Valera y la Historia Universal de Nicolao de Damasco", en *Revista de Filología Hispánica*, 1942, págs. 274-281.

Loliée, Frédéric: *Les femmes du second Empire (Papiers intimes)*, Paris, 1906.

López Estrada, F.: "Epistolario de don Juan Valera a don Servando Arbolí, 1877-1897", en *Studia Philologica* (Homenaje a Dámaso Alonso), II, pp. 387-400.

Lott, Robert E.: "*Siglo de Oro*". *Tradition and Modern Adolescent Psychology in Pepita Jiménez. A Stylistic Study*, Washington, The Catholic University Press, 1958.

— *Pepita Jiménez* (Prólogo estudio a...), Washington D. C., 1958.

— "Pepita Jiménez and Don Quixote: A Structural Comparison", en *Hispania*, XLV, 1962, pp. 395-401.

Louis Lande, L.: "Un roman de moeurs espagnol", en *Revue des Deux Mondes*, 15 de enero 1875.

Marías, Julián: "La historia de la literatura empieza a ser historia", en *Ínsula*, n. 127, junio 1957.

— "Las noches de este mundo", en *La Nación*, Buenos Aires, 22 de febrero 1959. Publicado también en *Ínsula*, n. 154, setiembre 1959, bajo el título "Libertad y convivencia en Valera".

— "Una tradición olvidada", en *Ínsula*, n. 151, 15 de junio 1959.

Marichalar, Antonio: *Riesgo y fortuna del Duque de Osuna*, Madrid, 1942.

Martínez Kleiser, L.: *Don Pedro Antonio de Alarcón*, Madrid, ed. Suárez, 1943.

— "Campoamor, Zorrilla y Valera escriben a don Leopoldo Alas", en *La estafeta literaria*, 20 de marzo 1944.

Marvaud, A.: "Don Juan Valera", en *La quinzaine*, LXVI, 1905.

Maura, Antonio: "Centenario de Valera", en *Boletín de la Real Academia Española*, XI, 1924, pp. 509-518.

Mazzei, P.: "Per la fortuna di due opere spagnole in Italia: La Celestina e Pepita Jiménez", en *Revista de Filología Española*, 1922, IX, páginas 384-389.

— *Dante nel pensiero di D. Juan Valera*, Ferrara, Tipo. Taddei, 1927.

— "La lirica di don Juan Valera", en *Bulletin Hispanique*, 1925, XXVII, páginas 131-163.

Melian Lafinur, A.: "Valera novelista", en *Boletín de la Academia Argentina de Letras*, XXII, 1957, pp. 427-466.

Menéndez Pelayo, M.: *Historia de los Heterodoxos Españoles*, Madrid, 1882.

— "Canciones, romances y poemas de Valera", en *Estudios y discursos de crítica histórica y literaria*, Madrid, Editora Nacional, Obras Completas, 1942.

Merchán, Rafael: "Cartas al Señor D. Juan Valera sobre asuntos americanos", en *La España moderna*, abril y mayo, 1890.

Mesonero Romanos, R.: *Tipos y caracteres*, Madrid, 1881.

Monguio, L.: "Crematística de los novelistas españoles del siglo XIX", en *Revista Hispánica Moderna*, XVII, 1951.

Montesinos, J. F.: "Una nota sobre Valera", en *Estudios dedicados a don Ramón Menéndez Pidal*, T. IV, Madrid, 1953.

— *Valera o la ficción libre*, Madrid, ed. Gredos, 1957.

Montoliu, Manuel: *Literatura Castellana*, Barcelona, ed. Cervantes, 1937.

Montoto, Santiago: "Las amarguras de don Juan Valera", en *El Sol*, 13 de octubre 1926.

— "Thebussem, Valera y Montoto", en *La Época*, 21 de febrero 1931.

— "El veraneo de don Juan Valera", en *Semana*, 7 de agosto 1943.

— "Celos de don Juan Valera", en *Semana*, 6 de octubre 1952.

— "Retrato de don Juan Valera", en *Semana*, 5 de julio 1953.

— *Valera al natural* (Obra en la cual se incluyen los artículos anteriores junto a otros seis más), Madrid, 1962.

Morby, E. S.: "Una batalla entre antiguos y modernos: Juan Valera y Carlos Reyles", en *Revista Iberoamericana*, México D. F., 1941.

Moreno, Enrique: *Juanita la larga* (Dramatización de la novela, que recibió el premio "Valera" en la ciudad de Cabra el año 1934), Cabra, 1934.

Muñoz Rojas, J. A.: "Notas sobre la Andalucía de don Juan Valera" en *Papeles de Son Armadans*, octubre 1956.

Navas, Conde de las (López Valdemoro, J.): *Don Juan Valera. Apuntes del natural*, Madrid, 1905.

— "Centenario de Valera", en *Boletín de la Real Academia Española*, Madrid, 1924, XI, pp. 484-508.

— *Valera íntimo*, Madrid, Tip. Revista Archivos y Museos, 1925.

Nelken, Margarita: "La madre de don Juan Valera, o, en folletín, la ambición de una madre", en *ABC*, 30 de marzo 1930.

Ocharán Mazas, L. de: *Incorrecciones deslizadas en las páginas de Pepita Jiménez*, Madrid, 1924.

Olguín, M.: "Valera's Philosophical Arguments against Naturalism", en *Modern Language Quarterly*, Washington, XI, 1950.

Olivar Bertrand, R.: *Confidencias del Bachiller de Osuna*, Valencia, ed. Castalia, 1952.

Oliver, M. S.: "Sobre Terapéutica social", en *Entre dos Españas*, Barcelona, 1906.

Oliver Brachfeld, F.: "Juan Valera et l'Autriche-Hongrie", en *Bulletin Hispanique*, XLI, 1939.

Ombuena, José: "Don Juan Valera en los Estados Unidos", en *Boletín de la Real Academia de Ciencias, Nobles Artes y Bellas Letras de Córdoba*, XXVII, 1956, pp. 143-160.

OPINIÓN, LA: Número especial del semanario egabrense dedicado exclusivamente a don Juan Valera, Cabra, 7 de setiembre 1927.

Ortega y Gasset, J.: "La crítica de Valera", "De la dignidad del hombre" y "Valera como celtíbero", en *Obras completas*, Madrid, 1946, vol. I.

Oteyza, Luis de: *Las mujeres en la literatura*, Madrid, 1917.

Ovejero, A.: *Don Juan Valera*, discurso leído con ocasión de la inauguración del monumento a Valera en Córdoba, 1 de julio 1928.

Oyuela, Calixto: *Apuntes de literatura castellana, siglos XVIII y XIX*, Buenos Aires, 1896.

Pacheco, F. de Asís: "Don Juan Valera", en *El Imparcial*, Madrid, 23 de noviembre 1878.

Pagano, León J.: *Al través de la España literaria*, Barcelona, Maucci, 1904.

Pageard, Robert: "L'oeuvre épistolaire de Juan Valera. Bibliographie critique", en *Bulletin Hispanique*, LXIII, 1961, pp. 38-45.

— "Pepita Jiménez en France", en *Bulletin Hispanique*, LXIII, 1961, páginas 28-37.

Palacio Valdés, Armando: "Los novelistas españoles: Don Juan Valera", en *Revista Europea*, abril y mayo 1878.

— "Semblanzas literarias", en *Los oradores del Ateneo*, Madrid, O. C., XI, 1925.

— *La literatura en 1881*, Madrid, 1882.

Palma, Ricardo: "Los sábados de don Juan Valera", en *El mercurio peruano*, Lima, 1919, III, p. 336.

Pardo Bazán, Emilia: "Una polémica entre Valera y Campoamor", en *Nuevo teatro crítico*, Madrid, febrero 1881.

— *La cuestión palpitante*, Madrid, 1891.

— *Retratos y apuntes literarios*, Madrid, 1908.

Pardo Canalis, E.: "Valera y la sátira", en *Revista de ideas estéticas*, X, 1952.

Pazos García, D.: "Los ataques que al regionalismo catalán dirige el Excelentísimo Sr. D. J. Valera", en *La España regional*, febrero 1888.

Peers, E. Allison: "Ángel de Saavedra, Duque de Rivas. A Critical Study", en *Revue Hispanique*, LVIII, 1923.

Pella y Forgas, J.: "Los ataques que al regionalismo catalán dirige don Juan Valera", en *La España regional*, octubre 1887.

Penedo, Fr. Manuel: "Epistolario inédito de don Juan Valera a don José María Carpio", en *Estudios*, T. III, 1947, pp. 415-429.

Peña López, A.: "Españolismo de Valera", en *La opinión*, Cabra, febrero 1932.

Peres, Ramón: *Críticas y semblanzas*, Barcelona, 1892.

Pérez de Ayala, R.: "Valera y Galdós. La incógnita y Realidad", en *La Prensa*, Buenos Aires, 13 de agosto 1939, y recogido luego en *Amistades y recuerdos*, Barcelona, Aedos, 1961.

— "Don Juan Valera o el arte de la distracción", en *El Sol*, 16, 17 y 18 de abril 1925.

— *Las máscaras*, Buenos Aires, Col. Austral, 1940.

— "Valera y el escepticismo político", en *ABC*, 21 de marzo 1956.

— "Valera y la oratoria", en *ABC*, 23 de marzo 1956.

— "Recuerdos: Valera y Menéndez Pelayo", en *ABC*, 19 de septiembre 1957.

— *Divagaciones literarias*, Madrid, Biblioteca Nueva, 1958.

Porcher, J.: "Juan Valera", en *Revue Bleue*, n. 25, Paris, 1897.

Puccini, M.: *Peppina Jiménez*, traducción y prólogo de..., Milano, editorial Verona, 1936.

*Qualia, C. B.: *The Platonism of Valera*, Texas Technological College.

*— *The Renaissance influence in the Novels*, Texas Technological College.

Quesnel, Leo M.: "La littérature espagnole", en *Nouvelle Revue*, Paris, 15 de setiembre 1887.

Ramos López, J.: *El sacro monte de Granada*, Madrid, 1883.

Ratazzi, Princesa de: "Don Juan Valera", en *L'Espagne moderne*, Paris, 1878.

Revilla, Manuel de la: "Las ilusiones del doctor Faustino", en *Revista Europea*, Madrid, 1875.

— "Revista crítica", en *Revista contemporánea*, Madrid, 30 de mayo 1876.

— "Análisis y ensayos", en *Revista contemporánea*, 30 de julio 1877.

— "Bocetos literarios", en *Revista contemporánea*, 15 de diciembre 1877.

— "Pasarse de listo", en *Revista contemporánea*, 15 de junio 1878.

— "Disertaciones y juicios literarios", en *Revista contemporánea,* 15 de octubre 1878.

— "Juicio sobre el escepticismo de Valera", en *Obras,* Madrid, ed. Sainz, 1883.

Revuelta y Revuelta, L.: "Valera estilista", en *Boletín de la Real Academia de Ciencias, Nobles Artes y Bellas Letras de Córdoba,* 1946, n. 55.

Ríos, L.: *Le illusioni del dottore Faustino,* introducción y versión de..., Milano, 1908.

Ríos de Lampérez, B. de los: *De la mística en la novela de don Juan Valera,* discurso leído en la Real Academia Española de la Lengua, Madrid, 1924.

Rivas Cheriff, C.: *Pepita Jiménez,* refundición de la novela del mismo título en forma teatral, Madrid, El teatro moderno, 1929.

Roca Franquesa, J. M.: "La personalidad poética de don Juan Valera", en *Revista de la Universidad de Oviedo,* 1947.

Rodríguez Marín, F.: *Don Juan Valera epistológrafo,* Madrid, 1925.

— *Centenario de Valera,* discurso pronunciado en la Real Academia, octubre 1924.

Romero Mendoza, P.: "Don Juan Valera", en *Alcántara,* Cáceres, XI, 1955.

— *Don Juan Valera: Estudio biográfico crítico* (Premio Valera, 1935), Madrid, 1940.

Romeu, R.: "Les divers aspects de l'humeur dans le roman espagnol moderne", en *Bulletin Hispanique,* XLVIII, 1956 y XLIX, 1957.

Ruiz Cano, Bernardo: *Don Juan Valera en su vida y en su obra,* Jaén, Imprenta Cruz, 1935.

Rundorff, D. E.: "The Philosophical Trends of Valera", Doctoral dissertation, Minnesota, 1958.

Sáinz de Robles, F. C.: *Ensayo de un diccionario de la literatura,* Madrid, Aguilar, 1949.

Sáinz de Tejada, C.: "Valera y los Bonaparte", en *Semana,* 29 de agosto 1958.

— "Las delicias de doña Mencía", en *Blanco y Negro,* 23 de agosto 1959.

— "Juan Valera en su correspondencia", en *ABC,* 30 de agosto 1959.

Sáinz Rodríguez, P.: "Don Bartolomé José Gallardo y la crítica literaria de su tiempo", en *Revue Hispanique,* 1921, y luego como libro con idéntico título, Madrid, 1921.

— "Documentos para la historia de la crítica literaria en España", en *Boletín de la Biblioteca Menéndez Pelayo*, 1921 y 1922.

— *Epistolario de Valera y Menéndez Pelayo*, Madrid, Espasa Calpe, 1946.

Sampaio Passos, L.: *Los cuentos de Valera*, tesis doctoral leída en la Facultad de Letras de Madrid en 1959.

Sampelayo, Juan: "Don Juan Valera en sus cartas", en *La estafeta literaria*, 6 de abril 1957.

Sánchez Mohedano, G.: *Don Juan Valera y doña Mencía*, Cabra, Córdoba, 1948.

Sánchez Pérez, A.: "Nota sobre la primera serie de Cartas Americanas", en *La España moderna*, agosto 1889.

Sánchez Rojas, J.: *Apostillas a una conferencia* (sobre el Valera mundano), Madrid, 1924.

— "Valera", en *El Adelanto*, Salamanca, 12 de octubre 1917.

Sánchez Romero, C.: "El cuento y don Juan Valera", en *Boletín de la R. A. de Ciencias... de Córdoba*, XXVII, 1956. (En el mismo volumen se incluye el artículo "Don Juan Valera Pedagogo", del mismo autor.)

Sandoval, Manuel de: "La tertulia de don Juan Valera", en *La Época*, 30 de octubre, 15 de noviembre, 1 y 16 de diciembre de 1920, y 1 y 15 de enero de 1921.

— "Valera poeta". Conferencia leída en la Real Academia Española el 9 de diciembre de 1924.

Santacruz, P.: "Ensayo sobre las ideas estéticas de don Juan Valera", en *Boletín de la Real Academia de Ciencias, Bellas Artes y Nobles Letras de Córdoba*, 1945, XVI, pp. 167-195.

Sbarbi, P. J. María: "Un plato de garrafales: Pepita Jiménez", en *Revista de Archivos, Bibliotecas y Museos*, IV, 1874, pp. 187-190 y 203-205.

— *Ambigú literario*, Madrid, 1897.

Schanzer, George D.: "Russia and the United States in the Eyes of a Nineteenth century Spanish Novelist", en *Thought Patterns*, vol. VI, New York, pp. 167-195.

Serrano y Sanz, M.: "Cartas de algunos literatos a don Emilio Arrieta, don Ruperto Chapí y don Adelardo López Ayala", en *Boletín de la Real Academia Española*, T. XIX, 1932.

Siboni, Luis: *Plaza partida*, Madrid, 1897.

Silva, César: *Don Juan Valera*, Valparaíso, 1914.

Simón Díaz, J.: *Semanario pintoresco español, Madrid, 1836-1857*, Madrid, 1945.

— *Manual de bibliografía de la literatura española*, Barcelona, 1963.

Soca, Juan: "Semblanza y fantasía del pueblo de don Juan Valera", en *Boletín de la Real Academia de Ciencias, Nobles Artes y Bellas Letras de Córdoba*, XXVII, 1956.

— *Perfiles Egabrenses*, Cabra de Córdoba, 1961. (Contiene seis artículos dedicados a don Juan Valera.)

Tannenberg, Boris de: *La poésie castillane contemporaine*, Paris, Librairie Académique, 1889.

— *La España literaria, retratos de ayer y de hoy*, Madrid, 1903.

*Tayler, N. H.: *Valera's Philosophy of Instincts as Expressed in El Comendador Mendoza*, University of Toronto.

Thompson, Frank R.: *The Classicism of don Juan Valera*, Doctoral Dissertation, University of Wisconsin, VII, 1944.

Torre, Guillermo de: "Valera hoy", en *Cuadernos*, n. 17, 1956.

— *Tres conceptos de la literatura Hispanoamericana*, Buenos Aires, Losada, 1963.

Torrente Ballester, G.: *Panorama de la literatura española contemporánea*, Madrid, Guadarrama, 1956.

Urmeneta, Fermín de: "Sobre la estética valerina", en *Revista de Ideas Estéticas*, XIV, 1956.

Valbuena, A. de: *Ripios académicos*, Madrid, 1890.

Valbuena Briones, A.: "Don Juan Valera y la idea de América", en *Acta Salmanticensia*, X, n. 2, Salamanca, 1956.

Valbuena Prat, A.: *Historia de la literatura española*, Barcelona, 1957.

Valera y Alcalá Galiano, Juan [1]: *Ensayos poéticos*, Granada, 1884.

— *Estudios críticos sobre literatura, política y costumbres de nuestros días*, Madrid, 1864.

— *Pepita Jiménez*, Madrid, 1874.

— *Las ilusiones del doctor Faustino*, Madrid, 1875.

— *El comendador Mendoza*, Madrid, 1877.

— *Disertaciones y juicios literarios*, Madrid, 1878.

— *Pasarse de listo*, Madrid, 1878.

---

[1] Damos a continuación la lista de las primeras ediciones de las obras de Valera publicadas en forma de libro. Varias habían aparecido previamente en periódicos o revistas.

— *Tentativas dramáticas,* Madrid, 1879.
— *Doña Luz,* Madrid, 1879.
— *Dafnis y Cloe,* Madrid, 1880.
— *Cuentos y diálogos,* Sevilla, 1883.
— *Algo de todo,* Sevilla, 1883.
— *Apuntes sobre el nuevo arte de escribir novelas,* Madrid, 1887.
— *Nuevos estudios críticos,* Madrid, 1888.
— *Cartas americanas,* Madrid, 1889.
— *Nuevas cartas americanas,* Madrid, 1890.
— *Ventura de la Vega, biografía y estudio crítico,* Madrid, 1891.
— *Las mujeres y las academias,* Madrid, 1891.
— *Pequeñeces, Currita Albornoz al P. Luis Coloma,* Madrid, 1891.
— *La metafísica y la poesía,* Madrid, 1891.
— *La buena fama,* Madrid, 1894.
— *Juanita la larga,* Madrid, 1895.
— *El hechicero,* Madrid, 1895.
— *Cuentos y chascarrillos andaluces,* Madrid, 1896.
— *Genio y figura,* Madrid, 1897.
— *A vuela pluma,* Madrid, 1897.
— *De varios colores,* Madrid, 1898.
— *Morsamor,* Madrid, 1899.
— *Ecos argentinos,* Madrid, 1901.
— *Florilegio de poesías castellanas del siglo XIX,* Madrid, 1902-1903.
— *El superhombre y otras novedades,* Madrid, 1903.
— *Terapéutica social y otras novedades,* Madrid, 1903.
— *Discursos académicos.* (Volúmenes I y II de la primera edición de Obras Completas, Madrid, Imprenta Alemana, 1905.)
— *Mariquita y Antonio.* (Fragmentos inéditos de una novela), Madrid, 1907.
— *Correspondencia* (2 vols.), Madrid, 1913.
— "Noticia autobiográfica" (escrita en 1863), en *Boletín de la Real Academia Española,* T. I, 1914.
— "Epistolario inédito de don Juan Valera" (publicado por Juan Domínguez Bordona), en *Revista de la Biblioteca, Archivo y Museo Municipal,* volúmenes II y III, Madrid, 1925 y 1926.
— *Epistolario de Valera y Menéndez Pelayo.* Publicado por P. Sáinz Rodríguez y M. Artigas Ferrando, Madrid, Espasa Calpe, 1946.
— "Epistolario a Tamayo y Baus", en *Boletín de la Real Academia Española,* T. XXXIX, 1959 (publicado por R. Esquer Torres).

— *Correspondencia de don Juan Valera*. Cartas inéditas publicadas, con una introducción y notas, por Cyrus C. de Coster, Valencia, ed. Castalia, 1956.

— *Obras completas de don Juan Valera* (3 volúmenes, con introducción de L. Araujo Costa), Madrid, Aguilar, 1943.

Vázquez Dodero, J. L.: "El bombo solicitado", en *Semana*, 2 de marzo 1948.

— "Las cartas de don Juan Valera", en *Nuestro tiempo*, Madrid, 1958, número 49.

Vega Baeza, A.: *Ensayo sobre la evolución de la novela española en los tiempos modernos y contemporáneos*, Tacua, Chile, 1914.

Vezinet, F.: *Les maîtres du roman espagnol contemporain*, Paris, 1907.

Vidart, Luis: "Recuerdos de una polémica acerca de la novela de don Juan Valera: Pepita Jiménez", en *Revista de España*, T. III.

Villaurrutia, Marqués de: "Don Juan Valera, diplomático y hombre de mundo", en *Boletín de la Real Academia de la Historia*, LXXXVI, 1925.

Vorrath, J. C.: *Literary and Social Aspects of Valera's novel*, Yale, 1956.

Warren, L. A.: *Modern Spanish Literature*, London, 1927.

Ximénez de Sandoval, F.: "Un flirt de don Juan Valera", en *ABC*, 16 de diciembre 1955.

Zamora, Antonio: "Estudio biográfico de don Juan Valera", en *Revista de la Universidad de Buenos Aires*, 1953.

Zamora y Romera, Alfonso: "La tristeza de estar ciego"; "Don Juan Valera y la gracia andaluza"; "Don Juan Valera en el siglo xix"; "Ideas estéticas de don Juan Valera"; "Estudio biográfico de don Juan Valera". Colección de artículos —propiedad de la "Sociedad Amigos de Valera"— por la cual su autor recibió el premio Valera, en Cabra de Córdoba.

Zaragüeta, Juan: "Don Juan Valera filósofo", en *ABC*, 20 de mayo 1955.

— "Don Juan Valera filósofo y sus relaciones con Menéndez Pelayo", en *Revista de filosofía*, Madrid, 1956, T. XV.

— "Don Juan Valera filósofo", en *Boletín de la Universidad de Madrid*, 1929.

Zayas, A. de: "Elogio de don Juan Valera", en *Ensayos de crítica histórica y literaria*, Madrid, 1909.

Zum Felde, Alberto: *Índice crítico de la literatura hispanoamericana*, México, ed. Guaranía, 1954.

Zúñiga, Ángel: "El cervantismo en Valera", en *ABC*, 19 de octubre 1954.

ÍNDICE DE AUTORES

ÍNDICE GENERAL

BIBLIOTECA ROMÁNICA HISPÁNICA

Director: DÁMASO ALONSO

I. TRATADOS Y MONOGRAFÍAS

1. Walther von Wartburg: *La fragmentación lingüística de la Romania.* Agotada.
2. René Wellek y Austin Warren: *Teoría literaria.* Con un prólogo de Dámaso Alonso. Cuarta edición. 432 págs.
3. Wolfgang Kayser: *Interpretación y análisis de la obra literaria.* Cuarta edición revisada. 594 págs.
4. E. Allison Peers: *Historia del movimiento romántico español.* Segunda edición. 2 vols.
5. Amado Alonso: *De la pronunciación medieval a la moderna en español.*
   Vol. I: Segunda edición: 382 págs.
   Vol. II: En prensa.
6. Helmut Hatzfeld: *Bibliografía crítica de la nueva estilística aplicada a las literaturas románicas.* Segunda edición, en prensa.
7. Fredrick H. Jungemann: *La teoría del sustrato y los dialectos hispano-romances y gascones.* Agotada.
8. Stanley T. Williams: *La huella española en la literatura norteamericana.* 2 vols.
9. René Wellek: *Historia de la crítica moderna (1750-1950).*
   Vol. I: *La segunda mitad del siglo XVIII.* 396 págs.
   Vol. II: *El Romanticismo.* 498 págs.
   Vol. III: En prensa.
   Vol. IV: En prensa.
10. Kurt Baldinger: *La formación de los dominios lingüísticos en la Península Ibérica.* 398 págs. 15 mapas. 2 láminas.
11. S. Griswold Morley y Courtney Bruerton: *Cronología de las comedias de Lope de Vega (Con un examen de las atribuciones dudosas, basado todo ello en un estudio de su versificación estrófica).* 694 págs.

II. ESTUDIOS Y ENSAYOS

1. Dámaso Alonso: *Poesía española (Ensayo de métodos y límites estilísticos).* Quinta edición. 672 págs. 2 láminas.
2. Amado Alonso: *Estudios lingüísticos (temas españoles).* Tercera edición. 286 págs.

26. José Ares Montes: *Góngora y la poesía portuguesa del siglo XVII.* Agotada.

27. Carlos Bousoño: *La poesía de Vicente Aleixandre.* Segunda edición, en prensa.

28. Gonzalo Sobejano: *El epíteto en la lírica española.* Agotada.

29. Dámaso Alonso: *Menéndez Pelayo, crítico literario. Las palinodias de Don Marcelino.* Agotada.

30. Raúl Silva Castro: *Rubén Darío a los veinte años.* 296 págs. 4 láminas.

31. Graciela Palau de Nemes: *Vida y obra de Juan Ramón Jiménez.* Segunda edición, en prensa.

32. José F. Montesinos: *Valera o la ficción libre (Ensayo de interpretación de una anomalía literaria).* Agotada.

33. Luis Alberto Sánchez: *Escritores representativos de América.* Primera serie. La segunda edición ha sido incluida en la sección VII, *Campo Abierto,* con el número 11.

34. Eugenio Asensio: *Poética y realidad en el cancionero peninsular de la Edad Media.* Agotada.

35. Daniel Poyán Díaz: *Enrique Gaspar (Medio siglo de teatro español).* 2 vols. 10 láminas.

36. José Luis Varela: *Poesía y restauración cultural de Galicia en el siglo XIX.* 304 págs.

37. Dámaso Alonso: *De los siglos oscuros al de Oro.* La segunda edición ha sido incluida en la sección VII, *Campo Abierto,* con el número 14.

39. José Pedro Díaz: *Gustavo Adolfo Bécquer (Vida y poesía).* Segunda edición corregida y aumentada. 486 págs.

40. Emilio Carilla: *El Romanticismo en la América hispánica.* Segunda edición revisada y ampliada. 2 vols.

41. Eugenio G. de Nora: *La novela española contemporánea (1898-1960).* Premio de la Crítica.
Tomo I: (1898-1927). Segunda edición. 622 págs.
Tomo II: (1927-1939). Segunda edición corregida. 538 págs.
Tomo III: (1939-1960). Segunda edición, en prensa.

42. Christoph Eich: *Federico García Lorca, poeta de la intensidad.* Segunda edición, en prensa.

43. Oreste Macrí: *Fernando de Herrera.* Agotada.

44. Marcial José Bayo: *Virgilio y la pastoral española del Renacimiento.* Agotada.

45. Dámaso Alonso: *Dos españoles del Siglo de Oro (Un poeta madrileñista, latinista y francesista en la mitad del siglo XVI. El Fabio de la "Epístola moral": su cara y cruz en Méjico y en España).* 258 págs.

46. Manuel Criado de Val: *Teoría de Castilla la Nueva (La dualidad castellana en la lengua, la literatura y la historia).* Segunda edición, en prensa.

IV. TEXTOS

1. Manuel C. Díaz y Díaz: *Antología del latín vulgar.* Segunda edición aumentada y revisada. 240 págs.
2. María Josefa Canellada: *Antología de textos fonéticos.* Con un prólogo de Tomás Navarro. 254 págs.
3. Sánchez Escribano y A. Porqueras Mayo: *Preceptiva dramática española del Renacimiento y el Barroco.* 258 págs.
4. Juan Ruiz: *Libro de Buen Amor.* Edición crítica de Joan Corominas. 670 págs.
5. Julio Rodríguez-Puértolas: *Fray Íñigo de Mendoza y sus "Coplas de Vita Christi".* 634 págs.

V. DICCIONARIOS

1. Joan Corominas: *Diccionario crítico etimológico de la lengua castellana.* Tomos I, II y III, agotados. Tomo IV y último. 1226 páginas.
2. Joan Corominas: *Breve diccionario etimológico de la lengua castellana.* Segunda edición revisada. 628 págs.
3. *Diccionario de autoridades.* Edición facsímil. 3 vols.
4. Ricardo J. Alfaro: *Diccionario de anglicismos.* Recomendado por el "Primer Congreso de Academias de la Lengua Española". 480 págs.
5. María Moliner: *Diccionario de uso del español.* 2 vols.

VI. ANTOLOGÍA HISPÁNICA

1. Carmen Laforet: *Mis páginas mejores.* 258 págs.
2. Julio Camba: *Mis páginas mejores.* 254 págs.
3. Dámaso Alonso y José M. Blecua: *Antología de la poesía española.* Vol. I: *Lírica de tipo tradicional.* Segunda edición corregida. LXXXVI + 266 págs.
4. Camilo José Cela: *Mis páginas preferidas.* 414 págs.
5. Wenceslao Fernández Flórez: *Mis páginas mejores.* 276 págs.
6. Vicente Aleixandre: *Mis poemas mejores.* Tercera edición aumentada. 322 págs.
7. Ramón Menéndez Pidal: *Mis páginas preferidas (Temas literarios).* 372 págs.
8. Ramón Menéndez Pidal: *Mis páginas preferidas (Temas lingüísticos e históricos).* 328 págs.

VII. CAMPO ABIERTO